Tamoxifen

Beyond the Antiestrogen

Cover: Cover design by David Gardner, Dorchester, MA.

Cover represents a schematic presentation of the estrogen-agonistic and antagonistic effect of Tamoxifen, expressed by the yin-yang symbol, as well as of the various non-steroidal actions of this compound. Figure by John A. Kellen, Istvan Berczi, and Patsy Cunningham.

Tamoxifen

Beyond the Antiestrogen

John A. Kellen

Editor

Birkhäuser
Boston • Basel • Berlin

John A. Kellen
89 Rameau Drive
Toronto, Ontario M2H 1T6
Canada

Library of Congress Cataloging-in-Publication Data

Tamoxifen: beyond the antiestrogen / John A. Kellen, editor.
    p.   cm.
    Includes bibliographical references and index.
    ISBN 0-8176-3842-3 (H : alk. paper). -- ISBN 3-7643-3842-3 (H:
alk. paper)
    1. Tamoxifen--Physiological effect.   I. Kellen, John A.
RC271.T36T36   1996   95-52783
  616.99'4061--dc20   CIP

Printed on acid-free paper
© Birkhäuser Boston 1996

Birkhäuser

ISBN 0-8176-3842-3
ISBN 3-7643-3842-3
Camera-ready text prepared by the editor.
Printed and bound by Quinn-Woodbine, Woodbine, NJ.
Printed in the U.S.A.

9 8 7 6 5 4 3 2 1

Contents

PREFACE

Tamoxifen has persisted as a widely accepted and administered drug for almost 25 years. Following the many scientific papers and books on the subject, it has remained a very intriguing substance. This, perhaps, is the reason for another monograph on Tamoxifen. It is regrettably true that overviews, even when up to date after exhaustive research - the shibboleth of our cultures -, rapidly lose relevance with the passage of time. Scientists can sometimes be pictured as deep sea divers, who plunge into the unknown in search of a hitherto unknown world. Their descent is exciting, but eventually they must come up for air and integrate their experiences with others who also had to resurface.

This book intends to collect and, where possible, to collate recent, but sometimes seemingly unrelated information. To quote Stephane Mallarmé: "Everything in the world exists to end up in a book". Even if this is a tad cynical, it might not be far from the truth. If a little knowledge is a dangerous commodity, one can also add - tongue in cheek - that a vast amount of knowledge can be truly hazardous. It is likely that what might seem as entangled data is confusing, especially for those satisfied with the comfortable interpretation of Tamoxifen as an antiestrogen which has long been found insufficient. The complexity of its mechanisms and effects defies simple explanations and may even seem capricious, but only because of our ignorance. Clearly, Tamoxifen is far from being an ideal antiestrogen, yet concerted efforts to introduce other, potent non-steroid substances with equal or greater therapeutic success have, so far, been disappointing.

We have knowingly avoided the issue of Tamoxifen as a preventive agent. Some of the already available data are contentious, insufficient and tainted by "scientific politics". To analyze - prematurely - sins or omission and commission without solid statistical basis would force us to take sides. At the time of going to print, we chose watchful waiting.

Tamoxifen, whether used in prevention or as adjuvant therapy in various cancers, requires long-term or perhaps indefinite administration. Any prolonged exposure to a substance whose wide range of effects and potency are still being clarified and only partially understood is necessarily fraught with problems and risks, known and unknown.

The authors hope that their contributions will permit readers to weigh the problems and promises, the hurdles and the hopes of Tamoxifen with more insight. Allow me to end on a cautious (and sceptical) note: "The world always makes assumptions that the exposure of an error is identical with the discovery of a truth - that error and truth are simply opposite. They are nothing of the sort. What the world turns to when it has been cured of one error, is usually another error..."(H.L. Mencken).

John A. Kellen
Toronto, December 1995

List of Contributors

Marku Ahotupa, Ph.D., MCA Research Laboratory, BioCity, University of Turku, Finland

Edward Baral, M.D., Ph.D., Depts. of Internal Medicine and Oncology, University of Manitoba, Winnipeg, Manitoba, Canada

Istvan Berczi, Ph.D.,Dept. of Immunology, University of Manitoba, Winnipeg, Manitoba, Canada

Marc E. Bracke, M.D., Ph.D., Lab. Experimental Cancerology, University Hospital, University of Ghent, Belgium

Myles C. Cabot, Ph.D., Breast Cancer Res. Program, John Wayne Cancer Institute, St. John's Hospital and Health Center, Santa Monica, California, USA

Vincent Castronovo, M.D., Ph.D., Metastasis Res. Laboratory, Sart-Tilman, University of Liège, Belgium

Robert Clarke, Ph.D., Lombardi Cancer Center, Georgetown University, Washington D.C.,USA

Mitchell Dowsett, M.D.,Biochemical Endocrinology, Royal Marsden Hospital, London, England

Isabelle Gendre, B.Sc., Program of Epidemiology for Cancer Prevention, International Agency for Research on Cancer, WHO, Lyon, France

Armando E. Giuliano , M.D.,John Wayne Cancer Institute, St. John's Hospital and Health Center, Santa Monica, California, USA

Pirkko L. Härkönen, M.D.,Ph.D.,Inst. of Biomedicine, University of Turku, Finland

Taisen Iguchi, D.Sc., Dept. of Biology, Yokohama City University, Japan

Stephen R.D. Johnston, MA MRCP, Dept. of Academic Biochemistry, Royal Marsden Hospital, London England

John A. Kellen, M.D., Ph.D., Dept. of Clinical Biochemistry, Sunnybrook Health Science Centre, University of Toronto, Ontario, Canada

David Kupfer, Ph.D., Worcester Foundation of Biomedical Research, Shrewsbury, Massachusetts, USA

Marc E. Lippman, M.D., Lombardi Cancer Center, Georgetown University, Washington D.C. USA

Marc M. Mareel, M.D., Ph.D., Lab. of Experimental Cancerology, University of Ghent, Belgium

Leigh C. Murphy, Ph.D., Dept. of Molecular Biology and Physiology, Unversity of Manitoba, Winnipeg, Manitoba, Canada

Liam J. Murphy, M.B., Ph.D., Depts. of Internal Medicine and Physiology, University of Manitoba, Winnipeg, Manitoba, Canada

Eva Nagy, M.D., Dept. of Immunology, University of Manitoba, Winnipeg, Manitoba, Canada

Yasuhiko Ohta, professor, Laboratory of Animal Science, Dept. of Veterinary Science, Faculty of Agriculture, Tottori University, Tottori, Japan

Michael N. Pollak, M.D. Ph.D., Depts. of Medicine and Oncology, The Sir Mortimer B. Davis - Jewish General Hospital, McGill University, Montreal, Quebec, Canada

Charles Rowlatt, BM, BCh, Ph.D., Dept. of Surgery, University College, London, England

Annie J. Sasco, M.D., Dr.P.H., Program of Epidemiology for Cancer Prevention, International Agency for Research on Cancer, WHO, Lyon France

Frans M. Van Roy, Ph.D., Laboratory of Molecular Biology, University of Ghent, Belgium

Anni M. Wärri, Ph.D., Cancer Research Laboratory, Orion Corp. Farmos, Turku, Finland

Helen Wiseman, M.D., Dept. Nutrition and Dietetics, King's College, London, England

1. INTRODUCTION: THE ENIGMA OF TAMOXIFEN

J.A. Kellen

> *"To single out causes,*
> *one must make loose*
> *assumptions"*
> *(G.B. Levy, 1995)*

The antiestrogen effect of Tamoxifen remains the basic rationale for its general acceptance and wide use. Estrogens play a definite role in the etiology and growth of a variety of cancers, including the breast, endometrium, prostate and probably others; interference with their action, prevention of estrogen effects, has been a promising goal long before the introduction of chemical castration by antiestrogens. However, the straightforward interpretation that antiestrogens operate by competitive binding to estrogen receptors alone had soon to be abandoned. Tamoxifen was found to be cytocidal at high concentrations and tumoristatic at serum levels achievable *in vivo*. The evaluation of physiological and pharmacological actions of Tamoxifen in humans is an increasingly complex issue, not in the least because of its mixed estrogen agonistic and antagonistic effects.

The synthesis of a great number of proteins and other substances is regulated both by estrogens and their antagonists. Transcriptional activation of various subsets of genes results in an increase or decrease of growth factors, their binding proteins, enzymes and steroid receptors themselves. Difficulties in understanding these complex, interrelated processes are compounded by the lack of appropriate models; obviously, *in vitro* studies can not reflect the heterogeneity and continuous dynamics characteristic of solid tumours. Animal models suffer from sometimes unpredictable species-specific variations of Tamoxifen action; the drug exerts varying degrees of estrogenic effects in different laboratory animals (White et al., 1995) and in different tissues (Gottardis et al., 1988). Even in human cell cultures, tumour cells exhibit receptor heterogeneity, differences in estrogen binding avidity, receptor localization and responses, varying with the level and duration of exposure.

Because of the preoccupation with the "antihormone" concept, thought to directly counteract the action of natural estrogens and other steroids, telling details which pointed to new directions were underestimated. Yet, successful treatment of receptor-negative breast cancer as well as treatment failures in receptor-rich tumours were inconsistencies encountered at an early stage. The nemesis of chemotherapy, the development of resistance to Tamoxifen, also made its inexorable entry on the scene, together with the estrogen-like activity able to stimulate certain tumours and even lead to dependency (Zimniski and Warren, 1993). In certain circumstances, Tamoxifen may act as a carcinogen, since it causes adduct formation to DNA and proteins, *in vivo* and *in vitro* (Jordan, 1995; Pongracz et al., 1995; Pathak et al., 1995) which is a signal usually sufficient to ring alarm bells (Pathak and Bodell, 1994; Carther et al., 1995; Rutquist et al., 1995).

The following is a tentative effort to arrange the colourful spectrum of Tamoxifen actions into some resemblance of a system.

In situations where a recurrent or metastatic tumour responds to Tamoxifen, prolonged and persistent administration of the drug is mandatory. Long-term biological effects of Tamoxifen, on a wide range of lipids and hormones, on bone density and hemostatic factors has been reported (Cuzick et al., 1993). In sum, low density cholesterol was found to decrease, together with some increase in triglyceride levels. Thyroid hormone levels were higher and sex hormone globulins almost doubled. Bone density increase was insignificant, however clotting times were shorter and fibrinogens as well as antithrombin III levels decreased. These potentially desirable effects appear to be reversible on cessation of treatment.

Perhaps the most diverse array of effects, directly caused by Tamoxifen, is the stimulation or inhibition of enzymes - their synthesis, inactivation or repression. Numerous mechanisms cause these changes, which may be early and profound. The regulation of signal transduction, leading to gene transcription with ensuing protein synthesis, allows for many modulations along these complex pathways. Binding of a variety of cellular effectors to receptors (other than those for steroids) can affect membrane phospholipid hydrolysis with products functioning as second messengers to innumerable events (Phaneuf et al., 1995).

A conspicious example is the distinct inhibitory effect of Tamoxifen on Protein Kinase C (PKC). This enzyme has specific, direct triphenylethylene-binding sites at the ATP-binding region. There is evidence that PKC inhibition (as well as of calmodulin) by both cis- and trans-Tamoxifen may contribute to their antitumour activity (O'Brian et al., 1985, 1986, 1988a, 1988b, 1990). This inhibition has been documented *in vivo* at therapeutic concentrations, is obviously independent of estrogen or estrogen receptors and is not reversible by estrogen. Since PKC is a recognized tumour promotor receptor protein and a key enzyme in the regulation of cellular growth, its specific inhibition may have a definite antiproliferative effect.

Tamoxifen influences drug-metabolizing as well as antioxidant liver enzymes (Ahotupa et al., 1994) and inhibits significantly the hexose monophosphate shunt, decreases the hepatic content of reduced glutathione and glutathione-S-transferases and the potential for microsomal peroxidation. Most of these effects are less desirable, but have been observed mostly in rats and after relatively long exposure and high doses. In women, some liver toxicity has been observed after long-term therapy (Blackburn et al., 1984) as well as steatohepatitis (Pinto et al., 1995). In the rat, Tamoxifen is a weak, phenobarbital-like, xenobiotic metabolizing enzyme-inducer in the liver (Nuwaysir et al., 1995).

Various proteases contribute to tumour growth and invasiveness by allowing cancer cells to digest and traverse basement membranes. In this process, the involvement of plasminogen activators and collagenases has been well documented. Some tumours, such as the R3230AC rat mammary adenocarcinoma, show estrogen-dependency in the synthesis of plasminogen activators, which can also be stimulated by Tamoxifen (Ng et al., 1986). Urokinase-type plasminogen activator(s) (uPA) also play a role in tumour cell invasiveness and nidation capability; breast cancer patients with uPA-negative tumours exhibit a more favourable outcome and better response to Tamoxifen treatment (with tumour regression or at least stability), compared to those with uPA-negative tumours. The determination of uPA levels in surgical specimens may be useful in predicting the therapeutic success of antisterodial therapy (Foekens et al., 1995). In MCF-7 human breast cancer cells, there is good correlation between suppression or stimulation of cell growth (Katzenellenbogen et al., 1984).

The collagenolytic activity of K562 leukemic cells is strongly inhibited (75%) by Tamoxifen; these cells do not have demonstrable binding sites for estrogen, but show high-affinity binding for ^{3}H-Tamoxifen (which does not affect cellular differentiation (Akeli et al., 1991).

These observations are mostly based on *in vitro* studies; *in vivo* antiestrogen effects of fibrinolytic and collagenolytic factors may differ, by their simultaneous association with other steroid hormones brings about novel, unexpected responses. There is an indication of increased incidence of venous thrombophlebitis complicating Tamoxifen therapy, at least in some, mostly menopausal individuals; this effect is unlikely to be caused by changes in the protein S and C activity levels in the anticoagulant pathway (Mamby et al., 1994).

Maping of MCF-7 cells in G_1 phase by morphology of prematurely condensed chromosomes clearly demonstrated that Tamoxifen-exposed cells accumulate in early G_1, thus provoking a transition delay which results in proliferation decrease (Osborne et al., 1983). Tamoxifen inhibits key enzymes, such as DNA polymerase and Na/K transporting ATPase (Repke and Matthes, 1994). Synchronisation in certain cell phaes may be accompanied by alterations in cell membrane morphology.

The CG-5 cell line, an estrogen supersensitive variant of the MCF-7 model, shows marked changes in the cell surface after exposure to Tamoxifen. With scanning electron microscopy, reduction in the length and number of microvilli together with rounding up and flattening of the cells themselves have been observed. These changes are more pronounced in cells plated at low density, but they can also be seen in nearly confluent monolayers and they appear early after exposure. Parallel modifications in membrane functions may be responsible for alterations which affect transport mechanisms (Sica et al., 1984). In MCF-7 cell cultures, Tamoxifen influences cellular shape and cytoskeletal arrangement in a mode similar to estrogen. Both re-organize intermediate and actin filaments, as documented by fluorescence, phase contrast and interference reflection microscopy (Sapino et al., 1986). Tamoxifen also significantly decreases membrane fluidity, both in MCF-7 and MDA-MB-436 cell cultures, accompanied by apparently non-estrogen receptor-mediated cytotoxicity. This may be the result of antiestrogen association with hydrophobic domains within the cell membranes. Since this effect is approximately parallel to the action of estrogens and may result in increased invasive and metastatic potential, it belongs among the estrogen-agonistic characteristics of Tamoxifen (Clarke et al., 1990).

Among the apparently estrogen-independent antiproliferative effects of Tamoxifen belongs its stimulatory action on phosphatidylil kinase and phosphatidylinositol-4-phosphate kinase; both enzymes are normally inhibited by polyphosphoinositides. Tamoxifen binds to the latter and releases the kinases from production inhibition; it also inhibits phospholipase C activity, which is involved in cell proliferation. Blockage of phosphoinositide breakdown may represent one facet of the steroid-independent antitumour effects of Tamoxifen (Freidman et al., 1994).

Calmodulin, a calcium-dependent regulatory protein of numerous cellular processes, including proliferation, interacts directly with Tamoxifen which results in the inhibition of cAMP phosphodiesterase activation. Since this is a key component of the second messenger system and regulates the metabolism of cyclic nucleotides, calmodulin appears to be part of the antiestrogen-binding sites, distinct from estrogen receptors (Lopes et al., 1990).

Permanent or even temporary loss of cell adhesiveness, togethter with increased ability to migrate, is a fundamental property of invasive cancer cells. This has been and still is the topic of innumerable papers and a large number of factors have been implicated. One of them, reduced expression of E-cadherin, has been closely correlated with invasiveness (Sloane et al., 1994). Tamoxifen rapidly restores E-cadherin function in human breast cancer MCF-7 cells and thus activates the function of an invasion-suppressor molecule, a decidely desirable effect (Lipponen and Eskelinen, 1995; Bracke at al., 1994).

The attachment of cancer cells to the subendothelial matrix with the help of components such as collagen I and IV, laminin and fibronectin, plays a prominent role in cancer cell adhesion. The action of Tamoxifen was studied in ZR75-1 and estrogen-independent BT-20 cells; the results show a reducation of adhesiveness in the former line, but not in the BT-20 cells. Clearly, antiestrogens control, at least in part, the adhesive behaviour of hormone-responsive tumours cells, possibly by regulating the expression of the above cell adhesion proteins (Millon et al., 1989). Our understanding of Tamoxifen action on cell adhesion leaves much to be desired and we can only deduct that there is no uniform or predictable effect.

Another protein assumed to be involved in tumour dissemination, cathepsin D, is secreted by hormone-dependent breast cancer cells and stimulated by esterogens; it is also produced constitutively in estrogen-independent cell lines (Fernö et al., 1994). Cathepsin D, a lysosomal protease, in increasingly accepted as a prognostic indicator and a predictive marker for adjuvant therapy. Tamoxifen has been found to have a significant beneficial effect predominately in patients with node- and progesterone receptor-positive breast cancer whose tumours also had a high cathepsin D content. Treatment with Tamoxifen further increased the cytosolic cathepsin D content in estrogen receptor positive, primary breast carcinomas (Maudelonde et al., 1994).

Another vast teritory in which steroid reign or, at times, exert decisive control, are the growth factors - a complicated, unruly collection of locally acting go-betweens which influence cell growth. When secreted, they modulate the autocrine control of cells that produced them or influence their neighbours by paracrine mechanisms. It is to be expected that antiestrogens may serve as agonists or antagonists in this system (Jordon, 1993).

Epidermal growth factor (EGF), Transforming growth factor (TGF) alpha and beta, Insulin growth factor (IGF) I and II and the Platelet-derived growth factor (PDGF), all and others play a role starting at the fetal development phase and ending with malignant growth. All act in concert with hormones and most are modulated by steroids (which thus function as mitogens).

IGF-I induced growth of MCF-7 cells can be inhibited, in a dose-dependent manner, by Tamoxifen, in the absence as well as in the presence of estrogenic compounds. Tamoxifen decreased IGF-I in the serum of women with primary breast cancer, but has no effect on IGF-II (Pollak et al., 1993). This suggests that Tamoxifen may have an antiproliferative effect by decreasing the secretion of stimulatory growth factors; it is not clear whether this effect also takes place *in vivo*.

In Ishikawa (endometrial adenocarcinoma) cells, 4-hydroxytamoxifen significantly inhibits cell proliferation and simultaneously decreased both TGF-alpha mRNA and TGF-alpha secretion. In HEC-50 cells, neither estradiol nor antiestrogens modulate cell proliferation of TGF-alpha mRNA levels. The respons of human endometrial adenocarcinoma cells *in vitro* varies between cell lines and depends upon culture conditions (Gong et al., 1992). In the rat uterus, both estrgeons and Tamoxifen have analogous effects on both TGF-beta 1 and 2 (Sartor et al., 1995).

Expression of EGF receptors was found to be in inverse relationship with estrogen expression. ER-negative breast cancer cells, with high numbers of EGF receptors, do not show a mitogenic response to EGF. ER-negative cell lines also produce and secrete more TGF-alpha. MCF-7 cells in culture under stringent estrogen depletion respond to estradiol, TGF-alpha, EGF and insulin which a three to six-fold increase in IGF-I; synthesis of the latter is inhibited by antiestrogens (Dreicer and Wilding, 1992). Also, TGF-beta is induced in human breast cancer *in vivo* following Tamoxifen treatment (Butta et al., 1992), but can not be induced in Ly2 cells, a stable MCF-7 variant.

TGF-beta regulates other growth factors, has slight mitogenic effects on various fibroblast systems but has, in general, a negative growth modulatory influence. In human breast cancer, TGF-beta is inhibited by estrogen and insulin. TGF-beta from antiestrogen-treated MCF-7 cells inhibits the growth of the ER-negative MDA-MB-231 cell line.

Growth factors are increasingly gaining recognition in the pharmacological manipulation of the malignant process; together with antiestrogens, once their agonistic or antagonistic role is fully understood, thay may become an additional effective tool in chemotherapy.

Apart from the well-trodden path of estrogen action on (mainly breast cancer) cells by direct stimulation of enzyme systems involved in DNA synthesis - and thus in mitosis -, several other mechanisms have been recognized: estrogens affect the synthesis of great numbers of cellular and secretory proteins. Among them, polyamines play a substantial rol in cellular proliferation. Putrescine, spermidine and spermine are ubiquitous, small aliphatic amines which function as "second messengers" of hormonal stimulation (Manni, 1994).

Nitrosomethylurea (NMU) - induced rat mammary tumours are under multihormonal control; tumour colony formation is stimulated by estradiol, prolaction, growth hormone and progesterone. Administration of alpha-difluoromethylornithine (DFMO) which specifically inhibits ornithine decarboxylase (the enzyme responsible for the rate-limiting step of putrescine formation from ornithine), completely abolishes the growth promoting action of the above mitogens (Manni, 1989). On the other hand, polyamines when added to NMU tumours cells grown in soft agar are able to reverse the inhibitory effect of antiestrogens on colon formation, in a dose-dependent manner (Manni and Wright, 1984). It follows that polyamines mediate hormonal action resulting in cell proliferation. Also, Tamoxifen significantly inhibits the rise of ornithine decarboxylase which leads, in MCF-7 tumours, to a dose-related decrease of putrescine and spermidine (while spermine levels remain unaffected, Cohen et al., 1988). Administration of Tamoxifen to the hormone-independent MDA-MB-231 breast cancer cells does not suppress ornithine decarboxylase activity or decrease cellular polyamine content despite inhibition or proliferation.

It appears that at least one of the several antitumour effects of Tamoxifen is mediated through induction of polyamine depletion. This action has been recorded both *in vitro* and *in vivo* (Manni et al., 1988).

Another aspect of antiestrgeon action is their direct involvement in apoptosis. In the context of the widely accepted model, steroids act as tumour promoters by modulating oncogene expression in cells where the initiating carcinogen had already induced mutations in proto-oncogens or in their alignment to hormone-responsive elements. This topic has been extensively reviewed (Sekeris, 1991).

In experimental rat hepatocarcinomas, Tamoxifen was found to induce frequent mutations in exons 7 and 8 of the p53 gene (Vancutsem et al., 1994); it also regulates the expression of cytoplastmic c-erbB2 in estrogen receptor-positive breast cancer patients and increased erbB2 mRNA (Johnston et al., 1993). However, after long term adjuvant therapy with Tamoxifen, no significant trend in erbB2 or p53 or both has been observed (Jacquemier et al., 1994). In a human glioblastoma cell line, Tamoxifen induced p53-independent apoptosis *in vitro*, by a mechanism linked to protein kinase C inhibition (Toms et al., 1995).

This brief review would be incomplete without some anecdoctal references to unexpected and so far marginal observations. Tamoxifen and Clomiphene citrate have been investigated as to their effect on male infertility. Antiestrogens are expected to block the negative feedback of steroids on the hypothalamo-pituitary-testicular axis without interference with the action of circulating hormones. The results, so far, have been inconclusive: more studies are necessary to identify a subgroup of idiopathic infertile men responsive to this treatment (Sterzik et al., 1993; Kotoulas et al., 1994; Mascarenhas et al., 1994).

Retroperitoneal fibrosis is an idiopathic disorder characterized by ill-defined periaortic fibrotic masses, which gradually encircle the aorta, the inferior vena cava and the ureters. Treatment is primarily surgical, but glucocorticoids and immunosuppressants have been tried as adjuvant therapy. Tamoxifen has shown some efficacy; it has been assumed that it increased TGF-beta secretion by fibroblasts, which may decrease the size of the fibrous masses (Spillane and Whitman, 1995; Loffleld and van Weel, 1993; Antoniuk et al., 1993).

A beneficial therapeutic effect on experimental murine Systemic Lupus Erythematosus (SLE) after Tamoxifen treatment has been reported; the drug creased immune complex deposits in the kidneys together with proteinuria and protected from leukopenia and thrombocytopenia (Sthoeger et al., 1994; Tylan, 1995). Tamoxifen may correc the dysregulation of cytokines in SLE or otherwise interact with immunomodulatory steroids; the exact mode of action is not clear. Tamoxifen in combination with interferon-beta and retinoids shows an additive (or synergistic) antiproliferative effect on breast cancer cell lines and appears to prolong median survival in patients with metastasis; this effect was independent of receptor status (Recchia et al., 1995).

A possible influence of Tamoxifen on hair pigmentation via intermediate action of cholesterol has been described; diffuse growth of black hair (in a 68-year-old breast cancer patient) has been attributed to the antiestrogen. It is hard to envisage our grey-haired population flocking to this therapy for cosmetic reasons (Hampson et al., 1995).

Tamoxifen exerts a marked antifunal effect on Saccharomyces cerevisiae and Candida albicans. Since this drug inhibits peroxidation of liver microsomes, this effect may be the result of its interaction with and stabilization of cell membranes, leading to a growth-inhibitory reduction in membrane fluidity. On a mole for mole basis, the fungistatis and fungicidal efficacy of Tamoxifen is similar to miconazole (Beggs, 1994, 1995).

Tamoxifen has been found useful in the treatment of cyclical psoriatic arthritis (Stevens et al., 1993) and of autoimmune progesterone dermatitis (Nabai and Rahbari, 1994).

In the steroid receptor-positive breast carcinoma cell lines T-47D and MCF-7, the production of prostate-specific antigen (PSA) can be induced by a variety of steroids as well as by Tamoxifen. PSA synthesis has long been considered as a relatively rare event in tumours of non-prostatic origin. Recent, refined and highly sensitive determination procedures using immunofluorometry permit the detection of PSA in approximately 30% of breast tumours (Yu et al., 1994). Both uni- and multivariant analysis of human breast cancer patients suggests that PSA may be an independent favourable predictive marker, useful for the identification of subgroups of estrogen receptor-negative and/or node positive patients with good prognosis (Yu et al., 1995).

The many beneficial "side-effects" of Tamoxifen, mainly in women past the menopause, outscore by far the relatively few undesirable events. Delay in atherogenesis by suppression of homocysteine (Anker et al., 1993), prevention of bone mineral loss (Neal et al., 1993, Wright and Compston, 1995) and a generally cardioprotective effect have been extensively documented. On the negative side: some individuals show untoward immune responses, probably associated with Tamoxifen, such as inflammatory polyarthritis (Creamer et al., 1994); interference with the coagulation pathway may lead to thromboembolic accidents (Cutuli et al., 1993) and the affinity of the drug to block chloride channels has been implicated in cataract formation (Zhang et al., 1994, 1995). Retinopathy (Locher et al., 1994; Chern and Danis, 1993), superior ophthalmic vein thrombosis (Anja et al., 1993) and toxic optic neuritis (Gracia-Ruiz et al., 1994) have also been reported. Most visual symptoms were found to be reversible and dose-dependent (Szeczny and Steiner, 1994) and can be screened for (Heier et al., 1994).

In postmenopausal women, Tamoxifen therapy may result in an increase in thyroid-binding globulin, with secondary increases in T4 and thyroxine uptake; however, the women remain eumetabolic (Mamby et al., 1995).

Lists such as the above can not claim, out of necessity, completeness; Tamoxifen is being administered world-wide in truly large numbers of patients and for various indications. Because of the sheer numbers involved, side effects must necessarily occur. The problem of carcinogenesis will be discussed elsewhere in this book. Antiestrogens, by virtue of their negligible toxicity and paucity of unpleasant effects, are and obviously will be widely prescribed; anecdotal experiences and observations are usually of limited value and therefore not easily reproducible or generally accepted.

REFERENCES

Ahotupa M, Hirsimä P, Pärssinen R, Mantyla E (1994): Alternations of drug metabolizing and antioxidant enzyme activities during tamoxifen-induced hepatocarcinogenesis in the rat. *Carcinogenesis* 15:863-868

Akeli MG, Madoulet C, Rallet A, Jardillier JC (1991): Inhibition of collagenolytic activity in human leukemic K563 cells by tamoxifen. *Leukemia Res* 15:1153-1157

Anja S, Shekar GC, Rao DR, Mohandas S (1993): Superior ophthalmic vein thrombosis with tamoxifen. *Can J Neurol Sci* 20:S197

Anker G, Loenning PE, Ueland PM, Refsum H, Lien EA (1993): Tamoxifen suppresses the plasma level of atherogenic factor homocysteine. *Europ J Cancer* 29A:S110

Antoniuk P, Tjandra JJ, Lavery IC (1993): Diffuse intra-abdominal fibromatosis in association with bilateral ovarian fibromatosis and oedema. *Austral New Zealand J Surg* 63:315-318

Beggs WH (1994): Comparative activities of miconazole and the anticancer drug tamoxifen against Candida albicans. *J Antimicrob Chemother* 34:186-187

Beggs WH (1995): Growth phase in relation to the lethal action of tamoxifen on Candida albicans. *Res Com Mol Path Pharmacol* 88:115-117

Bracke ME, Charlier C, Bruyneel EA, Labit C, Mareel MM, Castronovo V (1994): Tamoxifen restores the E-cadherin function in human breast cancer MCF-7/6 cells and suppresses their invasive phenotype. *Cancer Res* 54:4607-4609

Butta A, MacLennan K, Flanders KC, Sacks PM, Smith I, McKinna A, Dowsett M, Wakefield LM, Sporn MB, Baum M, Colletta AA (1992): Induction of transforming growth factor beta1 in human breast cancer *in vivo* following tamoxifen treatment. *Cancer Res* 52:4261-4264

Carthew P, Martin EA, White INH, De Matteis F, Edwards RE, Dorman BM, Heydon RT, Smith LL (1995): Tamoxifen Induced Short-Term Cumulative DNA Damage and Liver Tumors in Rats: Promotion by Phenobarbital. *Cancer Res* 55:544-547

Chern S and Danis RP (1993): Retinopathy associated with low-dose tamoxifen. *Am J Ophthal* 116:372-373

Clarke R, van den Berg HW, Murphy RF (1990): Reduction of the Membrane Fluidity of Human Breast Cancer Cells by Tamoxifen and 17beta-Estradiol. *J Natl Cancer Inst* 82:1702-1705

Cohen FJ, Manni A, Glikman P, Bartholomew M, Demers L (1988): Involvement of the Polyamine Pathway in Antiestrogen-induced Growth Inhibition of Human Breast Cancer. *Cancer Res* 48:6819-6825

Coradini D, Biffi A, Pirronella E, Di Fronzo G (1995): Tamoxifen and beta-Interferon: Effect of Simultaneous or Sequential Treatment on Breast Cancer Cell Lines. *Anticancer Res* 15:315-320

Creamer P, Lim K, George E, Dieppe P (1994): Acute inflammatory polyarthritis in association with tamoxifen. *Brit J Rheumatol* 33:583-585

Cutuli B, Abecassis J, Petit JC, Fricker JC, Schumacher C, Jung GM, Velten M (1993): Thromboembolic accidents in postmenopausal women treated by adjuvant Tamoxifen: 19 case reports. *Europ J Cancer* 29A:S72

Cuzick J, Allen D, Baum M, Barrett J, Clark G, Kakkar V, Melissari E, Moniz C, Moore J, Parsons V, Pemberton K, Pitt P, Richmond W, Houghton J, Riley D (1993): Long Term Effects of Tamoxifen. *Europ J Cancer* 29A:15-21

Dreicer R and Wilding G (1992): Steroid Hormone Agonists and Antagonists in the Treatment of Cancer. *Cancer Invest* 10:27-41

Fernö M, Baldetorp B, Borg A, Brouillet JP, Olsson H, Rochefort H, Sellberg G, Sigurdson H, Killander D (1994): Cathepsin D, Both a Prognostic Factor and a Predictive Factor for the Effect of Adjuvant Tamoxifen in Breast Cancer. *Europ J Cancer* 30A:2042-2048

Foekens JA, Look MP, Peters HA, van Putten WLJ, Portengen H, Klijn JGM (1995): Urokinase-Type Plasminogen Activator and Its Inhibitor PAI-1: Predictors of Poor Response to Tamoxifen Therapy in Recurrent Breast Cancer. *J Natl Cancer Inst* 87:751-756

Friedman ZY (1994): The Antitumour Agent Tamoxifen Inhibits Breakdown of Polyphosphoinositides in GH4C1 Cells. *J Pharmacol Experim Therapeut* 271:238-245

Garcia-Ruiz N, Sanchez MC, Valenzuela P, Jimenez P, Rodriguez E, Cortes-Prieto J (1994): Ocular toxicity of tamoxifen: a case of optic neuritis. *Oncologia (Madrid)* 17:64-66

Gong Y, Ballejo G, Murphy LC, Murphy LK (1992): Differential Effects of Estrogen and Antiestrogen on Transforming Growth Factor Gene Expression in Endometrial Adenocarcinoma Cells. *Cancer Res* 52:1704-1709

Gottardis MM, Robinson SP, Satyaswaroop PG (1988): Contrasting actions of tamoxifen on endometrial and breast tumour growth in athymic mouse. *Cancer Res* 48:812-815

Hampson JP, Donnelly A, Lewis-Jones MS, Pye JK (1995): Tamoxifen-induced hair colour change. *Brit J Dermatol* 132:483-484

Heier JS, Dragoo RA, Enzenhauer RW, Waterhouse WJ (1994): Screening for ocular toxicity in asymptomatic patients treated with tamoxifen. *Amer J Ophthal* 117:772-775

Jacquemiere J, Penault-Llorca F, Viens P, Houveenaeghel G, Hassouni J, Torrente M, Adelaide J, Birnbaum D (1994): Breast Cancer Response to Adjuvant Chemotherapy in Correlation with erbB2 and p53 Expression. *Anticancer Res* 14:2273-2278

Johnston SRD, McLennan KA, Salter J, Sacks NM, McKinna JA, Baum M, Smith IE, Dowsett M (1993): Tamoxifen induced the expression of cytoplasmic c-erbB2 immunoreactivity in oestrogen-receptor positive breast carcinomas *in vivo*. *The Breast* 2:93-99

Jordan VC (1995a): Tamoxifen and Tumorigenicity: a Predictable Concern. *J Natl Cancer Inst* 87:623-626

Jordan VC (1995b): What if tamoxifen (ICI 46, 474) had been found to produce rat liver tumors in 1993? *Ann Oncol* 87:623-626

Katzenellenbogen BS, Norman MJ, Eckert RL, Peltz SW, Mangel WF (1984: Bioactivities, Estrogen Receptor Interactions and Plasminogen-Activator-Inducing Activities of Tamoxifen and Hydroxytamoxifen Isomers in MCF-7 Human Breast Cancer Cells. *Cancer Res* 44:112-119

Knabbe C, Lippman ME, Wakefield LM (1987): Evidence that TGF-beta is a hormonally regulated negative growth factor in human breast cancer cells. *Cell* 48:417-428

Kotoulas IG, Mitropoulos D, Kardamakis E, Dounis A, Michopoulos J (1994): Tamoxifen treatment in male infertibility. I. Effect on spermatozoa. *Fert Steril* 61:914-922

Lipponen PK and Eskelinen MJ (1995): Reduced expression of E-cadherin is related to invasive disease and frequent recurrence in bladder cancer. *J Cancer Res Clin Oncol* 121:303-308

Locher D, Tang R, Pardo G, Hamlin M (1994): Retinal changes associated with tamoxifen treatment for breast cancer. *Invest Ophthalmol Visual Sci* 35:1526

Loffeld RJLF and Van Weel TF (1993): Tamoxifen for retroperitoneal fibrosis. *Lancet* 341:382

Lopes MCF, Vale MGP, Carvalho AT (1990): Ca^2-dependent Binding of Tamoxifen to Calmodulin Isolated from Bovine Brain. *Cancer Res* 50:2753-2758

Mamby CC, Love RR, Feyzi JM (1994): Protein S and protein C level changes with adjuvant tamoxifen therapy in postmenopausal women. *Breast Ca Res Treat* 30:311-314

Mamby CC, Love RR, Lee KE (1995): Thyroid Function Test Changes With Adjuvant Tamoxifen Therapy in Postmenopausal Women With Breast Cancer. *J Clin Oncol* 13:854-857

Manni A, Badger B, Luk G, Wright C, Caplan R, Rockette H, Bartholomew M, Ahmed SR (1988): Role of polyamines in the growth of hormone-responsive experimental breast cancer *in vivo*. *Breast Ca Res Treat* 11:231-240

Manni A (1989): Polyamines and Hormonal Control of Breast Cancer Growth. *CRC Crit Rev Oncogenesis* 1:163-174

Manni A (1994): The role of polyamines in the hormonal control of breast cancer cell proliferation. In: Dickson R and Lippman M (eds): Mammary Tumorigenesis and Malignant Progression. Kluwer Academ Publ pp 209-225

Mascarenhas MR, Garcia-e-Costa J, Galvao-Teles A (1994): Medical Therapy in Male Infertility. *Prog Reprod Biol Med* 16:9-17

Maudelonde T, Escot C, Pujol P, Rouanet P, Defrenne A, Brouillet JP, Rocherfort H (1994): *In vivo* Stimulation by Tamoxifen of Cathepsin D RNA Level in Breast Cancer. *Europ J Cancer* 30A:2049-2053

Millon R, Nicora F, Muller D, Eber M, Klein-Soyer C, Abesassis J (1989): Modulation of human breast cancer cell adhesion by estrogens and antiestrogens. *Clin Expl Metast* 7:405-415

Nabai H and Rahbari H (1994): Autoimmune Progesterone Dermatitis Treated with Tamoxifen. *Cutis* 54:181-182

Neal AJ, Evans K, Hoskin PJ (1993): Measurement of the effect of Tamoxifen on bone mineral density. *Brit J Radiol* 66:49-50

Ng R, Kellen JA, Wong AHC (1986): The effect of estrogens and anti-estrogens on plasminogen activator levels in an experimental tumor model. *J Nutr Growth Cancer* 3:177-181

Nuwaysir EF, Dragan YP, Jefcoate CR, Jordan VC, Pitot HC (1995): Effects of Tamoxifen Administation on the Expression of Xenobiotic Metabolizing Enzymes in Rat Liver. *Cancer Res* 55:1780-1786

O'Brian CA, Liskamp RM, Solomon DH, Weinstein IB (1985): Inhibition of Protein Kinase C by Tamoxifen. *Cancer Res* 45:2462-2465

O'Brian CA, Liskamp RM, Solomon DH, Weinstein IB (1986): Triphenylethlenes: A New Class of Protein Kinase Inhibitors. *J Natl Cancer Inst* 76:1243-1246

O'Brian CA, Ward NE, Anderson BW (1988a): Role of Specific Interactions Between Protein Kinase C and Triphenylethylenes in Inhibition of the Enzymes. *J Natl Cancer Inst* 80:1628-1633

O'Brian CA, Housey GM, Weinstein IB (1988b): Specific and Direct Binding of Protein Kinase C to an Immobilized Tamoxifen Analogue. *Cancer Res* 48:3626-3629

O'Brian CA, Ioannides CG, Ward NE, Liskamp RM (1990): Inhibition of Protein Kinase C and Calmodulin by the Geometric Isomers Cis and Trans-Tamoxifen. *Biopolymers* 29:97-104

Osborne CK, Boldt DH, Clark GM, Trent JM (183): Effects of Tamoxifen on Human Breast Cancer Cell Cycle Kinetics: Accumulation of Cells in Early G_1 Phase. *Cancer Res* 43:3583-3855

Pathak AU and Bodell WJ (1994): DNA adduct formation by tamoxifen with rat liver microsomal activation systems. *Carcinogenesis* 15:529-532

Pathak DN, Pongracz K, Bodell WJ (1995): Microsomal and perioxidase activation of 4-hydroxytamoxifen to form DNA adducts. *Carcinogenesis* 16:11-15

Phaneuf S, Europe-Finner GN, MacKenzie IZ, Watson SP, Lopex Bernal A (1995): Effects of oestradiol and tamoxifen on oxytocin-induced phospholipase C activation in human myometrial cells. *J Reprod Fertil* 103:121-126

Pinto HC, Baptista A, Camillo ME, deCosta EB, Valente A, de Moura MC (1995): Tamoxifen-associated steatohepatitis. *J Hepatol* 23:95-97

Pollak M, Powles TJ, Baum M, Sacks N (1993): Tamoxifen used as a chemopreventive agent lowers serum IFG-I levels. *Proc AACR* 34:255

Pongracz K, Pathak DN, Nakamura T, Burlingame AL, Bodell WJ (1995): Activation of the Tamoxifen Derivative Metabolite E to Form DNA Adducts. *Cancer Res* 55:3012-3015

Recchia F, Sica G, De Fipillis S, Discepoli S, Rea S, Torchio P, Frate L (1995): Interferon-beta, Retinoids and Tamoxifen in the Treatment of Metastatic Breast Cancer: A Phase II Study. *J Interferon Cytokine Res* 15:605-610

Repke KRH and Matthes E (1994): Tamoxifen in a Na-antagonistic Inhibitor of Na/K-transporting ATPase from tumour and normal cells. *J Enzyme Inhib* 8:207-212

Rutquist LE, Johansson H, Signomklao T, Johansson U, Fornander T, Wilking N (1995): Adjuvant Tamoxifen Therapy for Early Stage Breast Cancer and Second Primary Malignancies. *J Natl Cancer Inst* 87:645-651

Sapino A, Pietribiasi F, Bussolati G, Marchsio PC (1986): Estrogen- and Tamoxifen-induced Rearrangements of Cytoskeletal and Adhesion Structures in Breast Cancer MCF-7 Cells. *Cancer Res* 46:2526-2531

Sartor BM, Sartor O, Flanders KC (1995): Analogous tamoxifen and estrogen effects on transforming growth factors beta1 and 2 in rat uterus. *Reprod Toxicol* 9:225-232

Sekeris CE (1991): Hormonal Steroids Act as Tumour Promotors by Modulating Oncogene Expression. *J Cancer Res Clin Oncol* 117:96-101

Sica G, Natoli C, Marchetti P, Piperno S, Iacobelli S (1984): Tamoxifen-induced membrane alterations in human breast cancer cells. *J Steroid Biochem* 20:425-428

Simon R (1995): Discovering the Truth About Tamoxifen: Problems of Multipicity in Statistical Evaluation of Biomedical Data. *J Natl Cancer Inst* 87:627-629

Sloane B, Herman CJ, Padarathsingh M (1994): Molecular Mechanisms of Progression and Metastasis of Human Tumors. *Cancer Res* 54:5241-5245

Spillane RM and Whitman GJ (1995): Treatment of Retroperitoneal Fibrosis with Tamoxifen. *AJR* 164:515-516

Sthoegar ZM, Bentwich Z, Zinger H, Mozes E (1994): The Beneficial Effect of the Estrogen Antagonist Tamoxifen on Experimental Systemic Lupus Erythematosus. *J Rheumat* 21:2231-2238

Sterzik K, Rosenbusch B, Mogck J, Heyden M, Lichtenberger K (1993): Tamoxifen treatment of oligozoospermia: a re-evaluation of its effects invluding additional sperm function tests. *Arch Gyn Obstet* 252:143-147

Stevens HP, Ostler LS, Black CM, Jacobs HS, Pustin MHA (1993): Cyclical psoriatic arthritis responding to anti-oestrogen therapy. *Brit J Dermatol* 129:458-460

Szczensy PJ and Steiner R (1994): Reversibility of visual symptoms in tamoxifen toxicity depends on total cumulative dose. *Proc AACR* 35:250

Thylan S (1995): The beneficial effect of the estrogen antagonist tamoxifen on experimental lupus erythematosus. *J Rheumatol* 22:1606

Toms SA, Casey G, Hercbergs A, Zhoe P, Barnett GH, Barna BP (1995): Tamoxifen-induced p53 independent apoptosis in a human glioblastoma cell line. *Proc AACR* 36:8

Vancutesem PM, Lazarus P, Williams GM (1994): Frequent and Specific Mutations of the Rat p53 Gene in Hepatocarcinomas Induced by Tamoxifen. *Cancer Res* 54:3864-3867

Weckbecker G, Tolcsvai L, Stolz B, Pollak M, Bruns C (1994): Somatostatin Analogue Octreotide Enhances the Antineoplastic Effects of Tamoxifen and Ovarectomy on 7,12-Dimethylbenz (alpha)anthracene-induced Rat Mammary Carcinoma. *Cancer Res* 54:6334-6337

White INH, De Matthesis F, Gibbs AH, Lin CK, Wolf CR, Henderson C, Smith LL (1995): Species Differences in the covalent binding of tamoxifen to liver microsomes and the forms of cytochrome P450 involved. *Biochem Pharmacol* 49:1035-1042

Wright CDP and Compston JE (1995): Oestrogen or anti-oestrogen in bone? *Quart J Med* 88:307-310

Yu H, Diamandis EP, Zarghami N, Grass L (1994): Induction of prostate specific antigen production by steroids and tamoxifen in breast cancer cell lines. *Breast Ca Res Treat* 32:291-300

Yu H, Diamandis EP, Katsaros D, Sutherland DJA, Levesque MA, Roagna R, Ponzone R, Sismondi P (1995): Prostate-specific Antigen Is a New Favorable Prognostic Indicator for Women with Breast Cancer. *Cancer Res* 55:2104-2110

Zhang JJ, Jacob TJC, Valverde MA, Hardy SP, Mintenig GM, Sepulveda FV, Gill DR, Hyde SC, Trezise AEO, Higgins CF (1994): Tamoxifen Blocks Chloride Channels. A Possible Mechanism for Cataract Formation. *J Clin Invest* 94:1690-1697

Zhang JJ, Jacob TJC, Hardy SP, Higgins CR, Valverde MA (1995): Lens opacidication by antiestrogens: Tamoxifen vs ICI 182,780. *Brit J Pharmacol* 115:1347-1348

Zimniski SJ and Warren RC (1993): Induction of Tamoxifen-dependent Rat Mammary Tumors. *Cancer Res* 53:2937-2939

Tamoxifen in the treatment of tumours other than of breast

The mechansims of antitumour activity, clinical pharmacology, toxicity and efficacy of Tamoxifen therapy in women with early and advanced breast cancer as well as the possible role of this drug in prevention of breast cancer have been extensively reviewed (Jaiyesimi et al., 1995).

The importance of estrogens and necessarily of their antagonists is derived from the unmistakable role in the etiology and stimulation of many other cancers. The original concept that tumours containing steroid receptors, which respond to steroid stimulation, can be inhibited by competitive binding of substances mimicking some structural peculiarities of the hormones but lacking their stimulative action, appears logical, pragmatical and promising. In real life, such straightforward logic rarely works; in cancer therapy, almost never.

There are many tissues in which steroid receptors have been detected; the gastrointestinal system (including liver, pancreas, stomach, colon and rectum) and probably many if not most other organs. The function of estrogens is obvious in some, such as the larynx in puberty and difficult, if not impossible to interpret in others. It is to be expected that treatment with Tamoxifen can be of some benefit in tumours of these organs. Furthermore, in view of the "multiple" unrelated effects of this drug, its generally antiproliferative action could be useful even in tumours which do not respond to hormones, particularly estrogens. There is scattered, but numerous literature on this subject; a table with a review of available data follows.

Table 1. Tamoxifen treatment in malignancies other than breast cancer

Tumour	Effect	Comment	Reference
GLIOBLASTOMA			
multiforme	promising	as adjuvant th	Vertosick et al, 1993 & 1994
			Toms et al., 1995
high grade (recurrent)	"	stabilizing effect	Baltuch et al., 1993

Table 1, cont.

in childhood (brainstem)	"	"	Pons et al., 1994
supratentorial	"	with BCNU	Lafitte et al., 1994
WiTG3 cells	"	with TNF-alpha	Iurasaki et al., 1995
ASTRO-CYTOMA	inconclusive beneficial	with antiepileptics	Shenouda et al, 1994 Rabinowicz et al. 1995
ENDO-METRIAL CA	promising tumour	In ER positive	Satyaswaroop et al., 1984
"	promising		Sismondi et al., 1994
CERVICAL CA	decrease in mitotic figures	invasive Ca	Vargas-Roig et al., 1993
OVARIAN CA	promising	In ER positive tumour	Lazo et al., 1984
"	growth inhibition	"	Langdon et al., 1994
"	palliation	chemoresistant epithelial Ca	Ahlgren et al., 1993
PANCREAS adenoCa	increased survival	with Octreotide	Rosenberg et al., 1995
" (unresectable)	"		Wong et al., 1987
" (advanced)	"	with Onconase	Constanzi et al., 1994
"	promising	with Leuprolide	Zaniboni et al., 1994
" (resectable)	"		Horimi et al., 1993

Table 1, cont.

PROSTATE CA	promising	with vinblastine	Pienta et al., 1995
MELANOMA sk-30 CELLS (*in vitro*)	growth inhibition	with cis-Pt, DTIC, Interferon-alpha2b, vitamins	Prasad et al., 1994
Melanoma cells	with quercetin	growth inhibition	Piantelli et al., 1995
metastatic	promising	with chemotherapy	Gasparini, 1995
metastatic	promising	with Fotemustine	Punt et al., 1995
metastatic	no improvement	"	Bajetta et al., 1993
metastatic	improvement	high-dose Tamoxifen	Spitler et al., 1994
stage 4	improvement	Cis-Pt, DTIC, BCNU	Reintgen and Saba, 1993
ocular	improvement	with calmodulin antagonists	MacNeil et al., 1994a MacNeil et al., 1994b
THYROID CA follicular, papillary "	growth inhib. dose-responsive	in cell culture	Hoelting et al., 1995
medullary	no improvement		Garcia-Pascual et al., 1993
HEPATO-CELLULAR CA	promising	double-blind, placebo-controlled	Bruix et al., 1994
" (advanced)	improvement	with VP-16	Cheng et al., 1993

Table 1, cont.

DESMOID TU	partial response		Gouyon et al., 1994
"	"		
"			
(abdominal)	promising	with Sulindac	Dean et al., 1994
RENAL CA advanced	promising	with Tegafur, Adriamycin, Methotrexate	Wada et al., 1995
BLADDER CA	chemosensitization		Pu et al., 1995
LARYNX CA			
UM-SCC cells	growth inhib.	*in vitro*	Shapira et al., 1986
"			
SQUAMOUS CA	inconclusive	recurrent Ca	Urba et al., 1990
SQUAMOUS CA (head and neck)	growth inhib.	*in vitro*	Grenman et al., 1987
ADENOCA, eccrine	promising	in E-receptor positive tu	Sridhar et al., 1989

REFERENCES

Ahlgren JD, Ellison N, Lokich J, Ueno W, Gottlieb R, Laluna F, Wampler G, Fryer J, Fryer D (1993): High-dose tamoxifen: Extended palliation in patients with chemoresistant epithelial ovarian cancer. *Proc Amer Soc Clin Oncol* 12:258

Bajetta E, Zampino M, Nole F, Zilembo N (1993): Tamoxifen does not improve response when added to chemotherapy in metastatic melanoma. *Proc Amer Soc Clin Oncol* 12:393

Baltuch G, Shenouda G, Langleben A, Villemure JG (1993): High Dose Tamoxifen in the Treatment of Recurrent High Grade Glioma. *Can J Neurol Sci* 20:168-170

Bruix J, Castells A, Bru C, Ayuso MC, Boix L, Roca M, Rodes J (1994): Treatment of advanced hepatocellular carcinoma with tamoxifen. *Hepatology* 20:297A

Cheng AL, Chen YC, Sheu JC, Chen BR, Hsu HC, Lkai MY, Yeh KH, Chen DS (1993): Chronic oral VP-16 plus tamoxifen in the treatment of far-advanced hepatocellular carcinoma. *Proc Amer Soc Clin Oncol* 12:204

Chmielowska E, Potemski P, Pluzanska A (1995): Three-drug combination of cisplatin, dacarbazine and tamoxifen in metastatic malignant melanoma. *J Clin Oncol* 13:2146

Constanzi J, Chun H, Mittelman A, Puccio C, Coombe N, Panella T, Mesches D, Shogen K, Mikulski S (1994): Phase I/II clinical trial of onconase plus tamoxifen in patients with advanced pancreatis carcinoma. *Proc Amer Soc Clin Oncol* 13:205

Dean PA, Penna C, Camillari MJ, Dozois RR (1994): Prospective evaluation of the association of sulindac-tamoxifen in the treatment of abdominal desmoid tumors in familial adenomatous polyposis. *Gastroent Clin Biol* 18:B313

Garcia-Pascual L, Millan M, Anglada J, Garau (1993): Tamoxifen failure in medullary thyroid carcinoma. *Tumori* 79:357-358

Gasparini G (1994): Tamoxifen and Chemotherapy in the Treatment of Metastatic Melanoma: Are There Other Possible Mechanisms Explaining Their Potentiation? *J Clin Oncol* 12:1994-1995

Goldin BR (1994): Nonsteroidal Estrogens and Estrogen Antagonists: Mechanism of Action and Health Implications. *J Natl Cancer Inst* 86:1741-1742

Grenman R, Virolainen E, Shapira A, Carey T (1987): *In Vitro* Effects of Tamoxifen on UM-SCC Head and Neck Cancer Cell Lines: Correlation with the Estrogen and Progesterone Content. *Int J Cancer* 39:77-81

Gouyon B, Ducreux M, Rougier P, Berthelot G, Lasser P (1994): Desmoid tumour: partial response with tamoxifen therapy. *Gastroent Clin Biol* 18:792-794

Hoelting T, Siperstein AE, Duh QY, Clark OH (1995): Tamoxifen Inhibits Growth, Migration and Invasion of Human Follicular and Papillary Thyroid Cancer Cells *in Vitro* and *in Vivo*. *J Clin End Metabol* 80:308-313

Horimi T, Morita S, Takasaki M, Yormitu Y, Takahashi I (1993): Hormone therapy of Tamoxifen in resectable carcinoma of the pancreas. *J Jap Soc Cancer Ther* 28:494

Iwasaki K, Toms SA, Barnett GH, Estes ML, Gupta MK, Barna BO (1995): Inhibitory effects of tamoxifen and tumour necrosis factor alpha on human glioblastoma cells. *Cancer Immunol Immunother* 40:228-234

Jaiyesimi IA, Buzdar AU, Decker DA, Hortobagyi GN (1995): Use of Tamoxifen for Breast Cancer: Twenty-Eight Years Later. *J Clin Oncol* 13:513-529

Laffite C, Li YJ, Ameri A, Chauveinc L, Poisson M, Delattre JY (1994): Treatment of Malignancy Supratentorial Gliomas With the Association of BCNU and Tamoxifen: A Phase II Study. *Neurology* 44:A308

Langdon SP, Crew AJ, Ritchie AA, Muir M, Wakeling A, Smyth JF, Miller WR (1993): Growth inhibition of ER-positive ovarian carcinoma cells by antiestrogens *in vitro* and *in vivo*. *Proc AACR* 34:244

Lazo JS, Schwartz PE, MacLusky NJ, Labaree DC, Eisenfeld AJ (1984): Antiproliferative Actions of Tamoxifen in Human Ovarian Carcinomas. *Cancer Res* 44:2266-2271

MacNeil S, Wagner M, Rennie IG (1994a): Investigation of the role of signal transduction in attachment of ocular melanoma cells to matrix proteins: inhibition of attachment of calmodulin antagonists including tamoxifen. *Clin Exp Metast* 12:375-384

MacNeil S, Wagner M, Rennie IG (1994b): Tamoxifen Inhibition of Ocular Melanoma Cell Attachment to Matrix Proteins. *Pigment Cell Res* 7:222-226

Piantelli M, Maggiano N, Ricci R, Larocca LM, Capelli A, Scambia G, Isola G, Natali PG, Ranelletti FO (1995): Tamoxifen and quercetin interact with type II estrogen binding sites and inhibit the growth of human melanoma cells. *J Invest Dermatol* 105:248-253

Pienta KJ, Replogie T, Lehr JE (1995): Inhibition of prostate cancer growth by vinblastine and tamoxifen. *Prostate* 26:270-274

Pons M, Hetherington M, Massey V, Hanson EJ, Egelhoff J, Zwick D, Convy L, Freemand A (1994): Preliminary Results: Recurrent Intrinsic Brainstem Gliomas of Childhood Respond to Tamoxifen. *Ann Neurol* 36:514

Prasad KN, Hernandez C, Edwards-Prasad J, Nelson J, Borus T, Robinson WA (1994): Modification of the Effect of Tamoxifen, cis-Platin, DTIC and Interferon-alpha2b on Human Melanoma Cells in Culture by a Mixture of Vitamins. *Nutr Cancer* 22:233-245

Pu YS, Hsieh TS, Tsai TC, Cheng AL, Hsieh CY, Su IJ, Lai MK (1995): Tamoxifen enhances the chemosensitivity of bladder carcinoma cells. *J Urol* 154:601-605

Punt CJA, Tytgat JH, van Liessum PA, Gerard B (1995): Fotemustin and Tamoxifen Combination Therapy in Metastatic Malignant Melanoma. A Phase II Study. *Europ J Cancer* 31A:421-422

Rabinowicz AL, Hinton DR, Dyck P, Couldwell WT (1995): High-Dose Antiepileptic Drugs. *Epilepsy* 36:513-515

Reintgen D, Saba H (1993): Chemotherapy for Stage 4 Melanoma: A Three-Year Experience with Cisplatin, DTIC, BCNU and Tamoxifen. *Sem Surg Oncol* 9:251-255

Rosenberg L, Barkun AN, Denis MH, Pollack M (1995): Low Dose Octreotide and Tamoxifen in the Treatment of Adenocarcinoma of the Pancreas. *Cancer* 75:23-28

Satyaswaroop PG, Zaino RJ, Mortel R (1984): Estrogen-Like Effects of Tamoxifen on Human Endometrial Carcinoma Transplanted into Nude Mice. *Cancer Res* 44:4006-4010

Shapira A, Virolainen E, Jameson J (186): Growth inhibition of laryngeal UM-SCC cell lines with Tamoxifen, comparison with effects on the MCF-7 breast cancer line. *Arch Otolaryngol Head Neck Surg* 112:1151-1158

Shenouda G, Preul M, Langleben A, Villemure JG, Bahary JP, Wainer I, Pollak M, Leyland-Jones B, Tsatoumas A, Choi A (1994): A phase I/II trial of high dose tamoxifen in patients with recurrent high grade cerebral astrocytomas. *J Neuro Oncol* 19:181

Sismondi P, Biglia N, Volpi E, Gail M, DeGrandis T (1994): Tamoxifen and Endometrial Cancer. *Ann NY Acad Sci* 734:310-321

Spitler L, Good J, Jacobs M, Gilyon K (1994): The use of high-dose tamoxifen to potentiate the anti-tumor effects of cytotoxic chemotherapy in patients with metastatic melanoma. *Proc Amer Soc Clin Oncol* 13:397

Sridhar KS, Benedetto P, Otrakji CL, Charyulu KK (1989): Response of Eccrine Adenocarcinoma to Tamoxifen. *Cancer* 64:366-370

Toms SA, Casey G, Hercberg A, Zhou P, Barnett GH, Barna BP (1995): Tamoxifen-induced p-53 independent apoptosis in a human glioblastoma cell line. *Proc AACR* 36:8

Urba S, Carey T, Kudla-Hatch V (1990): Tamoxifen therapy in patients with recurrent laryngeal squamouc carcinoma. *Laryngoscope* 100:76-78

Vargas Roig LM, Lotfi H, Olcese JE, Lo Castro G, Ciocca DR (1993): Effects of Short-Term Tamoxifen Administration in Patients with Invasive Cervical Carcinoma. *Anticancer Res* 13:2457-2464

Vertosick FT, Selker RG, Arena V (1994): A Dose-Escalation Study of Tamoxifen Therapy in Patients with Recurrent Glioblastoma Multiforme. *J Neurosurg* 80:385A

Wada T, Nishiyama K, Maeda M, Hara S, Tanaka N, Yasutomi M, Kurita T (1995): Combined Chemoednocrine Treatment with Tegafur and Tamoxifen for Advanced Renal Cell Carcinoma. *Anticancer Res* 15:1581-1584

Wong A, Chan A, Arthur K (1987): Tamoxifen Therapy with Unresectable Adenocarcinoma of the Pancreas. *Ca Treat Rep* 71:749-750

Zanboni A, Meriggi F, Arcangeli G, Alghisi A, Huscher C, Marini G (1994): Leuprolide and Tamoxifen in the Treatment of Pancreatic Cancer. A Phase II Study. *Europ J Cancer* 30A:128

2. ASSESSING NEOPLASIA

Charles Rowlatt

This chapter is based on the premise that the current clinical paradigm of neoplasia, which rests on descriptions of neoplastic phenomena in the clinic (Gatter, 1994; Cotran et al., 1994) has been overtaken by analytical methods available in the laboratory (Salomon, 1987). Yet the scientist is still dependent on clinical judgements which appear subjective in the absence of a unifying hypothesis. A reasoned perspective is presented which attempts to account for the whole range of neoplastic phenomena, and goes some way towards providing common ground for the various disciplines involved. Such an enormous field can only be presented in the most general terms, but even these can provide guidelines for assessing neoplasia. This introduction is followed by summary of the basic principles, how they account for neoplastic phenomena, how this applies in practice and what consequences might follow.

Need for assessment

Clearly assessing each case precisely is fundamental in the management of any disease process. If a lesion may be neoplastic, the assessment should allow its future behaviour to be predicted and hopefully controlled. In principle the lesion is allocated to a specific place in the established course of the disease. But in practice its future route is often uncertain, and the diagnostician collates its previous course and current appearances with a probable final outcome. The diagnosis combines their original training, subsequent advice from clinical and laboratory specialists and their own lay and professional experience. Each practitioner has learnt the current paradigm (Kuhn, 1972) of neoplasia and adds their own experience. In the pressing need for management decisions, clinico-pathological experience and laboratory-derived concepts mix uneasily.

Clinical versus scientific paradigms

Present perceptions of neoplasia have evolved from the historical recognition and description of the lesions in the nineteenth century (Triolo, 1964), through identification of the various phenomena in experimental animals in the present century (Foulds, 1969, 1975), to detailed analyses of particular mechanisms mainly in the last three decades (Pitot, 1986; Sirica, 1989; Hodges and Rowlatt, 1994). General studies of the phenomena by physicians, epidemiologists and pathologists tend to generate hypotheses within a unified clinical paradigm of neoplasia with the diagnosis standardised on nineteenth century technology. Meanwhile more specific hypotheses based on supposedly key mechanisms underlying the various processes have provided a succession of mechanistic paradigms. Each has reflected contemporary adademic and technical approaches, from metabolic processes through to cell and molecular biology (for details, discussion and references see Rowlatt 1994a).

The difficulty is that the lesions have eluded scientific definition (Foulds, 1969; Rowlatt, 1989; Rowlatt et al., 1990; Sirica, 1969; Sporn, 1991), and descriptions of typical cases provide the parameters for laboratory models. But specific aberrations of behaviour form an uncertain basis for generalisations in cancer research, and more than a century of investigation has failed to reveal the single cause or a specific marker of neoplasia.

Current perceptions

It is generally accepted that neoplastic lesions are operationally irreversible foci (or fields) of tissue disorganisation, and that various structural and functional characteristics may contribute to recognising them (e.g. Gatter, 1992; Cotran et al., 1994). The foci may grow (growth). The disorganisation may change in nature (progression). The lesions may be found widely distributed (metastasis). Those whose appearance suggests a fatal outcome on past experience are called malignant: others with characteristics known to be innocuous are described benign. There is an uncertain middle ground. The confidence in predicting eventual outcome (or prognosis) varies with organ or origin, and prognosis for epithelial lesions appears less uncertain than for the rest. For ease of communication lesions are typically assessed for treatment or trials by organ (e.g. mammary), tumour type (ductal adenocarcinoma), extent of spread (stage number) and aberrations of cell organisation (numerical grade).

In this pragmatic classification dissimilar classes of activity are grouped together. Behavioural differences between cases which might suggest a different route to the final outcome are not necessarily recorded. Thus stage IV does not distinguish sites of distant metastasis and the grades pool information on intercellular organisation, cytoplastic organisation, intranuclear organisation and cell turnover criteria. The approach masks distinctions between growth and malignancy in assessing prognosis. A scheme is proposed in which individual lesions and experimental models share common classification criteria. Although entirely compatible with present practice, it provides a supplementary framework allowing comparison of like with like both within the clinic and between clinic and laboratory.

Basic principles

The approach is to treat the phenomena of neoplasia as defects of biological organisation (Smithers, 1962; Dilman, 1971; Rubin, 1990; Rowlatt, 1989, 1990, 1994a,b). The whole range of lesions and processes can and indeed must be included. Each lesion is considered to represent escape from normal biological organisation, with the aberrant behaviour reflecting failure of one or more controls. Recognising limits set by methods of investigation is fundamental. Change with time is examined, including the assumption that an expected outcome is inevitable. Specific criteria for malignancy vary between lesions, and the concept of relative malignancy between lesions which emerges from the thesis forms the basis for scientific analyses. The term malignant is reserved for its clinical use for conveying the outcome to the patient.

Relevant characteristics of biological organisation

Biological organisation is complex, dynamic, hierarchical, interactive and self-replicating (Foulds, 1969) (Table 1). These familiar characteristics often escape notice, but when defective they provide the identifying characteristics of neoplasia. In summary: complexity underlies the heterogeneity; defective dynamics underlie growth; the level in the hierarchy which is defective determines the quality of the aberrant behaviour; complementary normal behaviour at interactive faces is reflected in contrasting aberrant behavious from the two sides; and defective self-replication underlies changed behaviour.

Table 1.   Main characteristics of normal and defective biological organisation in neoplasia

Character	Effect of Defect	Practical Considerations
complex	heterogeneity	uniqueness
*dynamic**	*growth*	*arhythmia?*
hierarchical	relative malignancy	level of study
interactive	contrasting behaviour	extrapolation?
*self-replicating**	*changed behaviour*	*single/ongoing?*

time dependent, presenting a structure/function dilemma in analysis

Constraints on investigation

Each characteristic imposes practical constraints on investigation (Elsasser, 1981; Rubin, 1985; Albrecht-Buehler, 1990) (Table I).   The consequence of heterogeneity is that spontaneous lesions must, as a first approximation, be treated as unique.   Functional dynamics can only be studied over time in intact running systems, while most structural analysis requires samples taken at a moment in time.   Thus the physician observes the growth of a tumour in the patient while pathologist analyses the tissue disorganisation in a fixed specimen for its malignancy.   The level in the biological hierarchy reproduced in a laboratory model dictates the level of disorganisation for which the model is relevant (Table II). Moreover extrapolation back from a model to the whole organisms may produce contrasting effects if the tissue type differs. When self-replication fails, the practical consideration is whether the behaviour change is a single episode or an on-going process.

Table II. Hierachy of supra-cellular organisation underlying relative malignancy in neoplasia

Level	Control Lost	Diagnostic Stigmata	Model
cells	like cell interaction	dissociation, dissemination	cell culture
tissues	tissue-tissue interaction	invasion by coherent tissues	organ culture
functional units of organs	functional unit mass	expansive well-organized tumour	in vivo

Simultaneity

These characteristics are necessary and indivisible aspects of living material. Each can be recognised but, as they are qualitatively different, attempts to study any one in detail reduces or obliterates the others. Two, dynamics and self-replication, can only be studied directly over time in intact systems: in fixed material they can only be inferred. Two more, hierarchy and interaction, can be considered as structural coordinates of the lesions, as the hierarchial nature of biological organisation is one aspect of the increasingly elaborate interactive processes. Complexity qualifies these coordinates and underlies much of the uncertainty between lesions with similar defective behaviour.

Some neoplastic phenomena

One route through this multidimensional system is to consider neoplastic phenomena successively in these terms.

The nature of relative malignancy at a moment in time. Developmental biology reveals the fundamentally hierarchial and interactive nature of biological organisation (Gilbert, 1991). The successive stages from a single cell through multiple cells, tissue sorting, organ rudiments to the full range of developed organs in the individual are well established. Moreover differential cellular differentiation, in part pre-programmed, arises largely from interactions between complementary components at the various levels in the system.

Turning to neoplasms, histopathological analysis correlated with subsequent clinial behaviour has allowed the outcome of broad categories of epithelial neoplasms to be established from fixed samples (Ewing, 1940; Nicholson, 1950; Willis, 1967). An apparently expansive mass of glandular tissue retaining most of its normal cell types can be judged benign. When tongues or sheets of abnormal epithelial cells are invading adjacent tissues the prognosis is more serious. More seriously still, these invading neoplastic cells are dissociated, or neoplastic cells or tissue masses are found to be established at distant sites. This sequence clearly reflects the level of supra-cellular organisation (cell-cell, tissue-tissue, or control of organ functional units) for which control has become defective. As these criteria underlie the severity of the process, we can infer that the relative malignancy of the neoplasm is determined by the level of supra-cellular organisation for which control has been retained.

This rule was established for the epithelial neoplasms, adenomas and carcinomas, but is much less clear for neoplasms or non-epithelial mesenchymal tissues, the sarcomas and neoplasms of the haemopoietic system. However it also clear both from developmental biology (Gilbert, 1991) and cytology (Alberts et al., 1994) that, while epithelial tissues normally express coherence and polarity, non-epithelial tissues can exist as relatively discrete cells within the extracellular matrix, and may normally move independantly in response to a variety of stimuli. If our inference is correct that the relative malignancy of a neoplasm depends on the level of organisation which is retained, we can conclude that neoplasms of mesenchymal cells which have dissociated or become established at a distant site need not have a serious prognosis provided the normal control has been retained. But they would have been considered malignant by the criteria for epithelial neoplasms. So the basis for contrasting carcinoma/sarcoma behaviour can be attributed to complementary tissue types.

These criteria for histopathological diagnosis were established by and depend on fixed tissue sections studied by light microscopy. But the analysis of three dimensional tissues in two dimensional samples entails loss of information. Epithelial sheets are seen as cords of cells, cords are seen as isolated cells, and single cells may be sampled or missed. Epithelial organs are recognised in sections by their supra-cellular organisation into coherent epithelial cell sheets or pockets surrounded by mesenchymal components. Neoplastic variants of this structure are recognised by retained epithelial properties. By contrast the supra-cellular organisation of mesenchymal tissues is difficult to determine in sectioned material, and it is virtually impossible to see the distinctions in breakdown of control described for epithelial neoplasms. As the significance of the neoplastic cellular behaviour often differed, histopathologists agreed to assess neoplastic prognosis organ by organ, with criteria differing between groups of organs. When the supra-cellular organisation cannot be seen, diagnosis depends on the secondary evidence of cellular abnormalities rather than the primary parameter of relative malignancy.

Origins of neoplasms in functional units. The study of pathology often unmasks normal function. Although the normal behaviour that is lost in carcinomas is self-evident (e.g. normal epithelial coherence lost by dissociated carcinoma cells), the normal counterpart of benign adenomas is less evident. While their focal nature shows local escape from overall control or organisation, their excess of neoplastic functional units shows that the organ of origin must consist of normal functional units (Rowlatt, 1993).

A functional unit of an organ can be defined as the domain comprising those interacting cells for various lineages necessary to provide a part of its (physiological) function. Any organ is therefore an array of functional units, and, extrapolating, the whole organism is composed of interacting functional units. Their collective functions are those of the whole organism, with some excluding or maintaining the internal environments and others providing the structural components within it.

Although any functional unit is to some extent indeterminate because its function depends on other functional units and their domains overlap, the concept provides a useful analytical tool. An epithelial component in a functional unit identifies the domain of associated mesenchymal cells and supporting systems (vessels, endocrine system, and so forth) necessary to maintain its differentiation and function, but these are hard to see. With hormone sensitive tissues, withdrawal leads to balanced involution. Evidence for the tissue interactions underlying mesenchymal functional units is accumulating indirectly from cytokine studies, but the units are difficult to identify anatomically in the plane sections required for microscopy.

If cells exist by virtue of their contribution to a functional unit, the functional unit is where neoplasms arise. Specific genetic or epigenetic abnormalities, which allow escape from tissue homeostatic controls in the hierarchy, need not suppress the whole function. The behaviour of the neoplasm is dictated by the cell types that survive, and by the properties they still express, irrespective of level of organisation. For example dissociated malignant cells may still express factors involved in higher-level tissue interactions. It is because neoplasms are lesions of the supra-cellular organisation, the functional unit, that the light microscope is still the best tool for analysing the disorganisation.

Distinction between growth and malignancy. Growth and malignancy are often treated as interdependant; in fact, growth is net increase in mass of biological material over time, while malignancy is the attribute of a neoplasm when it has a fatal outcome. Growth occurs normally during development. Cells produce more cells, tissues produce more of the same, organs acquire new functional units. Neoplastic growth reflects loss of normal homeostatic control, and this can be observed at any level of organisation. In contrast the indications for a fatal outcome are so numerous and varied that the adjective malignant, when unqualified, is virtually useless to specify neoplastic tissues for scientific comparisons. However its use is justified clinically when advising the patient. Here, the term relative malignancy is employed to grade the severity of the disorder in supra-cellular tissue organisation at the moment it is observed.

Growth can be assessed histologically by evidence of previous growth (the mass) and parameters indicating rapid cell turnover (mitotic figures, and other parameters or probes). Relative malignancy for the functional unit involved can be assessed by the level or organisation for which control is retained. With epithelial tissues, local invasion of neoplastic tissues or dissociated cells in a sample reveals a serious tendency to spread, while samples from distant sites confirm this. As each level of organisation must have different cytological controls, markers for them should provide firm evidence of the relative malignancy of a tissue sample. Convertional staging only provides a crude measure of relative malignancy. Grading, relying on conventional cytological stigmata of malignancy, combines evidence of tissue disorganisation, parameters of rapid cell turnover and evidence of disordered cell replication.

Change with time. Neoplasms are recognised and classified by their abnormal behaviour over time, and this traditionally includes apparently inexorable growth and/or risk of progression.   However these generalisations are by no means inevitable and the time related processes can be usefully subdivided, and separate accounts made of the underlying phenomena (Table III).

Table III. An outline of time related changes in biological self-replication

Class	Implications
no change	status quo maintained
change may be:	
reversible	changed status quo
	- dependent on conditions
	- reverts with appropriate conditions
irreversible	determination (as in embryo), mutation
and change may be:	
single	status quo changed
successive	multiple changes in status quo
	uncertain selection for
	- altered relative malignancy
	- advantagenous properties*
continuous	status quo lost
	rapid selection for:
	- the lowest common denominator,
	'malignant cell'
	- advantageous properties*

*advantageous properties include: neovascularisation, metastatic phenotypes, metabolic shifts, etc.

Biological systems are dominated by reversible change with time. The normal structure of an organ reflects its physiological and biochemical activity and the current state of development from conception to senescence of the component functional units. The smooth transition in expression of normal properties over time demonstrate the elaborate controls covering all levels of organisation.

Neoplastic change may be reversible when retained normal biological properties provide conditional support (such as growth stimulation) for the aberrant behaviour, and secondary modulation becomes possible through physiological manipulation of these retained supporting processes (such as down-regulating growth). An irreversible change may be physiological determination in the cell lineage or an error in self-replication, a mutation, which is expressed in the new phenotype.

While a single change would lead to a uniformly altered phenotype, successive changes would give variations in phenotype. If this involves controls at a lower level of organisation, a stepwise increase in relative malignancy can be expected, the phenomenon known as progression (Foulds, 1954). The more serious form of behaviour takes precedent by pre-empting the more highly organised tissues rather than by increased vitality. However there may also be uncertain slection for advantageous properties such as neovascularisation, metastasis or metabolic shifts.

However when continuing change occurs, the neoplasm rapidly degenerates into undifferentiated dissociated cells which will have been selected for cell turnover alone, lowest common denominator cells (LCD-cells). However in this scenario, LCD-cells can be very poorly adapted, and this is found in many transplantable tumour cell models. However if they retain or acquire advantageous properties for net growth, they become what is generally thought of as 'malignant cells'.

Both clinical observations and experimental carcinogenesis have provided evidence of progression in Foulds' (1954) sense of stepwise irreversible change for the worse. But if defects of control are acquired independently, any pattern of aberrant behavious may emerge at any time and reversible and irreversible expression need not be mutually exclusive. Historically, conditional neoplastic states appeared irreversible until analysis suggested modulation could work (Beatson, 1896; Pierce and Verney, 1961; Seilern-Aspang and Kratochwil, 1962; Huggins, 1967).

Although genetic aberrations dominate the picture in terminal cancer, identifying neoplasia as failure of organisation leaves open the possibility that dynamic considerations may precipitate or influence carcinogenesis (Rowlatt, 1993). If organs and their functional units are organised at distinct levels with separate feedbacks at each level these may breakdown when appropriate parameters shift critically. As each functional unit operates independently, the organ would provide a field in which independent neoplasms of eqivalent relative malignancy would develop. This is well recognised and is a criterion of non-genotoxic carcinogenesis (Butterworth and Slaga, 1987). It also occurs at the different levels of relative malignancy. For example in the colon, the onset of polyposis coli occurs in the second decade. With experimental alteration of cholesterol intake, a generalised alteration of malignancy occurs in dimethylhydrazine-induced colon carcinomas (Cruse et al., 1984). In longstanding ulcerative colitis, the presence of carcinoma in the colon is predicted by dysplastic glands in the rectum (Morson and Pang, 1967).

Applying these concepts to assessment

In the previous sections we have identified some major characteristics of biological organisation and proposed how defects in this can account for observed neoplastic phenomena. Unfortunately the methods of investigation can unduly emphasise particular characteristics of neoplasia for the discipline using them. Research requires comparison of like with like: the characteristics of compared materials should correspond. However, a series of questions based on their biological characteristics can provide a biological profile of the clinical lesion or material for the laboratory (Table IV). This could help to compare of like with like, and avoid unnecessary generalisations.

Table IV. Questions to establish the biological profile of normal or neoplastic material for comparative studies

Interaction
1. Which functional unit or organisation is involved?
2. On which side of any tissue interaction do the cells primarily involved lie?
3. What are their states of differentiation?

Hierarchy
4. For which level of organisation is expression of control defective?

Dynamics
5. Is net growth expressed?
6. Do differences in samples taken over time reflect aberations of the normal biorhythms?

Self-replication
7. Is there evidence of change in behaviour?

Complexity
8. How is the case different from apparently similar cases?

Although the detail is potentially vast, initially approximate answers are acceptable, and may only need re-evaluation of histopathological material. Specific markers, as they become available, should eventufally fill in supplementary detail. In general abnormal characteristics indicate that a lesion is neoplastic, but retained normal characteristics of living tissues drive the aberrant behaviour.

Interaction. Questions 1-3 specify organ and cell type of origin in more detail than is normal for tumour diagnosis. Histopathology has always provided an approximate assessment, but the development of many normal differentiation probes allows more specific qualities to be identified for research purposes. The answers specify what behaviour the tissues involved should express normally.

Hierarchy. Question 4 addressed the relative malignancy of the neoplasm. In practice, the level of organisation which is defective is recognised by the (lower) level of organisation for which control is still retained. As the control of tissue homeostasis is qualitatively different at each level of biological organisation, escape from control can be expected to have characteristic molecular properties at each level of relative malignancy. However the evidence may be indirect, reflecting reversible properties in the past, as well differentiated metastases express a higher level of organisation than that expressed when (dissociation and) spread occurred.

Dynamics. Question 5 assesses growth. Histopathological evidence for net growth at a moment in time is provided by the expanded mass(es) of neoplastic tissue. The proportion of cells fixed in mitosis, or bearing equivalent molecular markers provides evidence of excessive cell turnover, and by implication net growth. As balanced cellular proliferation is a pre-requisite or self-replication at higher levels of biological organisation, molecular markers of cell growth control derived from simple culture systems are still relevant in more organised tissues. Question 6 alerts the investigator to problems in sampling fluctuating dynamic systems where parameters alter over time.

Self-replication. Many neoplasms are remarkably homogeneous, with the same patterns of supra-cellular organisation repeating across many microscope fields. Histopathologists routinely store their specimens, to assess whether a later sample from a patient is from the same neoplasm or a new lesion. Evidence for change in the patterns (for which there is no microenvironmental explanation) is sought diligently as evidence of change in behaviour (question 7). Evidence for probable change in behaviour is provided by cytological signs of genetic instability, i.e. variability in cytological and nuclear structure and abnormal mitoses.

Complexity. Question 8 reminds the observer that the defects may be random and that each lesion should be treated as unique, despite the broad diagnostic categories employed at present. For research purposes biological subsets within conventional categories of cancer must provide one source of new therapeutic strategies (Rowlatt and Loizidou, 1995).

Consequences

Cancer is such a large field that multidisciplinary collaboration is essential. The present synthesis suggests a unifying approach based on analysis of normal biological organisation. Scienfitic analysis normally attempts to limit variables and compare like with like. The proposed common scheme for classification identifies unusual categories, embracing not only a very wide range of neoplastic phenomena but also constraints in the methods available to investigate them. This should allow correlation of particular scientific models and comparable clinical lesions. By specifying applicability it should strengthen laboratory findings and reduce the risk that unwarranted generalisations mask real effects in particular subsets. It should help communication between scientist and clinician.

The assumption that each case may be unique obliges the investigator to look beyond dysfunctional phenomena, as any several preceding steps may have become defective. The more specific the mechanisms for the dysfunction in the laboratory, the greater the onus to demonstrate applicability in the clinic. And the broader the insult in carcinogenesis, the wider the spectrum of lesions developed.

Most investigators treat cancer as an exclusively cellular disorder, despite pleas for a broader view (e.g. Smithers, 1962; Dilman, 1971;

Rubin, 1985). Here we argue strongly that neoplasms must arise as consequence of defective supra-cellular organisation in the functional units which make up the organs in the body. If so, laboratory models should match the supra-cellular organisation of the neoplastic lesions they represent. This includes both the level of complexity of intercellular interactions, which models the relative malignancy, and also the differentiation of the cell types involved, which dictates which of the potential behaviour in the genotype is likely to be expressed.

Interactions with their complementary thrusts occur at all levels: the yin-yan of biological organisation. The contrast between carcinoma and sarcoma was attributed to their respective tissue types. But contrasting effects when a balance is disturbed underlie other paradoxes, from misplaced cytokine therapy to control of neoplasia in secondary sex organs with complementary steroids.

Treatment of malignancy is normally assessed by time to eventual outcome. But unsuspected conditional neoplasia is indistiguishable from irreversible change and must be actively sought (Beatson, 1896; Pierce and Vernay, 1961; Seilern-Aspang and Kratochwil, 1962; Huggins, 1967). Identifying specific parameters in the biological profile may allow effects of suspected modulators on growth and relative malignancy to be distinguished and monitored. Each lesion is treated as unique, and the chosen parameters followed over time, irrespective of the overall picture. If withdrawal is permissable, checking for reversibility may be possible. Despite practical difficulties, potential rewards should make this theoretical approach worth considering.

This concept of neoplasia has been developed over years, but, as the concept of arhythmia as a defect only dawned while writing this chapter, chronobiology, a key field for the future, is only briefly introduced here. A review from a Festschrift for Franz Halberg (Cornelissen et al., 1989) indicates its extent. His recognition of rhythm structure in biology has led to a proper description of functional dynamics. Chronobiologis have identified circadian, circaseptan, circatrigentan, circannual and infradian (less than 24 hours) rhythms. Measurable rhythms with multiple frequencies must now replace putative set points in physiology. Roles of steroids, peptides and indoleamines in biological time measurement have been worked out. The implications for health and the prediction and management of a variety of chronic disease processes, including cancer, have absorbed Halberg's school for forty years.

This strongly suggests (and may well have already shown) that control of tissue homeostasis is dynamically as well as qualitatively different according to the hierarchy of biological organisation, and we would predict that the dynamics would alter accordingly as progression occurs. Intriguingly a shift from the circatrigintan to the circaseptan range of breast surface temperature is reported in women at high risk of breast cancer (Simpson et al., 1989). More practically, the need for time-specified interpretation of the single measurement within a parameter's rhythm should be emphasised here.

Conclusion

The scheme presented in this chapter attributes the phenomena of neoplasia to disorder in biological organisation, and the analysis bridges technological gaps which easily open between disciplines. For the investigators who accept the scheme, a biological profile of their material will position their work in the framework with any degree of precision they choose. A reader from any discipline can then compare their materials and conclusions. Could this cross-disciplinary approach crack the enigma of Tamoxifen?

REFERENCES

Alberts B, Bray D, Lewis J, Raff M, Roberts K, Watson JD (1994): Molecular Biology of the Cell (3rd ed.), New York: Garland Publishing Inc.
Albrecht-Buehler G (1990): In defense of "nonmolecular" cell biology. *International Rev of Cytology* 120:191-241
Beatson GT (1896): On the treatment of inoperable cases of carcinoma of the mamma: suggestions for a new method of treatment, with illustrative cases. *Lancet* ii:104-107,162-165
Butterwoth BE, Slaga TJ (eds), (1987): Nongenotoxic Mechanisms in Carcinogensis. Cold Spring Harbor: Cold Spring Harbor Laboratory.
Cornelissen G, Halberg E, Halberg F, Sampson M, Hillman D, Nelson W, Sanchez de la Pena S, Wu J, Delmore P, Marques MD, Fernandez JR, Hermida RC, Guillaume F, Caradente F (1989): Chronobiology: a frontier in biology and medicine. *Chronobiologia* 16:383-408
Cotran RS, Kumar V, Robbins SL (1994): Robbins' Pathologic Basis of Disease (5th ed.). Philadelphia: WB Saunders Company
Cruse JO, Lewin MR, Clark CG (1984): An investigation into the mechanism of co-carcinogenesis of dietary cholesterol during the induction of colon cancer in rats by 1,2dimethylhydrazine. *Clin Oncology* 10:213-230

Dilman VM (1971): Age-associated elevation of hypothalamic threshold to feedback control and its role in development, ageing and disease. *Lancet* i:1211-1219

Elsasser WM (1981): Principles of a new biological theory: a summary. *J Theorectical Biology* 89:132-150

Foulds L (1954): The experimental study of tumour progression: a review. *Cancer Res* 14:327-339

Foulds L (1969): Neoplastic Development 1. London: Academic Press

Foulds L (1975): Neoplastic Development 2. London: Academic Press

Gatter KC (1992): Morphology of neoplasms. In: JO McGee, PG Isaacson and NA Wright (eds.), Oxford Textbook of Pathology (vol. 1 Principles of Pathology, pp. 577-589). Oxford: Oxford University Press

Gilbert SF (1991): Developmental Biology (3rd ed.). Sunderland, MA: Sinauer Associates Inc.

Hodges GM, Rowlatt C (eds.) (1994): Developmental Biology and Cancer. Boca Ratton, FL: CRC Press Inc.

Huggins C (1967): Endocrine-induced regression of cancers. *Science* 156:1050-1054

Kuhn TS (1972): The Structure of Scientific Revoluations (2nd ed.). Chicago: University of Chicago Press

Morson BC, Pang L (1967): Rectal biopsy as an aid to diagnosis in ulcerative colitis. *Gut* 8:423-434

Nicholson GWDP (1950): Studies on Tumour Formation. London: Butterworth & Co.

Pierce GB, Verney EL (1961): An in vitro and in vivo study of differentiation in teratocarcinomas. *Cancer* 14:1017-1029

Pitot HC (1986): Fundamentals of Oncology (3rd ed.). New York: Dekker

Rowlatt C (1989): Defining Neoplasm. *The Cancer Journal* 2(11):363-368

Rowlatt C, Cruse JP, Hodges GM (1990): The neoplasm as tissue disorganisation: an hypothesis of neoplasia. *The Cancer Journal* 3(5):283-287

Rowlatt C (1993): Some consequences of defining the neoplasm as focal self-perpetuating tissue disorganisation. In: OH Inverson (ed.), New Frontiers in Cancer Causation: Proceedings of the Second International Conference on Theories of Carcinogenesis (pp. 45-58). Washington DC: Taylor and Francis

Rowlatt C (1994a): Relative malignancy and ontogeny. In: GM Hodges, C Rowlatt (ed.), Developmental Biology and Cancer (pp. 29-60). Boca Raton FL: CRC Press Inc

Rowlatt C (1994b): Applying molecular biology to neoplasia. *The Cancer Journal* 7:99-102

Rowlatt C, Loizidou M (1995): Biological subsets within conventional diagnostic categories of cancer. *The Cancer Journal* 8:32

Rubin H (1985): Cancer as a dynamic developmental disorder. *Cancer Res* 45:2935-2942

Rubin H (1990): On the nature of enduring modifications induced in cells and organisms. *American Journal of Physiology* 258:L19-L24

Salomon JC (1987): Cancer Classification. *The Cancer Journal* 1(6):286-289

Seilern-Aspang F, Kratochwil K (1962): Induction and differentiation of an epithelial tumour in the newt (Triturus cristatus). *Embryol Experim Morphology* 10:337-356

Simpson HW, Pauson A, Wilson DW (1989): The chrono-bra: the "electrocardiogram" of the breast? Proc 2nd Ann IEEE Symp on Computer-based Medical Systems (pp. 214-225). Minneapolis: Computer Society Press, Washington DC

Sirica AE (1989): Classification of neoplasms. In: AE Sirica (ed.), The Pathobiology of Neoplasia (pp.25-38). New York: Plenum Press

Smithers DW (1962): Cancer: an attack on cytologism. *Lancet* i:493-499

Sporn MB (1991): Carcinogenesis and cancer: different perspectives of the same disease. *Cancer Res* 51:6215-6218

Triolo VA (1964): Nineteenth century cancer research: origins of experimental research. *Cancer Res* 24:4-27

Willis RA (1967): Pathology of Tumours (4th ed.). London: Butterwoths

3. INTERACTIONS OF TAMOXIFEN WITH LIPID SIGNAL TRANSDUCTION CASCADES

Myles C. Cabot and Armando E. Giuliano

Background

Triphenylethylenes are extremely useful drugs with therapeutic potential beyond breast cancer. In light of this broad utility we must also begin to address important questions regarding Tamoxifen side effects, as concern has been expressed for participants in prophylactic clinical trials, and for those already taking Tamoxifen for breast cancer (Fisher et al., 1994; Magriples et al., 1993). The multiple effects of Tamoxifen certainly indicate the need for more intensive studies on cell-specific actions of this drug and related synthetic antiestrogen-based agents. Elucidation of nongenomic pathways of triphenylethylene action is key to understanding the multimodal effects of these molecules.

   It cannot be disputed the efficacy of Tamoxifen resides in its ability to antagonize the actions of estrogen by binding competitively to the estrogen receptor (Ecker and Katzenellenbogen, 1983; Coezy et al., 1982). New research has pinpointed specific actions of Tamoxifen which are estrogen receptor-independent. The biological activities are impressive. Triphenylethylenes have broad utility for treatment of many cancers including melanoma (McClay et al., 1993) and brain cancer (Rabinowicz et al., 1995). Tamoxifen is an important component of the Dartmouth regimen for metastatic melanoma (Del Prete et al., 1984; McClay et al., 1989), where it has been shown to be synergystic and modulate cisplatin sensitivity (McClay et al., 1993). Tamoxifen synergy with cisplatin is not dependent on the presence of estrogen receptors. Favorable response with malignant glioma is believed to be linked to the interaction of Tamoxifen with protein kinase C (PKC) (Couldwell et al., 1992). Tamoxifen and related antiestrogens are, as well, potent biological response modifiers, independent of estrogen.

Table 1. Antiestrogens as response modifiers

Cell/Tissue	Response	Reference
breast cancer; fibroblasts	TGF-ß↑	Butta et al., 1992; Colletta et al., 1990
membranes; endothelium	angiogenesis↓	Gagliardi and Collins, 1993; Haran et al., 1994
MCF-7 cells; cell free	calmodulin↓	Rowlands et al., 1995
-"-	block IGF-I action	Kawamura et al., 1994
-"- membranes	lipid peroxidation↓	Wiseman et al., 1993
-"- whole cell; cell-free	PKC↓↑	Rowlands et al., 1995; Issandou et al., 1990; O'Brian et al., 1985; Bignon et al., 1991
leukemia, breast, gastric, colon and lung cancers	MDR↓	Hotta et al., 1995; Kirk et al., 1994; Berman et al., 1994; Callaghan and Higgins, 1995
Human glioma *in vitro*	growth↓	Vertosick et al., 1994
ER(-) MDA-MB-435 cells	growth↓	Charlier et al., 1995

There are a number of observations regarding Tamoxifen's effects which provide valuable information on alternate mechanisms of action. In many of these cases the integration of lipids is a common denominator. Lipids have been shown to play an important role in multidrug resistance (MDR) and in PKC biology, and Tamoxifen interacts with P-glycoprotein (P-gp) and PKC. For example, increased cellular P-gp correlates with increased drug resistance (Yeh et al., 1992) and with increased lipid metabolism (Welsh et al., 1994). MDR expression correlates with enhanced phosphatidylcholine (PC) translocation (Ruetz and Gros, 1994). Doxorubicin resistance parallels modified lipid composition and membrane lipid organization (Ramu et al., 1983), and circumvention of MDR in leukemia is associated with a rise in cell PC content (Ramu et al., 1991). The effect of lipids on P-gp associated ATP-ase activity has also been evaluated (Doige et al., 1993), and results show membrane phospholipids containing amino polar head groups like PC and phosphatidylethanolamine (PE) are necessary for P-gp activity. Tamoxifen also contains an amino grouping (dimethylethanolamine) similar with PC and PE.

PKC is a Ca^{2+} - and phospholipid-dependent enzyme which plays a major role in transmembrane signaling of a wide variety of agonists including growth factors and hormones (Nishizuka Y., 1995). The cellular activator of PKC is diacylglycerol (DG) which accumulates in cells upon receptor-mediated breakdown of phosphatidylinositol 4, 5 - *bis* - phosphate (PIP_2) (Divecha and Irvine, 1995) and PC (Huang and Cabot, 1990; Exton, 1994; Wen et al., 1995). Agents which provoke production of second messengers and agents which interact with PKC, such as 12-*0*-tetradecanoylphorbol-13-acetate (TPA), therefore have the potential to regulate cell homeostasis. In this respect, Tamoxifen has been shown not only to interact with PKC (Issandou et al., 1990; O'Brian et al., 1985; Bignon et al., 1991), but as well promote the formation of second messengers PA and DG and stimulate phospholipase D (PLD) (Cabot et al., 1995). Interaction with PKC, followed by formation of PA and DG is also a biochemical property of TPA (Cabot et al., 1989; Huang and Cabot, 1990). This shows phorbol diesters and Tamoxifen share biochemical actions. The findings are important and merit investigation.

There is a great deal of controversy surrounding the antagonist/agonist influence of Tamoxifen on PKC. Initial work demonstrated Tamoxifen inhibited PKC (O'Brian et al., 1985; Horgan et al., 1986) and proposed such action was central to antitumor activity. Subsequent studies have expanded our view of triphenylethylene interaction with PKC. PKC activation by triphenylethylenes has been demonstrated in intact cells and in cell-free systems (Bignon et al., 1991). SAR studies for PKC-triphenylethylene interaction suggest the basic amino side-chain interacts with the regulatory domain and the 1, 1-*bis* (p-hydroxyphenyl) ethylene moiety interacts with the catalytic domain of PKC (Bignon et al., 1991). Tamoxifen can be inhibitory for PKC when assayed in cell-free systems (O'Brian et al., 1985) but can have an opposite influence in intact cells (Issandou et al., 1990). This brings to light a major biological question, "is Tamoxifen antiproliferative because it inhibits PKC?" Activation of PKC is usually associated with a mitogenic response. However, this is not always the case as with i) PKC activated via PC breakdown products (Nishizuka, 1995), and ii) breast cancer. In human breast cancer cells it has been demonstrated that activators of PKC, such as TPA and cell permeable diacylglycerols, inhibit cell growth (Issandou et al., 1990; Issandou et al., 1988; Darbon et al., 1986; Issandou and Darbon, 1988). Therefore, we can say the generation of PC second messengers and/or activation of PKC by Tamoxifen will have a growth-negative influence in some cells, in particular, breast cancer cells.

In an effort to characterize mechanisms underlying the various nongenomic actions, we have tested the effect of Tamoxifen on signal transduction. To clearly divorce those aspects of estrogen receptor biology from estrogen receptor-independent events, we have utilized some cell lines which are estrogen receptor negative. Our experiments demonstrate Tamoxifen provokes transmembrane signaling of the type associated with phospholipase-lipid second messenger cascades. We show activation of both PLC and PLD, with generation of PA and DG, occurs in response to Tamoxifen treatment of cultured cells of various types. The parameters, biochemical pathways, and cell type-specificity of these lipid metabolic responses to Tamoxifen are presented.

Results

To understand the mechanisms underlying estrogen receptor-independent actions, we have been studying the impact of Tamoxifen on membrane-associated events of signal transduction. Initial experiments showed Tamoxifen, when added to the medium, promoted the formation of second messenger lipids in cultured fibroblasts. Due to the powerful regulatory role of second messengers, this finding was somewhat intriguing. We were prompted to determine whether this was a biochemical response specific to fibroblasts or a more broad-spectrum response. The data in Table 1 show, employing several dissimilar cell types, Tamoxifen, at a concentration of 10-20 micromoles, elicits rapid formation of PA and DG. In normal breast fibroblasts and in ovarian cancer cells both PA and DG were generated in response to Tamoxifen, whereas in breast and uterine cancer cells only PA was formed. The estrogen status of the cell did not influence the response to Tamoxifen.

Table 2. Human cells in which Tamoxifen activates formation of second messengers

Cell line	Cell type	ER status	Second messengers formed
CCD986SK	fibroblast	(-)	PA, DG
MDAA-MB-231	breast cancer	(-)	PA
RL95-2	uterine cancer	(+)	PA
NIH:OVCAR-3	ovarian cancer	(+)	PA, DG

Cells were prelabeled with tritiated fatty acid, equilibrated in isotope-free, serum-free medium for 2-4 hr, then challenged with Tamoxifen (10-20 micromoles) for 20-30 min.

The time course of Tamoxifen's influence on second messenger metabolism was investigated in several cell lines in order to gain insight into the temporal pattern of lipid formation and biochemical events underlying the response. Figure 1 demonstrates of the three cells explored, only the normal fibroblast (CCD986SK) exhibited increases in PA and DG. With PA formation occurring first, the pattern suggests Tamoxifen activates a PLD and DG arises either independently via PLC or by dephosphorylation of PA by PA phosphatase. In breast cancer cells (Fig. 1, middle) and uterine cancer cells (Fig. 1, right) the biochemical events underlying Tamoxifen-activated PA formation are more obvious.

In MDA-MB-231 and in RL95-2 cells, PA is generated in response to Tamoxifen, at the expense of cellular DG. This suggests in these cells Tamoxifen activates DG-kinase. In all cell lines the response to Tamoxifen was rapid, with increases in lipids occuring as early as 5-15 min post-treatment.

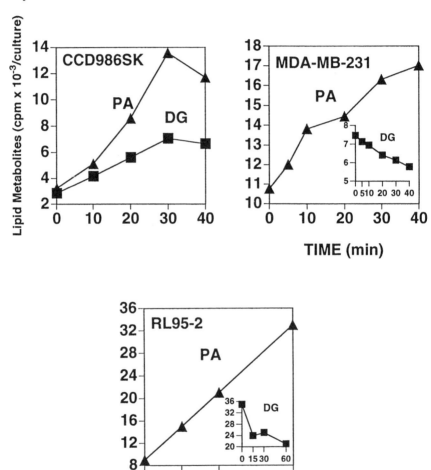

Figure 1. Tamoxifen Treatment of Cultured Cells Promotes Time-dependent Increases in Lipid Second Messengers. Fatty acid labeled ([3H] myristic acid) cells were treated with Tamoxifen (20 micromoles) for times indicated. CCD986SK, human breast fibroblasts; MDA-MB-231, human breast cancer cells; RL95-2, human endometrial carcinoma cells.

As with most work involving drug action, it was important to determine whether Tamoxifen activated transmembrane signaling at lower, pharmacological doses, in line with *in vivo* circulating and tissue-resident amounts of drug. The data of Figure 2 show lower dose Tamoxifen (0.1-2.5 micromoles) over extended time (three day exposure) causes dose-dependent elevation of PA in cultured uterine cancer cells (Fig. 2, left) and dose-dependent elevation of DG in normal fibroblasts (Fig. 2, right). At a concentration of 1.0 μM Tamoxifen caused a >50% increase in PA (RL95-2 cells) and a 25% increase in DG in CCD986SK fibroblasts.

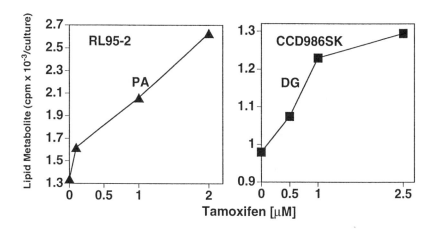

Figure 2. Effect of Low-dose Tamoxifen Over Extended Time on PA and DG Formation. Cells were grown with [3H]glycerol, +the indicated concentrations of Tamoxifen, for three days. Medium was phenol red-free plus 5% charcoal/dextran-treated FBS.

Using fibroblasts as a model, further experiments were conducted to delineate biochemical pathways and reveal the cellular lipid sources of PA and DG. The data of Figure 1, left, suggest Tamoxifen activates PLD and perhaps PLC. By prelabeling (48 hr) cells with [3H]choline and [3H]ethanolamine and examining the influence of Tamoxifen on the production of water-soluble phospholipid metabolites, it was possible to establish Tamoxifen activates PLD and PLC, and PC and PE are substrates. In labeled CCD986SK cells equilibrated in serum-free, isotope-free medium, Tamoxifen caused increases (in the medium and in the cytosol) of labeled choline, phosphorylcholine, ethanolamine and phosphorylethanolamine. The production of free base groups is indicative of PLD activity, and the production of phospho-bases is demonstrative of PLC activity.

To verify if Tamoxifen activates PLD and to evaluate the structure-activity relationship for activation, we compared several triphenylethylene-based agents, PKC agonists, and estrogen. These experiments were conducted with ethanol (1%) in the culture medium to measure PLD activity using the transphosphatidylation reaction. In the presence of a stronger nucleophile (ethanol as opposed to water), PLD catalyzes the production of a "phosphatidyl compound," in this case, phosphatidylethanol (PEt). As measured by the generation of PEt, Figure 3 clearly demonstrates Tamoxifen activates PLD in fibroblasts (7-fold increase in activity as opposed to control). Substitution at the 4-position, with a hydroxy group rendered the molecule nearly inactive as PLD agonist. Substitution of ethyl for methyl groups on the basic amino side-chain (Clomiphene) yielded activation of PLD (4-fold) but not to the extent of Tamoxifen. Estradiol was essentially without influence. Interestingly, agonists of PKC also activated PLD, as shown with TPA (3.5-fold) and DiC8 (2.5-fold increase). 4-*O-methyl*-TPA, which is inactive as a tumor promoter and PKC agonist, was void of activity.

The results with PKC agonists promoted us to further define the relationship between Tamoxifen, PLD, and PKC. To this end we employed PKC blocking agents and assessed the influence on Tamoxifen-induced PLD activity. Table 3 presents these results. Pretreatment of cells with phorbol dibutyrate, a protocol known to down-regulate PKC, resulted in an 80% inhibition of Tamoxifen ability to activate PLD. As a PKC control, we used TPA and showed down-regulation as well blocked, by 100%, TPA-induced PLD activity. The PKC inhibitor GF109203X retarded, by 60%, the activation of PLD by Tamoxifen.

Table 3. The influence of PKC blocking agents on Tamoxifen-induced PLD activity in fibroblasts

Agonist	Pretreatment protocol	Phospholipase activity (% inhibited)
Tamoxifen	+PDBu	80
	+GF109203X	61
TPA	+PDBu	100

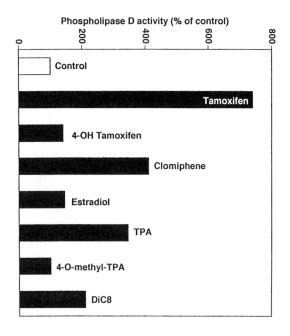

Figure 3. The Influence of Tamoxifen and Analogs, Estrogen, and PKC Agonists on PLD Activity in Fibroblasts. Fatty acid labeled CCD986SK cells were treated with triphenylethylenes (15 nM), estradiol (15 micromoles), phorbol esters (50 nM), and DiC8 (75 micromoles) for 30 min in medium containing 1% ethanol (to measure PLD by transphosphatidylation via PEt formation).

[^{3}H]Myristic acid labeled CCD986SK cells were exposed to 1.0 micromoles PDBu for 18 hr (control had no PDBu) and challenged with Tamoxifen (20 micromoles) or TPA (50 nM) for 20 min. GF109203X (5.0 micromoles) was added 2 min prior to Tamoxifen addition. PLD activity (PEt synthesized) is expressed as the percent activity inhibited, compared with controls in which PDBu and GF109203X were absent.

Discussion

Because Tamoxifen is being widely used for treatment and for prevention of breast cancer, and related triphenylethylenes are making an appearance in the clinical arena, careful consideration must be given to the biological activities of these agents. Studies on treatment of ovarian carcinoma (Lindner and Borden, 1995), efficacy for subduing MDR (Smith and Trump, 1995; and refer to Table) and synergy with combination chemotherapy (Warso et al., 1995; Cheng et al., 1995) are alone suggestive of the multimodal character displayed by Tamoxifen and analogs. In characterizing the biochemistry of Tamoxifen action we need also consider the potential hazards of these agents, especially as regards the endometrial-unfriendly effects (Dallenbach-Hellweg and Hahn, 1995; Sasco et al., 1995; Love, 1995). In an effort to unravel some of the mechanisms underlying Tamoxifen actions and to initiate a program aimed at demarking the benefits from the toxicities, we have focused attention on transmembrane signaling. Signal transduction at the plasma membrane is the initial control point for events regulated by extracellular agents. We have shown Tamoxifen, upstream from estrogen receptor interplay, initiates transmembrane signal transduction events common with other hormones and growth factors and tumor-promoting phorbol diesters.

The influence of Tamoxifen on formation of DG, the physiological activator of PKC (Nishizuka, 1995), and PA, a biological response modifier in its own right (for review, Cabot et al., 1995), has profound implications. Herein we show Tamoxifen activates phospholipid degradation by PLD and PLC. Phospholipid hydrolysis with formation of lipid second messengers is associated with sustained activation of PKC, which is influential in eliciting long-term responses such as differentiation (Nishizuka, 1995). The impact of Tamoxifen on phospholipases may lead to changes in cell homeostasis via second messenger lipid metabolites and PKC. Additionally, the ability of Tamoxifen to reverse MDR may be partially associated with plasma membrane lipid changes which could impact drug transport (efflux) and alter P-gp lipid microenvironments.

By using various cell lines our data clearly show the Tamoxifen transmembrane response is not an isolated phenomenon unique to a specific cell. We have shown that Tamoxifen has an impact on DG and/or PA metabolism in normal (noncancerous) cells, neoplastic cells, and in cells which are ER(+) and ER(-). This would imply that Tamoxifen, although a highly effective estrogen antagonist, has impact on numerous other cells and tissues of the body.

We have included work showing, at both relatively high doses (5-20 micromoles), and at lower doses over extended time (3 days), that

Tamoxifen elicits build-up of cellular PA and DG. This is of biological significance because these doses are comparable with *in vivo* situations. It is also important to consider even though test tube experiments show Tamoxifen has high affinity for the estrogen receptor, patients receiving tamoxifen do not have "test tube doses" in circulation. In patients taking tamoxifen, serum concentrations are around 0.1-$0.5\,\mu$M with intratumoral levels five to ten times higher (Johnston et al., 1993). The experiments raise important questions regarding DG levels in tamoxifen-responsive cells and tissues. Additionally in regard to pharmacokinetic dose, the new direction for high-dose Tamoxifen in treatment of cancer (Smith and Trump, 1995) is likely not founded upon pharmacokinetic relationships with the estrogen receptor.

The mechanism by which Tamoxifen activates phospholipases, in particular PLD, is not known. Although there have been mixed reports regarding Tamoxifen influence on PKC activity (O'Brian et al., 1985; Bignon et al., 1991), our data support the notion that Tamoxifen activates PLD through PKC. This is based on the following indirect evidence: i.) the PKC inhibitor GF109203X blocks (by 60%) PLD activation by Tamoxifen; ii.) pretreatment of cells with phorbol dibutyrate ("down-regulation") blocks TPA-induced PLD and Tamoxifen-induced PLD; iii.) addition of Tamoxifen to REF52 fibroblasts, a cell line which has been rigorously characterized (Cabot et al., 1989), does not interfere with TPA-induced PEt formation; iv.) known PKC agonists, TPA and cell-permeable DiC8, likewise activate PLD and 4-*O-methyl*-TPA, a poor promoter and PKC agonist, is void of activity. Previous work showing that Tamoxifen inhibits PKC (O'Brian et al., 1985) may be difficult to compare with our experiments using intact fibroblasts. Nevertheless, definitive answers await a more refined approach in which specific PKC isoforms can be studied.

In our preliminary look at structure activity relationships for PLD stimulation, it is noteworthy the hydroxylated form of Tamoxifen was inactive as a phospholipase effector. Droloxifene, a 3-hydroxylated analog, has been shown to have several advantages over Tamoxifen (Ke et al., 1995; Rausching and Pritchard, 1994; Hasmann et al., 1994), including decreased risk of endometrial cancer (Wiseman, 1994). It is tempting to speculate that some of the transmembrane signaling properties of Tamoxifen are associated with cell proliferative response; however, we have not as yet explored this biology. Further research on the nongenomic activities of triphenylethylenes is necessary for understanding the true potential of these compounds.

Summary

Tamoxifen and related compounds benefit breast and other cancers, reduce multi-drug resistance, and synergize with combination chemotherapeutics. Tamoxifen has also become a useful high-dose therapy in clinical trials for brain cancer, lymphoma, adenocarcinoma, and melanoma. These high-dose regimens are likely not based upon pharmacological doses which block estrogen, but rather based upon estrogen receptor-independent actions of Tamoxifen. It is now accepted Tamoxifen acts, in many instances, via estrogen receptor-independent pathways. The mechanisms for such actions remain obscure. The aim of our work on signaling properties of Tamoxifen is to provide insight into this poorly understood area of triphenylethylene action, for future application to the design of more patient-friendly, broad-scope pharmacologic agents. In this work we demonstrate Tamoxifen, in the low micromolar range, activates cellular phospholipases and thus potentiates the generation of lipid second messengers phosphatidic acid (PA) and diacylglycerol (DG). This nongenomic activity is very similar to the lipid signaling cascades initiated and utilized by many hormones and growth factors. Herein we characterize the biochemical pathways and cell type-specificity of the estrogen receptor-independent lipid metabolic responses provoked by Tamoxifen and provide information on the interplay of protein kinase C.

ACKNOWLEDGEMENTS

This work was supported by the Ben B. and Joyce E. Eisenberg Foundation and the Eisenberg-Keefer Breast Center, John Wayne Cancer Institute, Saint John's Hospital and Health Center. 4-OH-Tamoxifen was a gift from Dr. Dominique Salin-Drouin of Besins Iscovesco Laboratories (Paris, France). We are grateful to Christina Riley for preparing the figures and assembling the manuscript.

REFERENCES

Berman E, McBride M, Tong W (1994): Comparative activity of tamoxifen and N-desmethyltamoxifen in human multidrug resistant leukemia cell lines. *Leukemia* 8: 1191-6

Bignon E, Pons M, DorÄ JC, Gilbert J, Ojasoo T, Miquel JF, Raynaud JP, de Paulet AC (1991): Influence of di- and tri-phenylethylene estrogen/antiestrogen structure on the mechanisms of protein kinase C inhibition and activation as revealed by a multivariate analysis. *Biochem Pharmacol* 42:1373-1383

Butta A, MacLennan K, Flanders KC, Sacks NPM, Smith I, McKinna A, Dowsett M, Wakefield LM, Sporn MB, Baum M, Colletta AA (1992): Induction of transforming growth factor ß1 in human breast cancer *in vivo* following tamoxifen treatment. *Cancer Res* 52:4261-4264

Cabot MC, Welsh CJ, Zhang Z, Cao H (1989): Evidence for a protein kinase C-directed mechanism in the phorbol diester-induced phospholipase D pathway of diacylglycerol generation from phosphatidylcholine. *FEBS Lett* 245:85-90

Cabot MC, Zhang Z, Giuliano AE (1995): Tamoxifen elicits rapid transmembrane lipid signal responses in human breast cancer cells. *Breast Cancer Res Treat* 36:299-306

Callaghan R, Higgins CF (1995): Interaction of tamoxifen with the multidrug resistance P-glycoprotein. *Br J Cancer* 71:294-299

Charlier C, Chariot A, Antoine N, Merville M-P, Gielen J, Castronovo V (1995): Tamoxifen and its active metabolite inhibit growth of estrogen receptor-negative MDA-MB-435 cells. *Biochem Pharmacol* 49:351-358

Cheng AL, Yeh KH, Luo YJ, Chuang SE, Chen DS (1995): Synergistic effect of doxorubicin and tamoxifen in the treatment of hepatocellular carcinoma (HCC): *in vitro* and pilot clinical studies. *Proc Am Assoc Cancer Res* 36:347 Abst #2065

Coezy E, Borgna JL, Rochefort H (1982): Tamoxifen and metabolites in MCF-7 cells: correlation between binding to estrogen receptor and inhibition of cell growth. *Cancer Res* 42:317-323

Colletta AA, Wakefiels LM, Howell FV, van Roozendaal KEP, Danielpour D, Ebbs SR, Sporn MB, Baum M (1990): Antioestrogens induce the secretion of active transforming growth factor-ß from human fetal fibroblasts. *Br J Cancer* 62: 405-409

Couldwell WT, Antel JP, Yong VW (1992): Protein kinase C activity correlates with the growth rate of malignant gliomas: Part II. Effects of glioma mitogens and modulators of protein kinase C. *Neurosurgery* 31:717-724

Dallenbach-Hellweg G, Hahn U (1995): Mucinous and clear cell adenocarcinomas of the endometrium in patients receiving antiestrogens (tamoxifen) and gestagens. *Int J Gynecol Pathol* 14(1):7-15

Darbon JM, Valette A, Bayard F (1986): Phorbol esters inhibit the proliferation of MCF-7 cells: possible implication of protein kinase C. *Biochem Pharmacol* 35:2683-2686

Del Prete SA, Maurer LH, O'Donnell J, Jackson Forcier R, Le Marbre P (1984): Combination chemotherapy with cisplatin, carmustine, dacabarzine and tamoxifen in metastatic melanoma. *Cancer Treat Rep* 68:1403-1405

Divecha N, Irvine RF (1995): Phospholipid signaling. *Cell* 80:269-278

Doige CA, Yu X, Sharom FJ (1993): The effects of lipids and detergents on ATPase-active P-glycoprotein. *Biochim Biophys Acta* 1146:65-72

Ecker RL, Katzenellenbogen BS (1983): Physical properties of estrogen receptor complexes in MCF-7 human breast cancer cells. *J Biol Chem* 257:8840-8846

Exton JH (1994): Phosphatidylcholine breakdown and signal transduction. *Biochim Biophys Acta* 1212:26-42

Fisher B, Constantino JP, Redmond CK, Fisher ER, Wickerham DL, Cronin WM (1994): Endometrial cancer in tamoxifen-treated breast cancer patients: findings from the National Surgical Adjuvant Breast and Bowel Project (NSABP) B-14. *J Natl Cancer Inst* 86:527-527

Gagliardi A, Collins DC (1993): Inhibition of angiogenesis by antiestrogens. *Cancer Res* 53:533-535

Haran EF, Maretzek AF, Goldberg I, Horowitz A, Degani H (1994): Tamoxifen enhances cell death in implanted MCF7 breast cancer by inhibiting endothelium growth. *Cancer Res* 54:5511-5514

Hasmann M, Rattel B, Loser R (1994): Preclinical data for droloxifene. *Cancer Lett* 84:101-116

Horgan K, Cooke E, Hallett MB, Mansel RE (1986): Inhibition of protein kinase C mediated signal transduction by tamoxifen. *Biochem Pharmacol* 35:4463-4465

Hotta T, Tanimura H, Yamaue H, Iwahashi H, Tsunoda T, Tani M, Tamai M, Noguchi K, Mizobata S, Arii K, Terasawa H (1995): Adriamycin-resistance induced by P-glycoprotein is overcome by tamoxifen and cepharanthin. *Proc Am Assoc Cancer Res* 36:339 Abstr #2016

Huang C, Cabot MC (1990): Phorbol diesters stimulate the accumulation of phosphatidate, phosphatidylethanol, and diacylglycerol in three cell types. *J Biol Chem* 265:14858-14863

Huang C, Cabot MC (1990): Vasopressin-induced polyphosphoinositide and phosphatidylcholine degradation in fibroblasts: temporal relationship for formation of phospholipase C and phopholipase D hydrolysis products. *J Biol Chem* 265:17468-17473

Issandou M, Bayard F, Darbon JM (1988): Inhibition of MCF-7 cell growth by 12-O-tetradecanoylphorbol-13-acetate and 1,2-dioctanoyl-sn-glycerol: distinct effects of protein kinase C activity. *Cancer Res* 48:6943-6950

Issandou M, Darbon JM (1988): 1,2-Dioctanoylglycerol induces a discrete but transient translocation of protein kinase C as well as the inhibition of MCF-7 cell proliferation. *Biochem Biophys Res Commun* 151:458-465

Issandou M, Faucher C, Bayard F, Darbon JM (1990): Opposite effects of tamoxifen on *in vitro* protein kinase C activity and endogenous protein phosphorylation in intact MCF-7 cells. *Cancer Res* 50:5845-5850

Johnston SRD, Haynes BP, Sacks NPM, McKinna JA, Griggs LJ, Jarman M, Baum M, Smith IE, Dowsett M (1993): Effect of estrogen receptor status and time on the intra-tumoral accumulation of tamoxifen and N-desmethyltamoxifen following short term therapy in human primary breast cancer. *Breast Cancer Res Treat* 28:241-250

Kawamura I, Lacey E, Mizota T, Tsujimoto S, Nishigaki F, Manda T, Shimomura K (1994): The effect of droloxifene on the insulin-like growth factor-I-stimulated growth of breast cancer cells. *Anticancer Res* 14:427-431

Ke HZ, Simmons HA, Pirie CM, Crawford DT, Thompson DD (1995): Droloxifene, a new estrogen antagonist/agonist, prevents bone loss in ovariectomized rats. *Endocrinol* 136:2435-2441

Kirk J, Syed SK, Harris AL, Jarman M, Roufogalis BD, Stratford IJ, Carmichael J (1994): Reversal of P-glycoprotein-mediated multidrug resistance by pure anti-oestrogens and novel tamoxifen derivatives. *Biochem Pharmacol* 48:277-285

Lindner DJ, Borden EC (1995): An interferon ß and tamoxifen combination induces regression of established NIH-OVCAR-3 human ovarian carcinoma tumors in nude mice. *Proc Am Assoc Cancer Res* 36:264 Abstr #1575

Love RR (1995): Tamoxifen chemoprevention: public health goals, toxicities for all and benefits to a few. *Ann Oncol* 6:127-128

Magriples U, Naftolin F, Schwartz PE, Carcangiu ML (1993): High-grade endometrial carcinoma in Tamoxifen-treated breast cancer patients. *J Clin Oncol* 11:485-490

McClay EF, Albright KD, Jones JA, Christen RD, Howell SB (1993): Tamoxifen modulation of cisplatin sensitivity in human malignant melanoma cells. *Cancer Res* 53:1571-1576

McClay EF, Mastrangelo MJ, Sprandio JD, Bellet RE, Berd D (1989): The importance of tamoxifen to a cisplatin-containing regimen in the treatment of metastatic melanoma. *Cancer* 63:1292-1295

Nishizuka Y (1995): Protein kinase C and lipid signaling for sustained cellular responses. *FASEB* 9:484-496

O'Brian CA, Liskamp RM, Solomon DH, Weinstein B (1985): Inhibition of protein kinase C by tamoxifen. *Cancer Res* 45:2462-2465

Rabinowicz AL, Hinton DR, Dyck P, Couldwell WT (1995): High-dose tamoxifen in treatment of brain tumors: Interaction with antiepileptic drugs. *Epilepsia* 36:513-515

Ramu A, Glaubiger D, Magrath T, Joshi A (1983): Plasma membrane lipid structural order in doxorubicin-sensitive and -resistant P388 cells. *Cancer Res* 43:5533-5537

Ramu A, Ramu N, Rosario L (1991): Circumvention of multidrug-resistance in P388 cells is associated with a rise in the cellular content of phosphatidylcholine. *Biochem Pharmacol* 41:1455-1461

Rauschning W, Pritchard KI (1994): Droloxifene, a new antiestrogen: its role in metastatic breast cancer. *Breast Cancer Res Treat* 31:83-94

Rowlands MG, Budworth J, Jarman M, Hardcastle IR, McCague R, Gescher A (1995): Comparison between inhibition of protein kinase C and antagonism of calmodulin by tamoxifen analogues. *Biochem Pharmacol* 50:723-726

Ruetz A, Gros P (1994): Phosphatidylcholine translocase: a physiological role for the mdr2 gene. *Cell* 77:1071-1081

Sasco AJ, Raffi F, Satge D, Goburdhun J, Fallouh B, Leduc B (1995): Endometrial mullerian carcinosarcoma after cessation of tamoxifen therapy for breast cancer. *Int J Gynaecol Obstet* 48:307-310

Smith DC, Trump DL (1994): A phase I trial of high-dose oral tamoxifen and CHOPE. *Cancer Chemother Pharmacol* 35:65-68

Vertosick FT Jr, Selker RG, Randall MS, Kristofik MP, Rehn T (1994): A comparison of the relative chemosensitivity of human gliomas to tamoxifen and n-desmethyltamoxifen *in vitro*. *J Neurooncol* 19:97-103

Warso MA, Menini P, Das Gupta TK (1995): Synergistic effect of tamoxifen on cisplatinum toxicity. *Proc Am Assoc Cancer Res* 36:346 Abstr #2058

Welsh CJ, Yeh GC, Phang JM (1994): Increased phospholipase D activity in multidrug resistant breast cancer cells. *Biochem Biophys Res Comm* 202:211-217

Wen Y, Cabot MC, Clauser E, Bursten SL, Nadler JL (1995): Angiotensin II activated lipid signal transduction pathways in angiotensin II type 1 receptor transfected fibroblasts. *Am J Physiol* 269:435-442

Wiseman H (1994): Tamoxifen: new membrane-mediated mechanisms of action and therapeutic advances. *Trend Pharmacol Sci* 151:83-89

Wiseman H, Cannon M, Arnstein HR, Halliwell B (1993): Tamoxifen inhibits lipid peroxidation in cardiac microsomes. Comparison with liver microsomes and potential relevance to the cardiovascular benefits associated with cancer prevention and treatment by tamoxifen. *Biochem Pharmacol* 45:1851-1855

Yeh GC, Lopaczynska J, Poore CM, Poore CM, Phang JM (1992): A new functional role for P-glycoprotein: efflux pump for Benzo(a)pyrene in human breast cancer MCF-7 cells. *Cancer Res* 2:6692-6695

4. CARCINOGENICITY OF TAMOXIFEN

Annie J. Sasco and Isabelle Gendre

Tamoxifen, a synthetic antiestrogen, has been widely used for the treatment of breast cancer and has been shown to be effective in reducing overall mortality as well as mortality from breast cancer and the occurrence of contralateral breast cancer (Early Breast Cancer Trialists' Group, 1992). It is widely recognized as an important treatment modality for breast cancer, the indications of which have been progressively extended, from metastasis to less advanced carcinoma, from postmenopausal or premenopausal women, from some subsets of patients defined on the basis of nodal or hormonal receptor status to a large array of cases. This trend was supported by the good tolerance of Tamoxifen as a cancer treatment and its comparatively few serious side effects. The main surge in the prescription of Tamoxifen began in the mid 1970s when it was used in several randomized trails aiming at evaluating its efficacy in the treatment of breast cancer. By the mid 1980s, Tamoxifen represented one of the most strongly established treatment modalities and was listed by the World Health Organization as an essential drug for cancer chemotherapy (WHO, 1985). Yet reports had already appeared signaling some iatrogenic side effects on the female genital apparatus, the ovarian and non-ovarian endocrine system, as well as effects on bone metabolism, on the eye and liver, and cardiovascular and thromboembolic risks. In particular, concerns have been raised with regard to the potential carcinogenicity of this product. In the present paper, the criteria set out by the International Agency for Research on Cancer (IARC) Monographs on the evaluation of carcinogenic risks to humans have been applied to the review of available data obtained both from experimental and epidemological investigations. They suggest a strong presumption of the carcinogenicity of Tamoxifen.

The IARC criteria for the evaluation of carcinogenic risks to humans

The International Agency for Research on Cancer regularly publishes results of the evaluation of carcinogenicity of various compounds. A group of independent experts, the IARC Working Group, meets at IARC and critically reviews and evaluates published studies on a product or agent suspected of being carcinogenic. All available literature on the agent, *in vitro* and *in vivo*, for both experimental animals and humans is assessed. The evidence for carcinogenicity in humans and experimental animals is first described, along with supporting evidence. Then, other data relevant to the evaluation of carcinogenicity and it mechanisms are examined. The body of evidence thus assembled forms the basis for the classification of the product. The criteria used to assess agents are listed in Tables 1 to 3 and the overall evaluation is defined in Table 4. A fuller description of this material can be found in the preamble of the most recently published Monograph (IARC, 1995a).

For Tamoxifen, such an evaluation will be carried out at IARC in 1996. In the meantime, the present article will be limited to the evaluation by the authors of data available on this topic; the present paper is the sole responsibility of the authors. A previous review was published last year in French (Sasco, 1994). Since the time of that publication, new data have accumulated providing further evidence. They complete a review of the literature on the iatrogenic effects of Tamoxifen, excluding the aspect of carcinogenicity (Sasco et al., 1995a).

Table 1. Degrees of evidence for carcinogenicity in humans

- Sufficient evidence of carcinogenicity:
The Working Group considers that a causal relationship has been established between exposure to the agent, mixture or exposure circumstance and human cancer. That is, a positive relationship has been observed between the exposure and cancer in studies in which chance, bias and confouding could be ruled out with reasonable confidence.

- Limited evidence of carcinogenicity:
A positive association has been observed between exposure to the agent, mixture or exposure circumstance and cancer for which a causal interpretation is considered by the Working Group to be credible, but chance, bias or confounding could not be ruled out with reasonable confidence.

- *Inadequate evidence of carcinogenicity*:

The available studies are of insufficient quality, consistency or statistical power to permit a conclusion regarding the presence of absence of a causal association, or no data on cancer in humans are available.

- *Evidence suggesting lack of carcinogenicity*:

There are several adequate studies covering the full range of levels of exposure that human beings are known to encounter, which are mutually consistent in not showing a positive association between exposure to the agent, mixture or exposure circumstance and any studied cancer at any observed level of exposure. A conclusion of 'evidence suggesting lack of carcinogenicity' is inevitably limited to the cancer sites, conditions and levels of exposure and length of observation covered by available studies. In addition, the possibility of a very small risk at the levels of exposure studied can never be excluded.

In some instances, the above categories may be used to classify the degree of evidence related to carcinogenicity in specific organs or tissues.

IARC, 1995

Table 2. Degrees of evidence for carcinogenicity in experimental animals

- *Sufficient evidence of carcinogenicity*:

The Working Group considers that a causal relationship has been established between the agent or mixture and an increased incidence of malignant neoplasms or of an appropriate combination of benign and malignant neoplasms in (a) two or more species of animals or (b) in two or more independent studies in one species carried out at different times or in different laboratories or under different protocols.

Exceptionally, a single study in one species might be considered to provide sufficient evidence of carcinogenicity when malignant neoplasms occur to an unusual degree with regard to incidence, site, type of tumour or age at onset.

- *Limited evidence of carcinogenicity*:

The data suggest a carcinogenic effect but are limited for making a definitive evaluation because, e.g. (a) the evidence of carcinogenicity is restricted to a single experiment; or (b) there are unresolved questions regarding the adequacy of the design, conduct or interpretation of the study; or (c) the agent or mixture increases the incidence only of benign neoplasms or lesions of uncertain neoplastic potential, or of certain neoplasms which may occur spontaneously in high incidences in certain strains.

- *Inadequate evidence of carcinogenicity*:
        The studies cannot be interpreted as showing either the presence of absence of a carcinogenic effect because of major qualitative or quantitative limitations, or no data on cancer in experimental animals are available.

- *Evidence suggesting lack of carcinogenicity*:
        Adequate studies involving at least two species are available which show that, within the limits of the tests used, the agent or mixture is not carcinogenic. A conclusion of evidence suggesting lack of carcinogenicity is inevitably limited to the species, tumour sites and levels of exposure studied.

                                                                IARC, 1995

Table 3. Other data relevant to the evaluation of carcinogenicity and its mechanisms

Data on:
              - preneoplasic lesions
              - tumour pathology
              - genetic and related effects
              - structure-activity relationships
              - metabolism and pharmacokinetics
              - physiochemical parameters
              - analogous biological agents

Data relevant to mechanisms of carcinogenetic action:
              - strength of evidence for a particular mechanism
              - particular mechanism operative in humans

                                                                IARC, 1995

Table 4. Overall evaluation

-Group 1 - The agent (mixture) is carcinogenic to humans
The exposure circumstance entails exposures that are carcinogenic to humans.

        This category is used when there is *sufficient evidence* of carcinogenicity in humans. Exceptionally, an agent (mixture) may be placed in this category when evidence in humans is less than sufficient but there is *sufficient evidence* of carcinogenicity in experimental animals and strong evidence in exposed humans that the agent (mixture) acts through relevant mechanisms of carcinogenicity.

-Group 2

This category includes agents, mixtures and exposure circumstances for which, at one extreme, the degree of evidence of carcinogenicity in humans is almost sufficient, as well as those for which, at the other extreme, there are no human data but for which there is evidence of carcinogenicity in experimental animals. Agents, mixtures and exposure circumstances are assigned to either group 2A (probably carcinogenic to humans) or group 2B (possibly carcinogenic to humans) on the basis of epidemiological and experimental evidence of carcinogenicity and other relevant data.

-Group 2A - The agent (mixture) is probably carcinogenic to humans
The exposure circumstance entails exposures that are probably carcinogenic to humans.

This category is used when there is *limited evidence* of carcinogenicity in humans and sufficient evidence of carcinogenicity in experimental animals. In some cases, an agent (mixture) may be classified in this category when there is inadequate evidence of carcinogenicity in humans and *sufficient evidence* of carcinogenicity in experimental animals and strong evidence that the carcinogenesis is mediated by a mechanism that also operates in humans. Exceptionally, an agent, mixture or exposure circumstance may be classified in this category solely on the basis of limited evidence of carcinogenicity in humans.

-Group 2B - The agent (mixture) is possibly carcinogenic to humans
The exposure circumstance entails exposures that are possibly carcinogenic to humans.

This category is used for agents, mixtures and exposure circumstances for which there is *limited evidence* of carcinogenicity in humans and less than *sufficient evidence* of carcinogenicity in experimental animals. In may also be used when there is *inadequate evidence* of carcinogenicity in humans but there is *sufficient evidence* of carcinogenicity in experimental animals. In some instances, an agent, mixture or exposure circumstance for which there is *inadequate evidence* of carcinogenicity in humans but *limited evidence* of carcinogenicity in experimental animals together with supporting evidence from other relevant data may be placed in this group.

-Group 3 - The agent (mixture or exposure circumstance) is not classifiable as to its carcinogenicity to humans

This category is used most commonly for agents, mixtures and exposure circumstances for which the evidence of carcinogenicity is inadequate in humans and inadequate in experimental animals. Exceptionally, agents (mixtures) for which the evidence of carcinogenicity is inadequate in humans but sufficient in experimental animals may be placed in this category when there is strong evidence that the mechanism of carcinogenicity in experimental animals does not operate in humans.

Agents, mixtures and exposure circumstances that do not fall into any other group are also placed in this category.

-Group 4 - The agent (mixture) is probably not carcinogenic to humans

This category is used for agents or mixtures for which there is *evidence suggesting lack of carcinogenicity* in humans and in experimental animals. In some instances, agents or mixtures for which there is *inadequate evidence* of carcinogenicity in humans but *evidence suggesting lack of carcinogenicity* in experimental animals, consistently and strongly supported by a broad range of other relevant data, may be classified in this group.

                                                               IARC, 1995

Cell studies on Tamoxifen carcinogenicity

Many studies have been conducted to evaluate the effect of Tamoxifen on the growth of several cell lines, derived from human tumors. Most original studies were on the growth control Tamoxifen exerts on breast cancer cell lines (Furr and Jordan, 1984). We shall concentrate mainly on recent studies evaluating the stimulatory role of Tamoxifen on some specific cancer cell lines. Three kinds of studies will be considered depending on the cell being assessed and on whether the cell growth is studied *in vitro* or in experimental animals after implantation of human cancer lines.

In vitro studies of human cancer cell lines. Studies addressing the carcinogenicity of Tamoxifen have dealt mainly with endometrial cancer cell lines and selected breast cancer cell lines. Other studies looked at inhibition of growth in human breast cancer cell lines, but will not be considered here.

Trans-OH-Tamoxifen treatment of cells of the Ishikawa human endometrial cancer cell line resulted in a significant increase in cell number relative to controls, the effects of 4-OH Tamoxifen being greater than those obtained with estradiol, and the stimulation of growth being positively correlated with the OH-Tamoxifen concentration. In a variant of Ishikawa cells, the stimulatory effect was strong with OH-Tamoxifen and not observed with estradiol. The medium composition had marked effects on proliferation and on the antiestrogenic effects of OH-Tamoxifen (Anzae et al., 1989). An older study had by contrast found that Tamoxifen is capable of inducing growth inhibition of long-established endometrial cancer cell lines (HEC-1, KLE, RL95-2) and a new cell line (UM-EC-1), the effect being reversible and suppressed when Tamoxifen and estradiol were simultaneously added to the culture medium (Grenman et al., 1988). Only one study looked at cell proliferation of a cervical cancer cell line (SFR) which was stimulated by Tamoxifen at low concentrations (10^{-9} and 10^{-11}M). Tamoxifen also stimulated the gene transcription and E7 protein production of human papilloma virus type 16 (Hwang et al., 1992).

Although several studies have reported on the ability of Tamoxifen to limit the growth of breast cancer cell lines, some cell lines may not follow this pattern. In cell lines which have clear endocrine-insensitive behavior, such as MDA-MB 231 and BT20, the effect may be observed only at the highest (10^{-6}M) antiestrogen concentration and some such as T47D may even have an increased growth rate with antiestrogens. For MCF-7, 4-OH-Tamoxifen has a clear antiestrogen dose-dependent effect whereas Tamoxifen decreased the cell growth rate only at lower concentrations (10^{-8} and 10^{-7}M) (Coradini et al., 1991). In estrogen-receptor-positive MCF-7 cells, hormone independence may be linked to overexpression of exon 5 (Fuqua, 1994).

The culture of estrogen-receptor-negative multidrug resistant MDA-MB-A1 human breast cancer cell lines with or without a non-inhibitory concentration of Tamoxifen *in vitro* does not lead to inhibition or to stimulation (Maenpaa et al., 1993a). A clone of the estrogen-receptor-negative human breast cancer cell line MDA-MB-213 selected by Tamoxifen shows an altered chemosensitivity to Doxorubicin *in vitro* (Maenpaa et al., 1993b). Synergism of Tamoxifen and 12-0-tetradocanoylphorbol-13-acetate in the stimulation of retrovirus synthesis in an estrogen-receptor-negative (MaTu) but not in an estrogen-receptor-positive (MCF-7) human mammary carcinoma cell line has been reported (Wunderlich and Stein, 1994).

***In vitro* studies on hepatocytes and lymphocytes.** Several studies have addressed the ability of Tamoxifen to form DNA adducts in liver cells. This has been observed in microsomal preparations from phenobarbital pretreated rats as well as with female human liver (Pathak and Bodell, 1994). Distinct DNA adduct patterns were obtained with 4-OH-Tamoxifen and Tamoxifen (Pathak et al., 1995). The enzymatic activation of Tamoxifen produced several adducts (Pongracz et al., 1994).

The exposure of rat hepatocytes to Tamoxifen *in vitro* resulted in the induction of unscheduled DNA synthesis only in the rats which had been pretreated with Tamoxifen *in vivo* (White et al., 1992). One study, when looking at the effect of estrogen and Tamoxifen on hepatic proliferation, even found an inhibition of DNA hepatocyte synthesis as determined by [^{3}H]thymidine incorporation and labelling index on hepatocytes in primary culture and reversion of the stimulatory effect of estrogens, and explained this by the role Tamoxifen has on preventing the amiloride-sensitive NA+ influx necessary to initiate hepatocyte proliferation (Francavilla et al., 1989). A recent study found that Tamoxifen causes adducts in cultured human lymphocytes in a dose-dependent manner (Hemminki et al., 1995).

In vivo **studies of human cancer lines implants in experimental animals.** The effect of 17ßestradiol and Tamoxifen on growth rate and progestrone receptor concentration in a hormonally responsive endometrial tumor, EnCa 101, were evaluated in ovariectomized BALB/c, nu/nu athymic mice. Both compounds increased the growth rate with an increase in cytosol progesterone receptor concentration (Clarke and Satyaswaroop, 1985). An interesting study looked at the contrasting effects of Tamoxifen in two hormone-sensitive human tumors in athymic mice. An endometrial tumor EnCa 101 and a breast tumor MCF-7 were implanted on opposite sides of the same animal. Tamoxifen, either alone or in combination with estradiol, stimulated the growth of the endometrial tumor. Tamoxifen-treated tumors have higher progesterone and estrogen receptor levels than controls. Tamoxifen alone did not stimulate the growth of breast tumors and had an antagonist effect on estradiol-stimulated growth, suggesting that the host metabolism of Tamoxifen does not dictate tissue response (Gottardis et al., 1988). Subsequently, two variants of MCF-7 cells were compared *in vitro* and *in vivo* by subcutaneous implantation of MCF-7 cells in ovariectomized mice and rats. The animals were then treated with Tamoxifen, estradiol or control silastic capsules. A breast cancer cell variant stimulated to grow by Tamoxifen in athymic mice, MCF-7 Tam, was not stimulated compared to wild type MCF-7 cells *in vitro*. By contrast, Tamoxifen stimulated MCF-7 Tam *in vivo*, in both beige and athymic mice. Therefore, Tamoxifen was shown to stimulate growth *in* *vivo* and suppression of the immune function can facilitate this process. Other components of the host environment may play a role (Gottardis et al., 1989).

The Tamoxifen-stimulated growth of EnCa 101 in athymic mice may be inhibited by several steroidal and non sterodial antiestrogens, the degree of control varying according to the product (Gottardis et al., 1990). As later shown by the evaluation of growth of estrogen and progesterone-receptor-positive endometrial carcinoma, always in athymic mice, the ability of various antiestrogens to stimulate the growth of the EnCa 101 cell lines is related to their intrinsic estrogenic activity (Jordan et al., 1991). The predominant role of hormonal receptors had already been demonstrated earlier with human endometrial cell lines in nude mice. Whereas an estrogen-receptor-negative tumor grows at the same rate in the presence or absence of Tamoxifen or 17ßestradiol, an estrogen-receptor-positive tumor grows significantly more rapidly in the presence of Tamoxifen, albeit less than with estradiol. The progesterone receptor concentration was also elevated with Tamoxifen, and these receptors were functional, with subnuclear vacuolization of the tumors after progestin administration (Satyaswaroop et al., 1984). More recently, studies of the modulation of proto-oncogene expression in human endometrial carcinoma grown in nude mice showed that the induction of *c-fos* expression by Tamoxifen is consistent with its estrogen like effect on endometrial tumor growth (Sakakibara et al., 1992).

Several studies have evaluated the growth of specific breast cancer cell lines in mice. Development and growth of the MCF-7 human breast cancer is affected by hormonal manipulations. No tumor growth is seen in ovariectomized BALB/c athymic nude mice but the cells remain viable. There is minimal tumor growth in intact mice but this is dose-dependent both in ovariectomized and intact mice supplemented with 17ßestradiol. Treatment with Tamoxifen or LY156758 results in transient stimulation of tumor growth, followed by a prolonged stationary phase. For mice bearing an established MCF-7 tumor, estrogen withdrawal leads to cessation of tumor growth but not regression. Similarly, treatment by antiestrogens does not cause tumor regression but is associated with dose-dependent growth inhibition, without loss of viability of cells (Osborne et al., 1985). Long-term treatment by trans-Tamoxifen results in cessation of tumor growth suppression and indeed tumor progression occurs despite continued Tamoxifen administration. Resistant tumors are characterized by markedly lower intracellular Tamoxifen levels and by isomerization of the potent antiestrogenic metabolite, trans-4-OH-Tamoxifen to the less potent cis-isomer (Osborne et al., 1991). Tamoxifen effects on estrogen-receptor-negative, multidrug resistant MDA-MB-A1 human breast cancer cell line are different *in vitro* and *in vivo*. No inhibition or stimulation is seen *in vitro*, but *in vivo* Tamoxifen has a clear tumor growth-stimulating effect in mice and this is most marked in animals implanted with Tamoxifen-pretreated cells (Maenpaa et al., 1993a).

Several studies have demonstrated the ability of Tamoxifen to promote the growth of specific human tumor cancer cell lines, in particular endometrial carcinoma cell lines, but also selected human breast cancer cell lines. This effect is seen *in vitro* but is usually much clearer *in vivo*. Dose-response relationships can be observed as well as modification of effect by coacting agents or host factors. Synergism with other potential carcinogens such as viruses may exist although only a few studies are currently available. Normal cells, such as hepatocytes, are sensitive to Tamoxifen and are capable upon exposure of unscheduled DNA synthesis and proliferation.

In vivo studies on Tamoxifen carcinogenicity

The authors are only considering studies aimed at the evaluation of carcinogenic risk in experimental animals administered Tamoxifen by various routes and at different dosages, in several species. Studes analysing the effects of Tamoxifen on implants of human tumoral cell lines in animals were included in the above.

Most studies present data on the effect of Tamoxifen on the liver, and only one study has evaluated effects on the endometrium and one on the ovaries. Two main approaches have been used: one evaluating the induction and/or promotion of liver tumors, both benign and malignant, the second searching for DNA adduct formation mostly in hepatocytes. Finally, other data relevant to the evaluation of the carcinogenicity of Tamoxifen and its mechanisms will be briefly assessed.

Induction studies. The development of malignant liver tumors after treatment with Tamoxifen has been studied in female Sprague-Dawley, Alderley Park Wistar, LEW Ola (Lewis) and Fisher (F-344) rats. Few studies included male rats (Greaves et al., 1993). This induction is observed when Tamoxifen is administered by oral gavage, gastric intubation or by addition to a powdered diet, and results in the occurrence of both benign and malignant tumors.

One of the early effects of Tamoxifen administration on the liver is the appearance of altered foci, which are seen even after relatively short-term treatment with Tamoxifen (Ghia and Mereto, 1989; Hard et al., 1993; Carthew et al., 1995a) and become more frequent with increasing doses and latency (Meschter et al., 1991). The speed of appearance of foci as well as their number depends on the rat species (Carthew et al., 1995b). Liver adenomas appear in both male and female rats treated with Tamoxifen (Greaves et al., 1993). The frequency of benign tumor occurrence is dose and duration-dependent (Williams et al., 1991, 1993). Maligant liver tumors have been obtained in four species of rats: Sprague-Dawley, Alderley Wistart, Lewis Ola and Fisher F-344, albeit with different effectiveness. The lowest dose at which hepatocarcinoma occurred is 5 mg/kg/day of Tamoxifen for 2 years; in that group, hepatocellular tumors caused some early deaths although the overall survival was better than for controls. A dose-related increase in the incidence of hepatocellular tumors was observed with greater mortality in the 20 and 35 mg/kg/day exposed groups as compared to controls (Greaves et al., 1993). Several other studies compared doses of 11.3, 22.6 or 45 mg/kg/day. All found an increased incidence of hepatocellular carcinoma with rising Tamoxifen dose to 100% incidence at 12 and 15 months in the 22.6 dose category and 67 to 71% at 11.3 in one study (Hard et al., 1993). No increase in hepatocellular carcinoma was found at this last dose in two studies (Hirsimäki et al., 1993; Ahotupa et al., 1994), whereas a very high proportion of Sprague-Dawley rats developed liver cancer at 45 mg/kg/day, including some very large liver tumors. At high doses of Tamoxifen, the volume density of peroxisomes, mitochondria and residual bodies is elevated in non-neoplastic hepatocytes (Hirimäki et al., 1993). One study used 2.8, 11.3 or 45.2 mg/kg/day of Tamoxifen or equimolar quantities of Toremifene for up to 1 year with two recovery periods; 4 weeks after 6 months and 3 months after 1 year of exposure. In the intermediate dose group, it took one year for liver lesions to appear. At that time, 50% of animals had developed hepatocellular adenomas and 10% carcinomas. After a 3-month recovery period the proportion of carcinomas increased to 45%. At high does, the proportion of adenomas was similar at 50% at 12 months, but with 75% of animals having developed adenocarcinoma (Williams et al., 1993). Wistar rats fed 420 ppm of Tamoxifen in their diet for only 3 months developed liver tumors, mostly adenomas, but also one carcinoma. Following cessation of Tamoxifen administration, promotion was carried out with phenobarbital. This treatment increased the incidence of liver tumors, and the authors suggested that Tamoxifen DNA adducts may play a role in the ability of phenobarbital to promote liver carcinoma (Carthew et al., 1995a). In a recent study, different species of rats were also fed 420 ppm of Tamoxifen in their diet. Wistar and Lewis rats rapidly developed multiple liver nodules, and at autopsy performed at or before 11 months, all animals bore one or more liver carcinomas. The Fisher rats show similar results at 20 months (Carthew et al., 1995b).

The induction by Tamoxifen of tumors other than liver tumors has been poorly studied. However, Greaves et al. (1993) have found in male and female rats treated with Tamoxifen (20 and 35 mg/kg/day) an increase in the incidence of hepato/cholangiocellular carcinoma. In females, granulosa cell tumors of the ovaries have been observed in rats treated for 12 months but not for 15 months (Hard et al., 1993). In one study, the administration of 45 mg/kg/day daily by oral gavage induces squamous cell metaplasia of the endometrium in 9.6% of female Sprague-Dawley rats, with 2.9% dysplastic change and in 1.9% a focal invasive squamous cell carcinoma (Mäntylä et al., in press). Finally, when new-born female rats are exposed to Tamoxifen, gross abnormalities in the reproductive tract have been found without malignancy but with severe squamous metaplasia at only 4 months of age (Chamness et al., 1979). All these results indicate that in rats Tamoxifen induces malignant tumors in the liver and possibly other sites such as the ovaries and corpus uteri, and that the hepatocarcinogenicity is dose and time-dependent.

Promotion studies. Many experiments in female rats have been conducted to study the promotion by Tamoxifen of tumors after induction with a recognized carcinogen.

After initiation with diethylnitrosamine (DENA), the daily administration of Tamoxifen at 250 or 500 mg/kg acts as a promotor in the livers of Fisher F-344 rats, with an increase in size and number of altered hepatic lesions in promoted animals when compared to only initiated ones. The promotion index of Tamoxifen was lower than that of ethynil-estradiol but greater than phenobarbital (Dragan et al., 1991). In the same publication, it was reported that Tamoxifen used in a single intragastric dose at 40 mg/kg does not act as an initiator. If the initiation by DENA is associated with a partial hepatectomy, the treatment one week later with either Tamoxifen alone or in combination with ethynil-estradiol could enhance the appearance of foci in livers of Sprague-Dawley rats (Yager et al., 1986; Yager and Shi, 1991). Other studies have used dimethylbenzanthracene (DMBA) as an initiator of mammary tumors. The results show that the co-administration of Tamoxifen and

DNBA in animals results in a reduction of tumor incidence; however, rats later treated by Tamoxifen develop other tumors which regress after cessation and grow again after readministration of Tamoxifen (Zimniski and Warren, 1993). Several new tumors are found to be hormone-independent following ovariectomy and are more aggressive (Fendl and Zimniski, 1992).

DNA adducts. DNA adduct formation has been studied in various species of both female and male rats, mice and hamsters, with different dosages and routes of administration. (see also Chapter 9) The results differ accordingly to the sex of the experimental animal with only one DNA adduct spot being detected in a male rat liver in one study and four spots in a female liver (Han et al., 1990).

In hamsters, a single dose in the low mg/kg range (Han and Liehr, 1992) or a daily gavage (Montandon and Williams, 1994) induce the development of DNA adducts in the liver. Female ICR mice treated with Tamoxifen develop DNA adducts in the liver, but also kidney and lung (Randerath et al., 1994). The levels of DNA adducts in C57Bl/6J and DBA/2 mice are lower than those found in rats (White et al., 1992). DNA adducts are detected in the liver when Tamoxifen is administered by the intra-peritoneal route (Patnak et al., 1995) or by gavage (White et al., 1992). Adduct formation is dose-dependent with an adduct concentration increase after several injections of Tamoxifen (Han et al., 1990; Han and Liehr, 1992) and time-dependent (White et al., 1992). The level of adduct formation has been found to be greater with alpha-OH-Tamoxifen than with Tamoxifen (Phillips et al., 1994) and pyrrolidinoTamoxifen causes a similar level of adduct formation to Tamoxifen (White et al., 1992). Other studies have been conducted to evaluate the effect of antagonist products of DNA adducts induced by Tamoxifen, with a lack of effect with ascorbic acid and persistance of the induction of hepatic DNA damage by Tamoxifen (Han and Liehr, 1992). However, the association of Calcium Glutarate and Tamoxifen as a pretreatment of animals with tumors induced by DENA after partial hepatectomy inhibits the initiation phase of hepatocarcinogenesis (Oredipe et al., 1992).

Other relevant data. As seen above, data on carcinogenicity are much stronger in the rat than in the mouse. Several authors have addressed this issue. Evaluation of genotoxic potential of Tamoxifen and analogues suggest that Tamoxifen may induce enzymes responsible for its own activation (White et al., 1992). In particular, the induction of cytochrome P450-dependent activities by Tamoxifen may result in an accelerated liver metabolism of this drug with important implications for its metabolic conversion to genotoxic metabolites. The difference in inducibility of P450 between the rat and mouse may contribute to the differential carcinogenic response to Tamoxifen (White et al., 1993). A further study of species differences in the covalent binding of [^{14}C] Tamoxifen to liver microsomes suggests that the rat may be a better model than the mouse for human liver microsomal activation, both for kinetic parameters and for the pattern of metabolic products (White et al., 1995). A similar conclusion has also been reached by Robinson et al. (1991) who state that the rat is similar to the human in the way large oral doses of Tamoxifen are metabolized and may be more representative of the breast cancer patient than the mouse as far as toxicology and antitumor studies are concerned.

Other data relevant to the genotoxicity of Tamoxifen in rodents come from the fact that this product induces specific p53 mutations in a large proportion of rat hepatocellular carcinomas (Vancutsem et al., 1994).

Summary. The effects of Tamoxifen on the liver are complex: this product induces DNA adduct formation in rats, mice and hamsters, and produces hepatocellular carcinoma in rats. Experimental data therefore clearly support carcinogenic effect in the rat liver, either as a promotor or a complete carcinogen. In several independent studies (Ahotupa et al., 1994; Carthew et al., 1995a, 1995b; Greaves et al., 1993; Hard et al., 1993; Hirsimäki et al., 1993; Williams et al., 1993). Tamoxifen has been found to increase the incidence of malignant neoplasms (hepatocarcinoma) and a combination of benign (liver adenoma) and malignant tumors in all strains of rats tested. Extrapolation of animal data to humans is always problematic, in particular with regard to dose, as well as potentially different metabolic pathways. For Tamoxifen, several studies have used larger doses than those in clinical settings. Yet, according to Hard et al. (1993), the safety margin of Tamoxifen is low and differences in dose cannot fully reassure us. Furthermore, the serum levels observed in animal studies are not considerably different from those in human clinical studies (Hard et al., 1993; Robinson et al., 1991). In the past, the similarities between humans and rodents have often been found to be considerable and the concordance between lists of human and animal carcinogens is striking. Animal experiments have contributed much important data for the evaluation of carcinogenic risk and will continue to do so. In particular, given the different life spans of rodents and humans, they provide information which will take a long time to appear in humans. It takes twenty years or more for liver cancer to occur in humans, whereas in rodents, it only takes a few months.

Carcinogenicity of Tamoxifen: human evidence

There are currently many studies available on the effects of Tamoxifen in humans. The vast majority are studies on women having received Tamoxifen for breast cancer treatment. They comprise case reports, case series, randomized controlled trials (RCT) and case-control studies.

Case reports and case series. Numerous publications exist on Tamoxifen's effect on the histological and sonographical aspects of the endometrium, as well as the occurrence of several benign conditions such as endometrial polyps and effects on endometriosis. To our knowledge, the first report to appear on endometrial cancer was that of Killackey et al. in 1985 who described three cases of endometrial adenocarcinoma in women exposed to Tamoxifen. Since then, many others have followed. When looking at case reports and case series dealing with cancer, we noted that quite a number of these publications deal with somewhat rare forms of cancer. For cancer of the uterus, there have been reports of many adenocarcinomas as well as sarcomas (Altaras et al., 1993; Steward and Knight, 1989; Hardell, 1988a), mixed müllerian tumors (Clarke, 1993; Sasco et al., 1995c; Seoud et al., 1993), mucinous and clear cell adenocarcinomas of the endometrium (Dallenbach-Hellweg and Hahn, 1995), adenoacanthoma (Le Bouëdec et al., 1990) and serous papillary adenocarcinoma (Deprest et al., 1992). Reports also exist for other gynecologic cancers such as endocervical adenocarcinoma (LïVolsi et al., 1995) and primary Fallopian tube adenocarcinoma *in situ* (Sonnendecker et al., 1994). For the ovary, which may be particularly susceptible to Tamoxifen, benign pathologies have been described such as the occurrence of ovarian cysts (Terada et al., 1993) and cystic ovarian necrosis (Jolles et al., 1990), but malignant tumors can also occur, such as endometrioid carcinoma (Cohen et al., 1994) and granulosa cell tumors (Gherman et al., 1994). Finally, Johnstone et al. reported a hepatocellular carcinoma in 1991.

Most case reports reflect physiopathological mechanisms of Tamoxifen on the genital apparatus. They support Tamoxifen's agonist effect with the possibility of ovarian stimulation and induction of ovulation, as well as estrogenic effects on the vaginal epithelium and the endometrium. It is not possible to quantify these events from case reports although they do provide information of qualitative nature. If we try to add up published cases, we might end up with a few hundred (Jordan and Assikis, 1995). Unfortunately, this figure may only account for a small proportion of all cases occurring. For a case to be published, it needs to fulfill several criteria: the case must occur but it must also be correctly diagnosed, be recorded in the medical files (which will be a problem if several doctors are involved in the care of a single patient), be recorded in a cancer registry (if it exists) and also on study reporting forms (if part of a study protocol). Secondly, the case must be considered "interesting", which is more likely if a woman develops a rare tumor than if she gets a common endometrial tumor. The clinician must take the time to prepare a case report, the manuscript must be submitted and accepted for publication. In the event of publication bias, findings which are already considered as common knowledge may remain unpublished. Finally, other issues may play a role, such as choice of journal and language of publication. In populations where there is full national coverage by population-based cancer registries, there is more likelihood of cases being registered. In part, this explains why so much data come from Nordic countries. Therefore, it would seem that the figures which have been used to quantify the absolute risk of developing endometrial cancer are a clear underestimation. They may include cases from published randomized trials and isolated case reports and case series. The exposed cases found in case-control studies should be added and even that would not account for cases which occurred outside study settings throughout the world. For the time being, we do not know exactly how great the problem is.

Randomized controlled trials. When evaluating the carcinogenicity of a product, only very rarely are we in a position to have results from RCT. As Tamoxifen was widely used as treatment for breast cancer in the 70s and 80s, several trials on this product were conducted. Some, although not all, RCT indicate an increased risk of endometrial cancer among women receiving Tamoxifen. They will be presented briefly in alphabetical order by first author and year of publication.

♦ *Andersson et al., 1991*

The RCT was conducted in Denmark on a population of 3,538 postmenopausal women with breast cancer. They were divided into 1,828 low risk cases who did not receive any further treatment after surgery and 1,710 high risk patients defined as cases with histologically verified axillary lymph node metastases, primary tumors greater than 5 cm in diameter or tumors with invasion into the skin or underlying fascia. The high risk women were randomized to postoperative radiotherapy for 846 cases or radiotherapy and Tamoxifen at 30 mg/day for 48 weeks in 864 cases. Results are reported after a median observation time of 7.9 years. The comparison of the high risk group allocated to radiotherapy and Tamoxifen with the general population shows a standardized incidence ratio (SIR) of 1.8 (95% CI: 1.5-2.2) for all second cancers following breast cancer and, after exclusion of second breast cancer, of 1.2 (0.9-1.5). In particular, increased SIR were found for colon and rectum (SIR = 1.8; 1.1-2.9), breast (4.4; 3.3-5.8), corpus uteri (1.9; 0.8-3.9). The comparison Tamoxifen *versus* no Tamoxifen for the high risk patients shows the following rate ratios: corpus uteri (3.3; 0.6-32.4), ovary (2.8; 0.4-149.0); stomach (1.6; 0.7-3.7) and breast (1.1; 0.7-1.6).

♦ *Andersson et al., 1992*

Additional analyses were produced by the Danish group with a median follow-up time of eight years. Compared to the general population, all groups of women in the study had increased risk of second breast cancer occurring at any time after the first breast cancer diagnosis, with for the low risk, high risk - non-Tamoxifen and high risk - Tamoxifen women SIR of 1.4 (1.0-1.8); 4.2 (3.1-5.6) and 4.4 (3.3-5.8) respectively. In the analysis confined to breast cancer occurring more than a year after the first cancer, the SIR become 0.9 (0.6-1.4); 1.0 (0.4-1.9) and 1.1 (0.5-2.1). For cancer of the endometrium, only the women who had received Tamoxifen have an incrased risk with in the three groups SIR of: 1.1 (0.6-2.0); 0.6 (0.1-2.1) and 1.9 (0.8-3.9). Therefore, with Tamoxifen the risk of endometrial cancer is greater than in the general population, as well as compared to the low risk patients or high risk patients receiving radiotherapy only. A comparison of the cases of endometrial cancer occurring amoung women having received Tamoxifen with women considered low risk shows for exposed women an older age at diagnosis of breast cancer (68.8 vs. 65.4 years), a shorter interval between the two diagnoses of cancer (2.4 vs. 4.3 years) and finally a shorter survival after diagnosis of cancer of the endometrium (2.2 vs. at least 4.2 years).

♦ *Cummings et al., 1993*

A US study conducted on 181 women reports results of 168 eligible breast cancer cases aged 65 to 84 years with one or more histologically proven positive ipsilateral axillary lymph nodes, randomized to two groups; 83 receiving a placebo and 85 Tamoxifen at 20 mg/day for two years. After a median follow-up of ten years, there were fewer second breast cancers among the women exposed to Tamoxifen vs. the non-exposed (1 vs. 5) and an approximately equal number of non-breast cancers (6 vs. 7), including the same number of endometrial cancers (1 vs. 1).

♦ *Early Breast Cancer Trialists'Collaborative Group, 1992*

A meta-analysis of 133 randomized trials involving 31,000 recurrences and 24,000 deaths among 75,000 women was last reported in 1992. No results were shown for endometrial cancer and the issue was only mentioned briefly in the publication as follows "A Swedish study has also shown an excess of non-fatal endometrial cancer but, with specific causes thus far available for only about one third of all deaths without relapse, only two such deaths (both in the 1-year Tamoxifen group in an American trial) have in the present overview been ascribed to endometrial cancer". More recent results confirming the overall benefit to be expected from Tamoxifen in the treatment of breast cancer, but also indicating an increased risk of incidence and mortality from endometrial cancer should be available soon.

♦ *Fisher et al., 1994*

This publication presents results on endometrial cancer in the NSABP-B14 study. The total study population consisted of 2,843 patients at NSABP institutions in Canada and the USA. They were cases of invasive breast cancer with estrogen-receptor-positive (> 10fmol/mg) tumors and histologically negative axillary lymph nodes. 1,419 women were randomized to Tamoxifen at 20 mg/day for five years and 1,424 to placebo. Data are also present for Tamoxifen-treated women registered in the NSABP-B14 subsequent to randomization. The average study time was eight years for randomly assigned patients and five years for registered patients. The main results concerning second cancers as a first event in the randomized groups were as follows: the total number of second cancers, excluding breast, were 42 with Tamoxifen and 63 without, but there was a clear excess of cancer of the endometrium in the women allocated to Tamoxifen with 15 cases including 4 deaths from endometrial cancer vs. 0 among the women allocated to the control group. Including all originally reported endometrial cancers, the annual hazard rate is 1.6 in the randomized Tamoxifen-treated group vs. 0.2/1,000 in the placebo group for a relative risk (RR) of 7.5 (1.7-32.7). Allowing for a deficit of endometrial cancer in the reference group, other RR have been calculated at 2.2 using population-based cancer registry data and 2.3 using the NSABP-06 trial.

♦ *Fornander et al., 1989*

This publication from Swedent concerns 1,846 postmenopausal women under 71 years of age randomly allocated to Tamoxifen at 40 mg/day for two years for 931 women and 915 controls. Patients who were disease-free after two years (473 women) were further randomized by stopping Tamoxifen after two years for 237 women or continuing for three more years for 236. After a median follow-up time of 4.5 years, a statistically significant relative risk for cancer of the endometrium of 6.4 (1.4-2.8) is reported for women under Tamoxifen with a greater effect among women allocated to five years of treatment rather than two.

♦ *Fornander et al., 1991*

A further publication dealth with the hospital admissions in the same study population with a median follow-up time of 54 months. There was an increased risk of uterine cancer among Tamoxifen-exposed women of 2.7 (0.9-8.1) and of other gynecological diseases 3.2 (1.2-8.6), but interestingly enough there were no excess hospital admissions for uterine bleeding with an RR of 1.1 (0.7-1.9).

◆ *Fornander et al., 1993*

A study was conducted matching the 931 women who had been randomized to Tamoxifen at 40 mg/day for two years in the Stockholm trial to the Swedish Cancer Registry. 17 women were found to have subsequently developed endometrial cancer: 13 were still alive but 4 had died, 3 of them of endometrial cancer. 15 tumors were grades I or II, one was grade IV and there was a mixed mesodermal malignant tumor. The duration of Tamoxifen used varied from 6 to 60 months with a median at 24 months and a median cumulative dose of 29 g with a range of 7 to 72 g. The median time from start of Tamoxifen therapy to diagnosis of endometrial cancer was 32 months with a range of 6 to 13 months. The 10-year actuarial survival was 73%.

◆ *Rutqvist et al., 1995*

This publication, on behalf of the Stockholm Breast Cancer Study Group, reports data from both the Stockholm trial and a combined analysis of the Stockholm, Danish and South Swedish trials. In the Stockholm study, 2,749 postmenopausal women under 71 years of age with unilateral invasive breast cancer were randomized to either Tamoxifen at 40 mg/day for two years for 1,372 women or no treatment for 1,357 women. The median follow-up was nine years. The outcome of interest was the occurrence of second primary cancers. Increased RR were found for several cancer sites: stomach 2.4 (0.5-12.7), colon and rectum at 2.1 (0.8-5.6), liver and biliary tract at 2.9 (0.3-28.2), pancreas at 3.9 (0.4-34.9), lung at 2.4 (0.5-12.7), endometrial at 5.6 (1.9-16.2) and thyroid at 2.0 (0.2-21.5). A decreased RR was found for second breast cancers at 0.6 (0.4-0.9). Taking all sites together, there were 131 second cancers in the Tamoxifen group vs. 130 in the control group. When looking at these results, it is interesting to cite a quote from Powles and Hickish (1995) "Other organs potentially at special risk in humans are those with a high cellular proliferation rate, such as bone marrow, and those tissues that may be exposed to high levels of the carcinogenic metabolites, such as the liver, stomach and colon". These last three sites are exactly the same as those found by Rutqvist. In the combined anlysis of the three Scandinavian trials, statistically significant RR were found for cancer of the endometrium (4.1; 1.9-8.9), all gastrointestinal cancer (1.9; 1.2-2.9) and colorectal cancer (1.9; 1.1-3.3) with in general higher RR in the study center at 40 mg/day compared to 30.

◆ *Stewart, 1992*

This paper reports results from one center of the Scottish Cancer Trials Breast Group five years after the end of the trial which randomized 747 women with histological node-negative breast cancer to either Tamoxifen at 20 mg/day for five years or until relapse, or to Tamoxifen given for a minimum of six weeks upon confirmation of the first detection or recurrent or metastatic breast cancer. 236 disease-free patients on adjuvant therapy were randomly assigned at five years to either stop treatment or continue Tamoxifen until relapse. In this study, only two endometrial cancers were recorded, one in each arm of the trials.

♦ *Summary of the evidence in randomized controlled trials*
Most, although not all, RCTs report an increased risk of endometrial cancer for Tamoxifen-treated women with RR between 2 and 7.5. The risk is greater at 40 mg/day rather than 30 in the Nordic countries, but it should be noted that the highest risk was reported in the USA at 20 mg/day. Most of these studies find a decreased risk of second breast cancer. Finally, increased risks of several other second cancers are reported in a set of studies and the cancer sites concerned are those which could be expected based on physiopathological and metabolic considerations.

Results from the case-control studies. Five case-control studies are currently available, three as full publications, one as several letters to the editor and one as an abstract. They will all be reviewed here in chronological order of publication.

♦ *Hardell, 1988 (September)*
In a regional Swedish population-based cancer registry, 32 cases of uterine cancer diagnosed at least one year after breast cancer were identified during the period 1959-1988. Among these, 23 occurred subsequent to Tamoxifen being registered in Sweden. 11 or 48% had been treated with Tamoxifen including 6 who had also undergone therapeutic castration.

♦ *Hardell, 1988 (December)*
To the 23 cases described above were matched 4 controls with breast cancer per case chosen as the closest in age from the regional cancer registry. This constitues the first case-control study using a population-based cancer registry to evaluate the influence of Tamoxifen for subsequent endometrial cancer. Women having taken Tamoxifen had an odds ratio (OR) of 2.6 (0.7-9.6), women having undergone radiotherapeutic castration 4.7 (0.8-27.3) and women having had both 7.1 (2.3-22.1). If the analysis was restricted to women having received Tamoxifen for six months or more without pelvic irradiation, the OR was 3.3. If control women who died before diagnosis of uterine cancer in the case were excluded, there was a decrease in the exposure frequency among controls, therefore leading to a greater OR, both for Tamoxifen and radiotherapeutic castration.

♦ *Hardell, 1990*
Two additional cases were reported but not included in the analysis.

♦ *van Leeuwen et al., 1994*
This case-control study conducted in the Netherlands included 98 women with endometrial cancer diagnosed at least three months after breast cancer. Controls were 258 women matched to the cases on age (± three years), year of breast cancer diagnosis (± two years), pathology laboratory and survival time with uterus intact. The subjects were therefore recruited from population and hospital-based cancer registries. The overall OR for ever use of Tamoxifen is 1.3 (0.7-

2.4). There was a statistically significant p for trend for duration of treatment withTamoxifen at 0.049 with the following OR: for up to 12 months: 0.6 (0.2-1.7); 13 to 24 months: 1.9 (0.6-5.8); 25 to 60 months: 2.2 (0.8-6.5) and 60 months or more: 3.0 (0.6-15.8). The results were observed for a median daily dose of 40 mg. It is interesting to quote part of an ensuing letter to the editor by Baum et al. (1994) "van Leeuwen and colleagues raise concerns in a scientific and rational manner about the increased risk of endometrial cancer in patients taking Tamoxifen.....There now seems little doubt that there is a modest but important increase in the risk of endometrial cancer for women exposed to Tamoxifen therapy. van Leeuwen and colleagues' findings must be taken seriously because they suggest not only an increased risk of endometrial cancer in all Tamoxifen users (relative risk 1.3, 95% CI 0.7-2.4) but also that women who had used the drug for more than 2 years were at an even greater risk (2.3, 0.9-5.9).

♦ *Lutz et al., 1994*

For the time being, this is the largest population-based cancer registry case-control study even conducted. To date only an abstract has been published. The study was carried out in the United Kingdom at the Thames Cancer Registry. It included 248 women with endometrial cancer diagnosed at least one year after breast cancer. 644 controls were matched to cases on age at diagnosis of breast cancer, year of diagnosis of breast cancer and survival time. The OR for even use of Tamoxifen are 4.9 (0.8-29.9) for women under 50 when diagnosed with breast cancer and 1.8 (1.1-3.0) for women over 50.

♦ *Cook et al., 1995*

This represents the only case-control study currently available from the USA. Cases were women diagnosed with either ovarian or endometrial cancer at least six months after diagnosis of breast cancer. Controls were matched on age, stage and year of breast cancer diagnosis. There were 34 ovarian cancer cases with 89 controls and 36 endometrial cancer cases with 66 controls. All subjects came from the western Washington population-based cancer registry. Results were almost identical for both cancers with matched OR of 0.6 (0.2-1.8) for cancer of the ovary and 0.6 (0.2-1.9) for cancer of the endometrium for women having been exposed to Tamoxifen.

♦ *Sasco et al., 1995b, 1996*

This case-control study started in France in 1991. It concerns 43 cases of women having histologically proven endometrial cancer diagnosed at least one year after diagnosis of breast cancer during the period 1976-1992 in two French départements (Rhône and Côte d'Or). Controls were 177 women matched to the cases on age at diagnosis of breast cancer, date of diagnosis of breast cancer, residence and survival time with uterus intact. The case-control matching ratio was variable. The subjects were provided by population-based cancer registries and clinician surveys. Matched OR for ever use of Tamoxifen was 1.4 (0.60-3.5) and current or past use of Tamoxifen showed similar OR: 1.5 (0.58-3.8) for current use at time of endometrial cancer diagnosis and 1.4 (0.48-4.3) for past use. As in the van Leeuwen study, the *p* for trend was statistically significant with increasing OR for increased duration of use: less than 2 years: 1.5 (0.44-4.9); 2 to 5 years: 1.5 (0.42-5.5); more than 5 years 3.5 (0.94-12.7). This effect of duration became stronger in the multivariate analysis controlling for potential confounders by matched logistic regression. In the conditional model including castration, chemotherapy, radiotherapy, estrogen and progesterone receptor status, stage, menopausal status and being overweight, the matched OR for Tamoxifen use of up to five years is 2.8 (0.69-17.0) and for more than five years 4.4 (0.68-27.9). The median daily dose of Tamoxifen was identical for cases and controls at 20 mg, but the median duration of treatment was much greater for caes (63 months) than for controls (37 months). If the analysis is restricted to symptomatic cases, the overall OR becomes greater at 1.7 (0.59-5.0).

◆ *Summary of the evidence from the case-control studies*

We currently possess results from five case-control studies, four of which were carried out in Europe and which indicate an increased risk of endometrial cancer, and one in the USA which found a decreased risk. It is often stated that the increased risk found for endometrial cancer in fact only reflects surveillance bias. Several arguments can be put forward against such bias in the Europen setting. The authors excluded endometrial cancer diagnosis soon after breast cancer in order not to include cases which may just have been revealed rather than caused by Tamoxifen. The exclusion period is one year for Hardell, (1988), Lutz et al. (1994) and Sasco et al. (1995b, 1996) and three months for van Leeuwen et al. (1994). The strongest argument is duration effect. We see increasing risk with increasing duration of treatment, with values quite similar either at 20 mg/day (Sasco et al., 1995b, 1996) or at 40 (van Leeuwen et al., 1994) and in fact the value of the OR remains similar either for current or past use (Sasco et al., 1996). All studies (Hardell, 1988; Lutz et al., 1994; Sasco et al., 1995, 1996; van Leeuwen et al., 1994) were carried out in Europe in the period prior to 1993 at a time when there was still relatively little discussion on the iatrogenic effects of Tamoxifen. The cases were diagnosed by numerous physicians, most of them prior to the Tamoxifen controversy.

Another argument against other potential biases is the source of information as all studies were based on available clinical records or cancer registry data and there was no interview of either the women themselves or the clinicians in charge of the patients. If we compare the results from the US study to the European ones, there is no real disagreement. In fact the confidence intervals of all these studies overlap to a considerable extent. Therefore, from a purely statistical point of view, there is no significant contradiction. There were no major differences in study design between the USA and Europe except for two aspects: the minimum duration between the two diagnoses varied (one year for Hardell, 1988, Sasco et al., 1995, 1996 and Lutz et al., 1994; six months for Cook et al., 1995; three months for van Leeuwen et al., 1994) and matching with stage was only done in the USA, possibly leading to overmatching of cases and controls (Cook et al., 1995). On the other hand, a major difference was the very high proportion of ineligible controls in the US study. The proportion of potential controls considered ineligible due to hysterectomy was 43% in the USA (Cook et al., 1995), whereas in Europe it does not exceed 15% at the most. In the US conditions, the remaining controls were probably very highly selected low risk women, whereas a number of cases-to-be which were included in the potential controls disappear completely from the study design for a hysterectomy carried out for conditions which could have led rapidly to cancer of the endometrium or may already have been one but which remained undiagnosed and was therefore not counted. The issue of hysterectomy should also be mentioned within the context of the Fisher et al. study (1994) where the authors present several sets of results and comment on the lower than expected rate of cancer of the uterus among women in their study. With a proportion of women undergoing hysterectomy of the order of one third among the female US population over 50 or getting close to one half for women with breast cancer, the study of subsequent risk of endometrial cancer becomes very delicate. The situation is still different in Europe. However, the main difference between the US and European case-control studies is that the pattern of Tamoxifen use is different. When comparing Cook et al. (1995) and Sasco et al. (1996), two differences clearly emerge: the frequency of Tamoxifen use among controls is much lower than in Sasco and duration of Tamoxifen treatment is much shorter in the US (mean duration: 14 months for cases, 21 for controls) than in France (median duration: 63 months for cases, 37 for controls). Given the effect of duration on risk, it becomes clear that in Europe we are in a better position to observe risk than in the US, where, with the exception of women in clinical trials for which risk is very clearly seen, other breast cancer cases have not been treated long enough to observe the risk.

Comments on selected issues

Endometrial cancer. When this cancer occurs in the general female population, it usually has a favorable prognosis, but this may or may not apply to cases appearing under Tamoxifen as there is the possibility of more rate histological forms and more aggressive tumor progresion (Magriples et al., 1993). We cannot reject or confirm at the present time the role Tamoxifen may play in the occurrence of sarcomas, mixed müllerian tumors and other tumors. The issue of prognosis is still unsolved. Even after the exclusion of cases appearing early (less than a year after diagnosis of breast cancer) which may only have been revealed by Tamoxifen, the risk remains and in fact increased with treatment duration. When examining dose effect, there are two dose components which should be taken into account separately: daily dose and duration of treatment. In the present case, and in general in cancer epidemiology, duration seems more relevant to carcinogenic risk.

Liver cancer. A situation which may lead to underascertainment is lack of precise diagnosis of a condition. Where it has often been argued that some endometrial cancers may have been overdiagnosed due to the knowledge clinicians had of Tamoxifen's effects, it can just as well be argued that cases may be missed. An illustration of this is liver cancer in humans. Again, data come from the Nordic countries and case reports are very few. But how likely is it that a woman who has had breast cancer (known to be able to cause liver metastasis), who developed a primary tumor in her liver will be correctly diagnosed? If she is young, with just one image of her liver, she may undergo a biopsy and therefore may be correctly diagnosed. Otherwise, and considering that in most cases the therapy will not change much, no histological confirmation will be obtained and the patient will just be considered metastatic. Again, although liver cancer is very rare, this condition is also underdiagnosed. It would indeed by helpful to have data from randomized controlled trials on distribution of metastasis by site in Tamoxifen-treated and non-Tamoxifen-treated women. In addition, the evidence in rats in favor of liver cancer is extremely strong.

A study compared ^{32}P-postlabelling DNA extracted from liver samples, either post morten or as liver biopsies during abdominal surgery, of seven women receiving Tamoxifen at 20 or 40 mg/day, with liver DNA from seven women not receiving this drug, but it should be noted that most of the controls were taking dopamine at the time of sampling. In all women treated for whom sufficient material was available,

Tamoxifen and its metabolites were detected in liver samples, with higher concentrations in women receiving 40 mg/day rather than 20. No Tamoxifen was detected in the control samples. DNA adducts specific to Tamoxifen were not measured as the methodology is not currently available. The total level of DNA damage was not different in exposed and non-exposed women, and there was no significant difference in the total number of adducts (Martin et al., 1995).

Other cancers and general comments on data sources. When considering other cancer sites, the situation is even more complex. Where population-based cancer registries do not exist, the systematic recording of second cancers cannot be achieved in most circumstances. If results on this topic mostly come for the Nordic countries, it may be because the epidemiological surveillance system is much more systematic there. It is worth emphasizing that with systematic recording, the cancer sites seen in excess are in fact those which could be expected based on physiopathologic and metabolic considerations.

Strength of epidemiology. Epidemiology, as the Greek origin of the name indicates (demos), deals with people. Epidemiology findings are directly relevant to humans and even to whole populations. This is in particular the strength of population-based studies as opposed to clinical studies. Case-control studies based on population data sources provide information which cannot be easily discarded. We have five case-control studies, four in Europe, one in the USA. The number of cases included varies from 23 to 248 and the results of these studies are not in disagreement. The four European studies found an overall OR varying from 1.3 to approx. 3 (Hardell, 1988; Lutz et al., 1994; van Leeuwen et al., 1994; Sasco et al., 1995b, 1996). In two studies, where the duration of treatment was indicated, OR was found to increase with duration of treatment to attain or be greater than 3 after five years of Tamoxifen treatment (van Leeuwen et al., 1994; Sasco et al., 1995b, 1996). The US study found an OR of 0.6, but with exposure to Tamoxifen of low duration (the 75th percentile of treatment duration was at 44 months) (Cook et al., 1995) and in fact van Leeuwen et al. (1994) also reported an estimate of 0.6 for up to a year of Tamoxifen treatment.

We have a rare situation where we have evidence from RCT and if randomization was properly done, and mostly it was, there is no reason to believe women exposed and not exposed to Tamoxifen did differ in significant ways for variables such as reproductive history, weight, hormone replacement therapy or others. Therefore, the evidence from RCT is valid and good and is in favor of a positive association between endometrial cancer and Tamoxifen in humans, with an increased risk of endometrial cancer in several RCTs, although not all. Similarly, the evidence from case-control studies further reinforces the association of an increased risk of endometrial cancer in Tamoxifen users.

Additional information as compared to the RCT is the effect of duration. We have here a clear dose-response relationship: the longer the duration of treatment, the higher the risk. This is true even after adjustment for several potential confounders (Sasco et al., 1996).

Conclusions

Tamoxifen has been a very valuable and effective drug in the treatment for breast cancer and remains so. It is a complex product which has contrasting endocrinological effects as well as multiple other actions on many target tissues. For a drug used in cancer therapy it is extremely well tolerated. However, several chemotherapeutic drugs used for cancer treatment are recognized human carcinogens. Examples in the IARC "Group 1 compounds" include melphalan, cyclophosphamide, the MOPP protocol (IARC, 1995b). One could also add radiotherapy which is widely used for the treatment of cancer and is recognized as capable of inducing second cancers. The knowledge that these compounds are carcinogens does not lead to the products not being used but being used properly, with exact clinical indications and attention being paid to the issues of dose, timing and, most importantly, duration of treatment. Using a potentially toxic compound is perfectly acceptable for a potentially fatal disease such as breast cancer. This information must be made available to physicians, but also to women, who have the right to know. The same considerations may well apply to Tamoxifen which is a strong rat carcinogen and has repeatedly been associated with an increased risk of endometrial cancer in humans, both in RCT and in case-control studies.

Since completion of the manuscript (8 November 1995), the NCI press office issued a clinical announcement about long-term use of Tamoxifen in breast cancer treatment "recommending that physicians limit tamoxifen use in the treatment of early breast cancer to five years in clinical practive. The NCI action followed a decision by the NSABP to stop a clinical trial in which investigators were comparing five years to ten years of tamoxifen use after surgery in women with node-negative, estrogen receptor-positive breast cancer and found no additional benefit for women taking the anti-estrogen for more than five years."

This is the first official recognition that more than five years of Tamoxifen treatment may be associated with more risks than benefits. (National Institutes of Health, Press Office, November 30, 1995)
See also:
Jordan VC (editor): Long term tamoxifen treatment for breast cancer. University of Wisconsin Press, Madison 1994.

REFERENCES

Ahotupa M, Kirsimäki P. Pärssinen R, Mäntylä (1994): Alterations of drug metabolising and antioxidant enzyme activites during tamoxifen-induced hepatocarcinogenesis in the rat. *Carcinogenesis* 15:863-868

Altaras MM, Aviram R, Cohen I, Cordoba M, Yarkoni S, Beyth Y (1993): Role of prolonged stimulation of tamoxifen therapy in the etiology of endometrial sarcomas. *Gynecol Oncol* 49:255-258

Andersson M, Storm HH, Mouridsen HT (1991): Incidence of new primary cancers after adjuvant tamoxifen therapy and radiotherapy for early breast cancer. *J Natl Cancer Inst* 83:1013-1017

Andersson M, Storm HH, Mouridsen HT (1992): Carcinogenic effects of adjuvant tamoxifen treatment and radiotherapy for early breast cancer. *Acta Oncol* 31:259-263

Anzai Y, Holinka CF, Kuramoto H, Gurpide E (1989): Stimulatory effects of 4-hydroxytamoxifen on proliferation of human endometrial adenocarcinoma cells (Ishikawa line). *Cancer Res* 49:2362-2365

Baum M, Odling-Smee W, Houghton J, Riely D, Taylor H, on behalf of the Cancer Research Campaign Breast Cancer Trials Group (1994): Endometrial cancer during tamoxifen treatment. *Lancet* 343:1291

Carthew P, Martin EA, White INH, De Matteis F, Edwards RE, Dorman BM, Heydon RT, Smith LL (1995): Tamoxifen induces short-term cumulative DNA damage and liver tumors in rats: promotion by phenobarbitol. *Cancer Res* 55:544-547

Carthew P, Rich KJ, Martin EA, De Matteis F, Lim CK, Manson MM, Festing MFW, White INH, Smith LL (1995): DNA damage as assessed by ^{32}P-postlabelling in three rat strains exposed to dietary tamoxifen: the relationship between cell proliferation and liver tumour formation. *Carcinogenesis* 16:1299-1304

Chamness GC, Bannayan GA, Landry Jr LA, Sheridan PJ, McGuire WL (1979): Abnormal reproductive development in rats after neonatally administered antiestrogen (tamoxifen). *Biol Reprod* 21:1087-1090

Clarke CL, Satyaswaroop PG (1985): Photoaffinity labeling of the progesterine receptor from human endometrial carcinoma. *Cancer Res* 45:5417-5420

Clarke MR (1993): Uterine malignant mixed müllerian tumor in a patient on long-term tamoxifen therapy for breast cancer. *Gynecol Oncol* 51:411-415

Cohen I, Altaras MM, Lew S, Tepper R, Beyth Y, Ben-Baruch G (1994): Ovarian endometrioid carcinoma and endometriosis developing in a postmenopausal breast cancer patient during tamoxifen therapy: a case report and review of the literature. *Gynecol Oncol* 55:443-447

Cook LS, Weiss NS, Schwartz SM, White E, McKnight B, Moore DE, Daling JR (1995): Population-based study of tamoxifen therapy and subsequent ovarian, endometrial, and breast cancers. *J Natl Cancer Inst* 87:1359-1364

Coradini D, Cappelletti V, Granata G, Di Fronzo G (1991): Activity of tamoxifen and its metabolites on endocrine-dependent and endocrine-independent breast cancer cells. *Tumor Biol* 12:149-158

Cummings FJ, Gray R, Tormey DC, Davis TE, Volk H, Harris J, Falkson G, Bennett JM (1993): Adjuvant tamoxifen versus placebo in elderly women with node-positive breast cancer: long-term follow-up and causes of death. *J Clin Oncol* 11:29-35

Dallenbach-Hellweg G, Hahn U (1995): Mucinous and clear cell adenocarcinomas of the endometrium in patients receiving antiestrogens (tamoxifen) and gestagens. *Int J Gynecol Pathol* 14:7-15

Deprest J, Neven P, Ide P (1992): An unusual type of endometrial cancer, related to tamoxifen? *Eur J Obstet Gynecol Reprod Biol* 46:147-150

Dragan YP, Xu Y-D, Pitot HC (1991): Tumor promotion as a target for estrogen/antiestrogen effects in rat hepatocarcinogenesis. *Prev Med* 20:15-26

Early Breast Cancer Trialists' Collaborative Group (1992): Systemic treatment of early breast cancer by hormonal, cytotoxic, or immune therapy. 133 randomised trials involving 31,000 recurrences and 24,000 deaths among 75,000 women. *Lancet* 339:1-15,71-85

Fendl KC, Zimniski SJ (1992): Role of tamoxifen in the induction of hormone-independent rat mammary tumors. *Cancer Res* 52:235-237

Fisher B, Costantino JP, Redmond CK, Fisher ER, Wickerham DL, Cronin WM, Other NSABP Contributors (1994): Endometrial cancer in tamoxifen-treated breast cancer patients: findings from the National Surgical Adjuvant Breast and Bowel Project (NSABP) B-14. *J Natl Cancer Inst* 86:527-537

Fornander T, Rutqvist LE, Cedermark B, Glas U, Mattsson A, Skoog L, Somell A, Theve T, Wilking N, Askergren J, Rotstein S, Hjalmar ML, Perbeck L (1991): Adjuvant tamoxifen in early-stage breast cancer: effects on intercurrent morbidity and mortality. *J Clin Oncol* 9:1740-1748

Fornander T, Hellström AC, Moberger B (1993): Descriptive clinicopathologic study of 17 patients with endometrial cancer during or after adjuvant tamoxifen in early breast cancer. *J Natl Cancer Inst* 85:1850-1855

Francavilla A, Polimeno L, DiLeo A, Barone M, Ove P, Coetzee M, Eagon P, Makowka L, Ambrosino G, Mazzaferro V, Starzl TE (1989): The effect of estrogen and tamoxifen on hepatocyte proliferation *in vivo* and *in vitro*. *Hepatology* 9:614-620

Fuqua SAW (1994): Estrogen receptor mutagenesis and hormone resistance. *Cancer* 74:1026-1029

Furr BJA, Jordan VC (1984): The pharmacology and clinical uses of tamoxifen. *Clin Pharmacol Ther* 25:127-205

Gherman RB, Parket MF, Macri CI (1994): Granulosa cell tumor of the ovary associated with antecedent tamoxifen use. *Obstet Gynecol* 84:7171-719

Ghia M, Mereto E (1989): Induction and promotion of gamma-glutamyltranspeptide-positive foci in the liver of female rats treated with ethinyl estradiol, clomiphene, tamoxifen and their associations. *Cancer Lett* 46:195-202

Gottardis MM, Robinson SP, Satyaswaroop PG, Jordan VC (1988): Contrasting actions of tamoxifen on endometrial and breast tumor growth in the athymic mouse. *Cancer Res* 48:812-815

Gottardis MM, Wagner RJ, Borden EC, Jordan VC (1989): Differential ability of antiestrogens to stimulate breast cancer cell (MCF-7) growth *in vivo* and *in vitro*. *Cancer Res* 49:4765-4769

Gottardis MM, Ricchio ME, Satyaswaroop PG, Jordan VC (1990): Effect of steroidal and nonsteroidal antiestrogens on the growth of a tamoxifen-stimulated human endometrial carcinoma (EnCa101) in athymic mice. *Cancer Res* 50:3189-3192

Greaves P, Goonetilleke R, Nunn G, Topham J, Orton T (1993): Two-year carcinogenicity study of tamoxifen in Alderly Park Wistar-derived rats. *Cancer Res* 53:3919-3924

Grenman SE, Roberts JA, England BG, Grönroos M, Carey TE (1988): *In vitro* growth regulation of endometrial carcinoma cells by tamoxifen and medroxyprogesterone acetate. *Gynecol Oncol* 30:239-250

Han X, Liehr JG (1990): Genotoxicity of tamoxifen in rats and hamsters (abstract no. 1235) *Carcinogensis* 32:207

Han X, Liehr JG (1992): Induction of covalent DNA adducts in rodents by tamoxifen. *Cancer Res* 52:1360-1363

Hard GC, Iatropoulos MJ, Jordan K, Radi L, Kalternberg OP, Imondi AR, Williams GM (1993): Major difference in the hepatocarcinogenicity and DNA adduct forming ability between toremifene and tamoxifen in female Crl:CD(BR) rats. *Cancer Res* 53:4534-4541

Hardell L (1988): Tamoxifen as risk factor for carcinoma of corpus uteri. *Lancet* ii:563

Hardell L (1988): Pelvic irradiation and tamoxifen as risk factors for carcinoma of corpus uteri. *Lancet* ii:1432

Hardell L (1990): Tamoxifen as a risk factor for endometrial cancer. *Cancer* 66:1661

Hemminki K, Widlak P, Hou S-M (1995): DNA adducts caused by tamoxifen and toremifene in human microsomal system and lymphocytes *in vitro*. *Carcinogensis* 16:1661-1664

Hirsimäki P, Hirsimäki Y, Nieminen L, Payne BJ (1993): Tamoxifen induces hepatocellular carcinoma in rat liver: a 1-year study with two antiestrogens. *Arch Toxicol* 67:49-54

Hwang J-Y, Lin B-Y, Tang F-M, Yu WCY (1992): Tamoxifen stimulates human papillomavirus type 16 gene expression and cell proliferation in a cervical cancer cell line. *Cancer Res* 52:6848-6852

International Agency for Research on Cancer (1995): Preamble. In: IARC Monographs on the Evaluation of Carcinogenic Risks to Humans. Vol. 62 IARC, Lyon, pp. 9-30

International Agency for Research on Cancer (1995): IARC Monographs on the Evaluation of Carcinogenic Risks to Humans. List of IARC Evaluations. IARC, Lyon

Johnstone AJ, Sarkar TK, Hussey JK (1991): Primary hepatocellular carcinoma in a patient with breast carcinoma. *Clin Oncol* 3:180-181

Jolles CJ, Smotkin D, Ford KL, Jones KP (1990): Cystic ovarian necrosis complicating tamoxifen therapy for breast cancer in a premenopausal woman. *J Reprod Med* 35:299-300

Jordan VC, Gottardis MM, Satyaswaroop PG (1991): Tamoxifen-stimulated growth of human endometrial carcinoma. *Ann NY Acad Sci* 622:439-446

Jordan VC, Assikis VJ (1995): Endometrial carcinoma and tamoxifen: clearing up a controversy. *Clin Cancer Res* 1:467-472

Killackey MA, Hakes TB, Pierce VK (1985): Endometrial adenocarcinoma in breast cancer patients receiving antiestrogens. *Cancer Treat Rep* 69:237-238

Le Bouëdec G, De Latour M, Leillel V, Dauplat J (1990): Métrorhagies et tamoxifène. A propos de 22 patientes traitées pour cancer du sein. *J Gynecol Obstet Biol Reprod* 19:889-894

LiVolsi VA, Salhany KE, Dowdy YG (1995): Endocervical adenocarcinoma in tamoxifen-treated patient. *Am J Obstet Gynecol* 172:1065

Lutz JM, Chouillet AM, Coleman MP (1994): Endometrium cancer after tamoxifen treatment for breast cancer: a population-based case-control study (abstract no. C23). In: XIXème réunion du groupe pour l'épidémiologie et l'enregistrement du cancer dans les pays de langue latine. Granada, 12-13 May 1994, p. 24

Maenpaa J, Wiebe V, Koester S, Wurz G, Emshoff V, Seymour R, Sipila P, DeGregorio M (1993): Tamoxifen stimulates *in vivo* growth of drug-resistant estrogen receptor-negative breast cancer. *Cancer Chemother Pharmacol* 32:396-398

Maenpaa JU, Wurz GT, Baker WJ, Wiebe VJ, Emshoff VD, Koester SK, Seymour RC, Koehler RE, DeGregorio MW (1993): A breast cancer clone selected by tamoxifen has increased growth rate and reduced sensitivity to doxorubicin. *Oncol Res* 5:461-466

Magriples U, Naftolin F, Schwartz PE, Carcangiu ML (1993): High-grade endometrial carcinoma in tamoxifen-treated breast cancer patients. *J Clin Oncol* 11:485-490

Mäntylä ETE, Karlsson SH, Nieminen LS (1996): Induction of endometrial cancer by tamoxifen in the rat. *Horm Carcinogensis* (in press)

Martin EA, Rich KJ, White INH, Woods KL, Powles TJ, Smith LL (1995): ^{32}P-postlabelled DNA adducts in liver obtained from women treated with tamoxifen. *Carcinogenesis* 16:1651-1654

Meschter C, Kendall M, Rose D, Jordan K, Williams G (1991): Carcinogenicity of tamoxifen (abstract no. 695). *Toxicologist* 11:190

Montandon F, Williams GM (1994): Comparison of DNA reactivity of the polyphenylnitrosamine-induced hepatocarcinogenesis. *Toxicology* 74:209-222

Osborne CK, Hobbs K, Clark GM (1985): Effect of estrogens and antiestrogens on growth of human breast cancer cells in athymic nude mice. *Cancer Res* 45:584-590

Osborne KC, Coronado E, Allred DC, Wiebe V, DeGregorio M (1991): Acquired tamoxifen resistance: correlation with reduced breast tumour levels of tamoxifen and isomerization of *trans*-4-hydroxytamoxifen. *J Natl Cancer Inst* 83:1477-1482

Pathak DN, Bodell WJ (1994): DNA adduct formation by tamoxifen with rat and human microsomal activation systems (abstract no. 815). *Carcinogenesis* 35:136

Pathak DN, Pongracz K, Bodell WJ (1995): Microsomal and peroxidase activation of 4-hydroxy-tamoxifen to form DNA adducts: comparison with DNA adducts formed in Sprague-Dawley rats treated with tamoxifen. *Carcinogenesis* 16:11-15

Phillips DH, Carmichael PL, Hewer A, Cole KJ, Poon GK (1994): alpha-hydroxytamoxifen, a metabolite of tamoxifen with exceptionally high DNA-binding activity in rat hepatocytes. *Cancer Res* 54:5518-5522

Pongracz K, Pathak DN, Bodell WJ (1994): Investigation of DNA adduct formation by tamoxifen metabolites using ^{32}P-postlabeling (abstract no. 820). *Carcinogenesis* 35:137

Powles TJ, Hickish T (1995): Tamoxifen therapy and carcinogenic risk. *J Natl Cancer Inst* 87:1343-1345

Randerath K, Moorthy B, Mabon N, Sriram P (1994): Tamoxifen: evidence by ^{32}P-postlabeling and use of metabolic inhibitors for two distinct pathways leading to mouse hepatic DNA adduct formation and identification of 4-hydroxytamoxifen as a proximate metabolite. *Carcinogenesis* 15:2087-2094

Robinson SP, Langan-Fahey SM, Johnson DA, Jordan VC (1991): Metabolites, pharmacodynamics, and pharmacokinetics of tamoxifen in rats and mice compared to the breast cancer patient. *Drug Metab Disp* 19:36-43

Rutqvist LE, Johansson H, Signomklao T, Johansson U, Fornander T, Wiling N, for the Stockholm Breast Cancer Study Group. *J Natl Cancer Inst* 87:645-651

Sakakibara K, Kan NC, Satyaswaroop PG (1992): Both 17ß-estradiol and tamoxifen induce c-fos messenger ribonucleic acid expression in human endometrial carcinoma grown in nude mice. *Am J Obstet Gynecol* 166:206-212

Sasco AJ (1994): Quelques réflexions sur le rôle cancérogène potentiel du tamoxifène. *Bull Cancer* 81:706-714

Sasco AJ, Ah-Song R, Saez S, Kuttenn F (1995): Effets secondaires médicaux d'une intervention de chimioprévention: l'exemple du tamoxifène. *Bull Cancer* 82:186s-206s

Sasco AJ, Chaplain G, Saez S, Amoros E (1995): Case-control study of endometrial cancer following breast cancer. Effect of tamoxifen and radiotherapeutic castration (abstract no. 309). *Am J Epidemiol* 141:S78

Sasco AJ, Raffi F, Satgé D, Godurdhun J, Fallouh B, Leduc B (1995): Endometrial müllerian carcinosarcoma after cessation of tamoxifen therapy for breast cancer. *Int J Gynecol Obstet* 48:307-310

Sasco AJ, Chaplain G, Amoros E, Saez S (1996): Endometrial cancer following breast cancer: effect of tamoxifen and castration by radiotherapy. *Epidemiology* 7:9-13

Satyaswaroop PG, Zaino RJ, Mortel R (1984): Estrogen-like effects of tamoxifen on human endometrial carcinoma transplanted into nude mice. *Cancer Res* 44:4006-4010

Seoud MAF, Johnson J, Weed JC (1993): Gynecologic tumors in tamoxifen-treated women with breast cancer. *Obstet Gynecol* 82:165-169

Sonnendecker HEM, Cooper K, Kalian KN (1994): Primary Fallopian tube adenocarcinoma *in situ* associated with adjuvant tamoxifen therapy for breast carcinoma. *Gynecol Oncol* 52:402-407

Stewart HJ, Knight CM (1989): Tamoxifen and the uterus and endometrium. *Lancet* i:375-376

Stewart JF for the Scottish Cancer Trials Breast Group (1992): The Scottish trial of adjuvant tamoxifen in node-negative breast cancer. *J Natl Cancer Inst Monogr* 11:117-120

Terada S, Uchide K, Suzuki N, Akasofu K (1993): A follicular cyst during tamoxifen therapy in a premenopausal breast cancer woman. *Gynecol Obstet Invest* 35:62-64

Vancutsen PM, Lazarus P, Williams GM (1994): Frequent and specific mutations of the rat *p53* gene in hepatocarcinomas induced by tamoxifen. *Cancer Res* 54:3864-3867

van Leeuwen FE, Benraadt J, Coebergh JWW, Kiemeney LALM, Gimbrère CHF, Otter R, Schouten LJ, Damhuis RAM, Bontenbal M, Diepenhorst FW, van den Belt-Dusebout AW, van Tinteren H (1994): Risk of endometrial cancer after tamoxifen treatment of breast cancer. *Lancet* 343:448-452

White INH, De Matteis F, Davies A, Smith LL, Crofton-Sleigh C, Venitt S, Hewer A, Philipps DH (1992): Genotoxic potential of tamoxifen and analogues in female Fischer F344/n rats, DBA/2 and C57BL/6 mice and in human MCL-5 cells. *Carcinogenesis* 13:2197-2203

White INH, Davies A, Smith LL, Dawson S, De Matteis F (1993): Induction of CYP2B1 and 3A1, and associated monooxygenase activities by tamoxifen and certain analogues in the livers of female rats and mice. *Biochem Pharmacol* 45:21-30

White INH, De Matteis F, Gibbs AH, Lim CK, Wolf CR, Henderson C, Smith LL (1995): Species differences in the covalent binding of [^{14}C] tamoxifen to liver microsomes and the forms of cytochrome P450 involved. *Biochem Pharmacol* 49:1035-1042

Williams GM, Iatropoulos MJ, Hard GC, Djordjevic MV (1991): Hepatocarcinogenicity of tamoxifen but not toremifene in female rats. Abstracts of a satellite symposium at the Fourth International Congress on Hormones and Cancer, Amsterdam, September 1991

Williams GM, Iatropoulos MJ, Djordjevic MV, Kaltenberg OP (1993): The triphenylethylene drug tamoxifen is a strong liver carcinogen in the rat. *Carcinogenesis* 14:315-317

World Health Organization (1985): Essential drugs for cancer chemotherapy: memorandum from a WHO meeting. *Bull World Health Organization* 63:999-1002

Wunderlich V, Stein U (1994): Synergistic effect of tamoxifen and phorbol ester TPA on retrovirus synthesis in a human mammary carcinoma cell line. *Int J Cancer* 56:615-616

Yager JD, Roebuck BD, Paluszcyk TL, Memoli VA (1986): Effects of ethinyl estradiol and tamoxifen on liver DNA turnover and new synthesis and appearance of gamma glutamyl transpeptidase-positive foci in female rats. *Carcinogenesis* 7:2007-2014

Yager JD, Shi YE (1991): Synthetic estrogens and tamoxifen as promoters of hepatocarcinogenesis. *Prev Med* 20:27-37

Zimniski SJ, Warren RC (1993): Induction of tamoxifen-dependent rat mammary tumors. *Cancer Res* 53:2937-2939

ACKNOWLEDGMENTS

This work was supported by grants from the Caisse Primaire Centrale d'Assurance Maladie de Lyon, Caisse Nationale d'Assurance Maladie des Travailleurs Salariés - Institut National de la Santé et de la Recherche Médicale (Convention No. 3AM078) and the Ligue Nationale contre le Cancer. Isabelle Gendre was supported by a Special Training Award from the International Agency for Research on Cancer.

5. MECHANISMS OF RESISTANCE TO ANTIESTROGENS AND THEIR IMPLICATIONS FOR CROSSRESISTANCE

Robert Clarke and Marc E. Lippman

The first triphenylethylenes considered for clinical use were generated in the mid 1950's. These compounds were initially generated as fertility agents, e.g., ethamoxytriphetol (MER-25), and clomiphene. Their ability to induce favorable responses in some breast cancer patients was soon demonstrated (Kistner and Smith, 1960). Toxicity proved significant with these compounds (Herbst et al., 1964). However, in the early 1970's the first report of remissions in breast cancer following treatment with a new antiestrogen Tamoxifen (ICI 46474), was published (Cole et al., 1971). In the 17 years that followed, the total exposure to Tamoxifen reached 1.5 million patient years (Litherland and Jackson, 1988), with exposure now approaching 8 million patient years.

Perhaps one of the greatest enigmas of Tamoxifen is that, despite the substantial clinical experience and almost 25 years of basic science research, we still do not know the precise cellular and molecular mechanisms of action that predominate in patients (Fig. 1). The ability of Tamoxifen to function as a partial agonist through the estrogen receptor (ER) is clearly of central importance. It is estimated that approximately only 10% of tumors that do not express ER will respond to Tamoxifen treatment (Table 1).

The ER is not the only intracellular target for Tamoxifen. The function of the signal transduction molecules protein kinase C (O'Brian et al., 1986) and calmodulin (Lam, 1984) is inhibited by Tamoxifen as a result of direct interactions. Structural parameters of the plasma

TAMOXIFEN

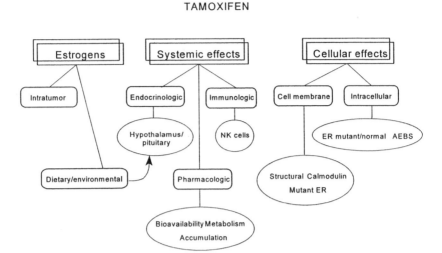

Figure 1. The diversity of mechanisms and targets implicated in mediating the effects of Tamoxifen.

membrane also are significantly altered by Tamoxifen (Clarke et al., 1990). The precise role of these targets is unclear, since less than 10% of ER-positive tumors respond to Tamoxifen, and the concentrations required to induce these *in vitro* effects approach the suprapharmacologic. There are clearly other sites of Tamoxifen action that are unrelated to targets within the tumor cells. These include endocrinologic effects on the pituitary-hypothalamic-gonadal axis in premenopausal patients, immunologic effects on certain effectors of the immune system and effects on serum growth factor concentrations.

We will review several of the potential mechanisms of action and resistance for Tamoxifen. We will touch only briefly on those specific targets that are described in greater detail elsewhere in this monograph.

Pharmacologic Mechanisms of Resistance

There are several pharmacologic properties of Tamoxifen that directly influence its biological activity and that, when significantly altered, could contribute to the emergence of an antiestrogen resistant phenotype. These include the classical pharmacokinetic parameters of absorption, distribution, biotransformation and excretion. We have previously reviewed several of these pharmacokinetic parameters in some detail (Clarke and Lippman, 1992).

Serum transport and intracellular influx/efflux. A significant proportion of Tamoxifen and its major metabolites ($\sim 98\%$)are either bound to serum albumin (Lien et al., 1989), or potentially sequestered in peripheral tissues (Daniel et al., 1981; Lien et al., 1989). Thus, the amount that is available to a tumor from extracellular sources could be significantly limited. For tumors to acquire a sufficient intracellular concentration, it seems likely that some degree of accumulation against a concentration gradient may be necessary. There are several observations that support this hypothesis. The plasma steady-state concentrations of Tamoxifen and its metabolites rarely exceeds 1 micromole in patients receiving 30 mg/day (Etienne et al., 1989), with the amount of bioavailable drug likely to be significantly lower. Concentrations approaching 1 micromole are often required to substantially inhibit MCF-7 cell proliferation *in vitro* (Clarke et al., 1990; Clarke et al., 1989c). The concentration of Tamoxifen appears higher in uterus (Fromson and Sharp, 1974) and other tissues (Daniel et al., 1981; Lien et al., 1989; Fromson and Sharp, 1974) than it is in serum.

The precise mechanism for intracellular uptake of Tamoxifen is unclear. A passive diffusion similar to steroids seems most likely. However, this would not readily account for an apparent ability to concentrate drug in tissues relative to serum (Fromson and Sharp, 1974; Daniel et al., 1981; Lien et al., 1989; Fromson and Sharp, 1974). In preliminary studies (unpublished), we have not found any significant accumulation of [3H] Tamoxifen in breast cancer cells growing *in vitro*. The high degree of lipophilicity of Tamoxifen and its major metabolites could result in sequestration of drug in adipose tissue and the plasma membrane of cells (Clarke et al., 1990). Thus, the presence of significant amounts of adipose, stromal and epithelial tissues could partly account of the ability of some sites to retain apparently high concentrations of drug.

The mechanism for drug efflux also is not known, although a passive diffusion again seems most likely. We and others (Leonessa et al., 1994; Ramu et al., 1984) have described the ability of Tamoxifen to interact with the gp170 efflux pump that is a product of the MDR1 (multidrug resistance 1) gene. However, it is apparent that Tamoxifen is not a classical substrate for this pump, and does not appear to be effluxed (Clarke et al., 1996b).

If the major mechanism for transport is passive diffusion, acquired resistance by an altered intracellular transport would seem an unlikely mechanism for resistance. Nevertheless, there is some evidence for lower intratumor levels of Tamoxifen in resistant versus sensitive tumors (Osborne et al., 1992; Osborne et al., 1991; Johnston et al., 1993)and in some cell lines (Kellen et al., 1986). Whether this reflects altered intracellular levels of Tamoxifen in tumors is unclear. A loss of either the stromal or adipose component of a tumor, or a redued degree of tumor vascularization, might be expected to also reduce a tumor's ability to apparently retain Tamoxifen. This could not explain the reduced accumulation of Tamoxifen in some cells growing *in vitro* (Kellen et al., 1986).

Bioavailability. The intracellular bioavailability of Tamoxifen is of critical importance in determining its ability to regulate cellular proliferation. There are at least three major intracellular binding compartments for Tamoxifen; partition into the cellular membranes, binding to antiestrogen binding sites (AEBS), and to a lesser extent binding to ER. Sequestration in the plasma membrane could significantly reduce intracellular bioavailability for ER binding. However, Tamoxifen's ability to inhibit membrane-associated signal transduction molecules, e.g., protein kinase C, may be largely unaffected.

One of the potentially more important intracellular binding components, at least for the triphenylethylenes, could be the AEBS. These are predominately microsomal proteins that exhibit a high affinity for triphenylethylenes but not for steroids (Katzenellenbogen et al., 1985). Overexpression could conceivably confer resistance in the presence of ER expression. The precise origin of the AEBS is unclear but they may represent novel histamine receptors (Brandes and Bogdanovic, 1986; Miller and Bulbrook, 1986). A basic alkylether side chain appears important in recognition of AEBS by triphenylethylenes (Murphy and Sutherland, 1985). The biological potency of antiestrogens does not correlate with their affinity for AEBS (Katzenellenbogen et al., 1985), implying the lack of an inherent signal transduction function. However, the ability of AEBS to sequester free drug could reduce intracellular bioavailability. This is of little importance for the new steroidal antiestrogens ICI 182,780 and ICI 164,384. Like the natural estrogens, these compounds do not bind to AEBS with a high affinity (Pavlik et al., 1992).

Metabolism. The metabolism of drugs to less active metabolites is a common mechanism for drug resistance. Tamoxifen is extensively metabolized in patients, and several metabolites have predominately estrogenic rather than antiestrogenic properties (Clarke, Lippman, 1992).

Osborne et al. (Osborne et al., 1991; Osborne et al., 1992) have described an increased isomerization of Tamoxifen to these estrogenic metabolites in breast tumors. It has been suggested that this metabolism could account for some of the Tamoxifen resistance that occurs in patients and for the Tamoxifen-stimulated phenotype that occurs in some human breast cancer xenografts (Gottardis et al., 1989; Osborne et al., 1987).

A series of elegant studies were performed by Jordan et al. to directly address the potential role of estrogenic Tamoxifen metabolites. Non-isomerizable Tamoxifen analogues were generated and used to determine their ability to inhibit the growth of the Tamoxifen-stimulated xenografts. It was predicted that these should inhibit tumor growth, since they could not be metabolized to estrogenic metabolites. However, the Tamoxifen-stimulated tumors were still stimulated by these derivatives (Wolf et al., 1993). This implied that the Tamoxifen-stimulated phenotype was unlikely to be explained by the result of significant metabolism to estrogenic metabolites. Subsequently, this group has identified a point mutation in the ER in the Tamoxifen-stimulated xenografts. This mutant receptor changes how the cell perceives Tamoxifen, which induces agonist rather than antagonist responses in cells transfected with the mutant ER (Catherino et al., 1995).

Altered target specificity. Since the ER is the major intracellular target for Tamoxifen, mutations in the ER protein could alter the sensitivity of the cell. Mutant ER mRNAs and proteins have been widely reported (Murphy and Dotzlaw, 1989; Dotzlaw et al., 1992; Murphy et al., 1995; Wang and Miksicek, 1991; Fuqua et al., 1992; Koehorst et al., 1994). For example, an alternatively spliced exon 4 deletion mutant in MCF-7 cells and meningiomas has been described that does not bind estradiol (Koehorst et al., 1994). Dominant negative mutant receptors also have been described, including an exon 3 deletion mutant (Wang and Miksicek, 1991). A truncated ER that lacks exon 7 has been described and is found in a significant proportion of ER-/PGR+tumors (Fuqua et al., 1992). This mutant is transcriptionally inactive and can prevent wild type ER from binding to an estrogen response element. It appears that mutant receptors are generally found coexpressed with significant levels of wild type receptor (Murphy and Dotzlaw, 1989), implicating dominant negative receptors rather than ligand-binding mutants.

While the precise contribution of mutant ER proteins to Tamoxifen resistance remains to be established, it seems likely that they will prove relevant. There is a well established role for mutant androgen receptors in disease, particularly those associated with androgen resistance/insensitivity (Tsukada et al., 1994; Kaspar et al., 1993). Androgen receptors also have been associated with breast cancer. For example, androgen receptor expression can predict for response to medroxyprogesterone acetate (Birrell et al., 1995), and an Arg to Lys mutation in this receptor is associated with male breast cancer (Lobaccaro et al., 1993b; Lobaccaro et al., 1993a).

Endocrinologic Mechanisms of Resistance

Blockade of the pituitary-hypothalamic-gonadal axis. Tamoxifen has proven to be of greater benefit when administered to premenopausal women when compared with postmenopausal women. A major mechanistic explanation may be the presence of high endogenous levels of estrogens in premenopausal women that effectively compete with Tamoxifen for ER binding. Paradoxically, Tamoxifen increases the circulating levels of estrogens (Ravdin et al., 1988; Szamel et al., 1994), further increasing this competition.

The explanation for the ability of Tamoxifen to increase serum estrogens is related to how estrogens regulate their own secretion (Fig 2). The release of estrogens from the ovaries is regulated by the hypothalamic-pituitary-ovarian axis, with the gonadotropins acting directly on the ovary. Estrogens regulate the release of gonadotropins at two levels, the release of gonadotropin releasing hormone (GnRH) from the hypothalamus and of LH and FSH from the anterior pituitary (Fig 2). Tamoxifen effectively blocks the ER in both the hypothalamus and anterior pituitary, disrupting the negative-feedback on GnRH and the gonadotropins, and producing a "hyperstimulation" of the ovaries (Ravdin et al., 1988). There also is some evidence to suggest that dehydroepiandrosterone, estrone and estradiol levels can be increased by antiestrogens in postmenopausal women (Szamel et al., 1994). The endocrinologic perturbation in these women likely reflects an effect mediated through the release of adrenal androgens.

Extragonadal de novo synthesis of estrogens. Breast tumor cells have been reported to possess most of the enzymes required to synthesize estrogens from the precursors in serum. The local production of estrogens could effectively compete with Tamoxifen for binding to ER (Pasqualini and Nguyen, 1991). Since there would likely be little sequestration of local estrogens by serum binding proteins like sex hormone binding globulin, it may only require a limited degree of de novo synthesis to impact Tamoxifen sensitivity. The two most important

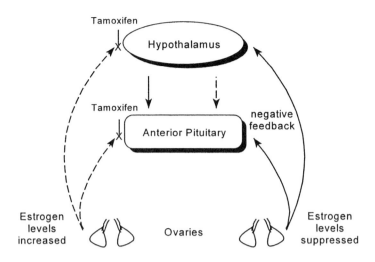

Figure 2. Endocrine perturbations in the hypothalamic-pituitary-ovarian axis induced by antiestrogens. The blockade of ER in the hypothalamus and anterior pituitary releases the normal negative feedback induced by estrogens.

enzymes in this regard are the P450 aromatase and the steroid sulfatase enzymes. In postmenopausal women, peripheral adipose tissue is the primary source of circulating estrogens (Brodie and Santen, 1985). The adipose tissues are capable of generating estrogens from the appropriate circulating adrenal androgen precursors.   The aromatase enzyme aromatizes the A-ring of the androgens, resulting in hydroxylation of the ketone at position 3. It is this conversion that is primarily responsible for conferring the ability of estrogens to recognize the ER (Clarke et al., 1996a). The major metabolite in postmenopausal women is estrone, which is generally present as the biologically inactive estrone sulfate. However, peripheral/local production of estrogens appears biologically significant in some breast tumors. Inhibitors of aromatase, e.g., aminoglutethimide, 4-hydroxyandrostenedione, can induce remissions in postmenopausal breast cancer patients, but their real value seems to be in premenopausal patients, where the primary target is ovarian aromatization.

The biological activity of the estrogens is regulated, at least in part, by the addition or removal of a sulfate at position 3. Thus, an increased activity of the steroid sulfatase enzyme, which releases the active estrogens by removal of this sulfate, could contribute to antiestrogen resistance. Many breast tumors express significant sulfatase activity (Reed et al., 1989). Unfortunately, there are relatively few effective inhibitors of this enzyme in clinical use. The most potent inhibitor used to date is danazol but it has significant toxicity, and can act as a relatively potent androgen. We have recently transduced MCF-7 cells with the full length cDNA for the steroid sulfatase enzyme, and generated a model in which to screen for novel inhibitors (James and Clarke, 1995).

It might be anticipated that a combination of an aromatase inhibitor, a sulfatase inhibitor and an antiestrogen would be a potent clinical strategy. Unfortunately, initial attempts have proved less than encouraging. In one of the initial studies, the overall response rate was comparable to Tamoxifen alone but the duration of response was shorter (Hardy et al., 1990). There are many unanswered questions in this area, including the possibility that scheduling is important and the complication that danazol may induce mitogenic effects through the androgen receptor. **Dietary and phytoestrogenic compounds.** If an increased exposure to endogenous estrogens, by either endocrinologic perturbations or local production can influence antiestrogen responsiveness, then exposure to other estrogenic stimuli could be problematic. The other major sources of such activities are those resulting from exposure through either diet or the environment. Many compounds in the western diet contain compounds known as "phytoestrogens". We have recently reviewed the properties of these compounds, and their potential mechanism(s) of action, in some detail (Clarke et al., 1996a).

Several phytoestrogenic compounds have relatively high affinities for the ER and can regulate gene transcription through activation of ER. For example, the mycotoxin zearalenone and its major metabolite zearalenol are present in barley, wheat, corn, corn flakes, rice and maize at concentrations varying from 35-115 g/kg (Hagler et al., 1984; Luo et al., 1990; Golinski et al., 1988; Schoental, 1985). Their estimated daily intake in humans is estimated at 100-500 ng per kg body weight (Kuiper-Goodman, 1990). These compounds bind to ER with relative affinities of 25% for zearalenol and 4% for zearalenone (Verdeal et al., 1980), and can regulate the expression of a reporter gene linked to an estrogen response element in an *in vitro* transcription assay (Mayr et al., 1992). Other compounds may function as partial agonists, in a manner similar to Tamoxifen (Mayr et al., 1992).

The ability of phytoestrogenic compounds to function as agonists or partial agonists could have important implications for patients receiving Tamoxifen. Depending upon the nature of the interaction, these compounds could interact additively, synergistically (if they are ER partial agonists) or as antagonists (if they are ER agonists). Consumption of a diet high in potent estrogenic activities could generate an apparent Tamoxifen resistance by directly competing for ER within tumors (Mayr et al., 1992).

Immunologic Mechanisms of Resistance

There is evidence implicating cell mediated immunity (CMI) in the control of breast cancer growth and metastasis (Head et al., 1993; Black et al., 1988). For example, there is a significant reduction in NK activity in patients with stage III and stage IV disease (An et al., 1987; Contreras and Stoliar, 1988; Akimoto et al., 1986) and in the axillary lymph nodes of patients with demonstrable metastatic disease (Horst and Horny, 1987; Bonilla et al., 1988). However, the incidence of breast cancer in women immunosuppressed following transplantation surgery is lower than that expected from the general population (Stewart et al., 1995).

ER negative tumors exhibit elevated levels of NK activity (Levy et al., 1990; Underwood et al., 1987), whereas low NK activity is associated with familial breast cancer (Strayer et al., 1986). Peripheral blood mononuclear cells, thymus and splenic cells (Danel et al., 1983) and CD8 + T-cells (Cohen et al., 1983; Stimson, 1980) all express ER. While the expression of ER per se is not sufficient evidence that estrogens are involved in the regulation of immune cell function, estrogens can increase IgM secretion (Myers and Peterson, 1985) and alter NK cell activation (see below).

There is clear evidence from studies in mice that estrogens can significantly influence several effectors of cell mediated immunity. Estrogen induces a biphasic response on NK cell activity. An initial increase in activity is generally followed by a subsequent reduction of activity to below pretreatment/untreated levels (Screpanti et al., 1987; Seaman et al., 1978; Hanna and Schneider, 1983; Seaman, Talal, 1980). In contrast, Tamoxifen stimulates NK activity both *in vitro* (Mandeville et al., 1984) and *in vivo* (Gottardis et al., 1989). NK cells are implicated in the host response to tumors, and may influence metastatic potential; see (Clarke, 1995) for recent review. A loss of responsiveness to Tamoxifen-induced NK cell activation could contribute to the appearance of resistance. However, there is little direct evidence supporting the clinical relevance of this in breast cancer patients. Tamoxifen also has been demonstrated to increase tumor necrosis alpha production by mononuclear cells (Teodorczyk-Injeyan et al., 1993), and to improve the persistent proteinuria and immune complex deposition in the kidneys of mice with experimental systemic lupus erythematosus (Sthoeger et al., 1994). A more detailed discussion of the role of immunological effects is provided by Baral et al. elsewhere in this monograph.

Alterations in Growth Factor Secretion

Growth factors may play a critical role in regulating the proliferative response of some breast cancer cells to estrogens and antiestrogens. Since these have been reviewed in detail elsewhere (Clarke et al., 1992; Clarke, Lippman, 1992), we will only briefly consider their potential role in antiestrogen resistance. In breast cancer cells, ER ligands alter the expression of two "classes" of growth factors, mitogens and growth inhibitors. In general, the effects of estrogens and antiestrogens are opposite in this regard. Thus, estrogens increase the secretion of mitogens such as TGF-alpha (Bates et al., 1988; Clarke et al., 1989a) and IGF-I (Huff et al., 1988), while decreasing the secretion of inhibitors including TGF-beta$_1$ (Knabbe et al., 1987). Tamoxifen appears to essentially produce the opposite effect upon the secretion of these factors (Bates et al., 1988; Knabbe et al., 1987; Huff et al., 1988; Colletta et al., 1990). There also is clinical evidence for some of these events. For example, patients receiving Tamoxifen have lower serum levels of IGF-I (Pollak et al., 1990).

Understanding the precise role of the various estrogen-regulated growth factors is often difficult. As with the study of many genes associated with growth regulation, it is important to determine which events are associative and which are functionally relevant. While estrogen can induce TGF-alpha expression, overexpression of this factor alone does not consistently confer a hormone-dependent or antiestrogen resistant phenotype (Clarke et al., 1989a). In contrast, the IGFs are potent mitogens for breast cancer (Yee et al., 1989) and there is limited evidence to suggest that inhibition of the type I IGF-receptor can inhibit breast cancer growth (Arteaga et al., 1989). It is likely that the role of growth factors is complex and interdependent in nature. It may require the concerted regulation of both mitogenic and inhibitory factors to significantly influence breast cancer cell growth. With the potential diversity of factors and the signal transduction pathways they regulate, it is conceivable that no single mix of growth factors will predominate in all breast cancers. However, the ability of estrogens and antiestrogens to differentially regulate growth factor expression/function, may contribute significantly to responsiveness and acquired resistance to antiestrogens.

Non-genomic events

The triphenylethylenes are generally considered to induce their growth effects through their interactions with ER. This gains considerable support from the associations among receptor expression and response in breast cancer patients (Ravdin et al., 1992; Stewart et al., 1982). Nevertheless, the triphenylethylenes appear to have several effects/targets that do not require interference with the transcriptional activities of ER. These are generally considered "non-genomic" effects, since the direct regulation of gene expression or direct interactions with nucleic acids are not involved. Estrogens have been known for many years to elicit responses that are inconsistent with a direct genomic involvement (Farhat et al. 1992; Duval et al., 1983).

Altered cell membrane structure and function. Triphenylethylenes are highly lipophilic compounds, and as such would be predicted to partition predominately into the hydrophobic domains of cellular membranes. Cellular membranes exist in a "liquid crystal" state, with fluidity representing a critical structural parameter. Compounds that partition into local domains within the membrane are likely to alter the fluidity of the membrane, at least within their immediate locality. Changes in the structural properties of local membrane domains could significantly alter the activity of integral and peripheral membrane proteins that are dependent upon their lipid environment for function (Lenaz et al., 1978). Thus, triphenylethylenes may have significant influences on membrane-mediated events, including signal transduction initiated by diverse pathways, e.g., G-proteins, phosphoinositide turnover, protein kinase C and growth factor receptor kinase activities.

Several years ago we demonstrated the ability of Tamoxifen to alter the physical attributes of breast cancer cells by assessing effects on gross membrane fluidity (Clarke et al., 1990). Fluidity was estimated by determining the steady-state polarization of fluorescence of the probe 1,6-diphenyl-1,3,5-hexatriene(DPH), which reflects the rotational ability of the probe resulting from the molecular packing of the lipids comprising the membrane domains into which the probe is inserted. We

introduced DPH into the membranes of both MCF-7 (ER-positive) and
MDA-MB-436 cells (ER-negative) in the presence and absence of
Tamoxifen.

Our data indicate that Tamoxifen decreases the membrane fluidity
of the cellular membranes in both the ER-positive and -negative cell lines
(Clarke et al., 1990). Similar effects have subsequently been reported in
artificial membranes (Custodio et al., 1993b) and liposomes (Custodio et
al., 1993a; Kayyali et al., 1994). These effects also are associated with
significant biological changes. In breast cancer cells, the changes in
membrane structure are accompanied by increasing cytotoxicity, and
clearly occur independent of receptor status (Clarke et al., 1990). There
also are effects on calcium ion influx (Morley and Whitfield, 1995),
gp170-mediated drug efflux (Leonessa et al., 1994), and membrane
phospholipid metabolism (Cabot et al., 1995).

It seems likely that the effects of Tamoxifen will reflect the
specific lipid domains into which it partitions. These domains may have
some specific physico-chemical characteristics, including size and degree
of lipophilicity. If so, then Tamoxifen may appear to have some degree
of specificity for effects on membrane-dependent events (Clarke et al.,
1990). Resistance could arise by cells switching to other pathways that
do not require these membrane-dependent events, or by altering local
membrane structure to reduce the stabilizing effects of Tamoxifen.

Protein kinase C. Protein kinase C is a membrane protein that has been
implicated as an important signal transduction molecule in several cellular
systems. Like many membrane-associated proteins, it is likely that the
function of protein kinase C is dependent upon its lipid environment.
The ability of Tamoxifen to alter the structural properties of membranes
(see above) could indirectly alter protein kinase C function. However, it
also is apparent that Tamoxifen can bind directly to protein kinase C in
a manner that can alter its function (O'Brian et al., 1986; O'Brian et al.,
1988). Thus, Tamoxifen inhibits protein kinase C activity with an IC50
=25 μM (O'Brian et al., 1986). While this concentration is significantly
higher than serum/plasma levels of Tamoxifen and its major metabolites,
the intracellular concentrations could exceed 1 micromole if cells can
selectively retain Tamoxifen against a concentration gradient.
Furthermore, if protein kinase C activity were rate limiting in
proliferation, any significant inhibition of its activity may be sufficient to
induce a reduction in cellular proliferation.

The inability of the 4-hydroxytamoxifen metabolite of Tamoxifen
to bind to protein kinase C (O'Brian et al., 1988) indicates that growth

inhibition from this compound may not involve this enzyme. Thus, whatever the functional role of protein kinase C inhibition by Tamoxifen, it is unlikely that this is solely responsible for the antiestrogenic effects of Tamoxifen in patients. The importance of protein kinase C in the regulation of mitogenic signals implies that, if Tamoxifen does regulate its function *in vivo*, this inhibition likely contributes to the overall effect on cellular proliferation. Perturbations in either the level of expression of protein kinase C, or its sensitivity to inhibition by Tamoxifen is modified, could contribute to acquired Tamoxifen resistance in some cells.

Calmodulin. Calmodulin is another signal transduction molecule that can be inhibited directly by Tamoxifen. The IC50 for this interaction (9 micromole) is significantly lower than that for protein kinase C (Greenberg et al., 1987). Calmodulin is primarily a calcium ion-binding protein, and is involved in cyclic nucleotide metabolism. Some aspects of ER-mediated gene transcription can be regulated by cAMP (Aronica and Katzenellenbogen, 1993). Thus, Tamoxifen could indirectly influence ER function by inhibiting calmodulin function. Alterations in the sensitivity of calmodulin to inhibition by Tamoxifen could also influence cellular response and contribute to the acquisition of resistance.

Conclusions. A major problem in general with the non-genomic effects is in determi ning their clinical relevance. It might be anticipated that protein kinase C and calmodulin are important molecules that function independent of the ER status of the cell. Thus, both ER-positive and ER-negative cells should be growth inhibited by antiestrogen-induced perturbations in their respective activities. It is not clear that this is the case. At best, only 10% of ER-negative tumors respond, and few of the ER-negative breast cancer cell lines *in vitro* respond, except at concentrations that are generally considered suprapharmacologic. There are several pieces of information that are required to support a likely important clinical/biological role for these nongenomic effects. It should be demonstrated that these targets are important for mediating the growth regulatory signals of antiestrogens/estrogens. For example, if protein kinase C activity is inhibited, does this alter response to Tamoxifen. Since ER-positive cells are more sensitive to antiestrogens, these cells should be more reliant upon protein kinase C and/or calmodulin. There is only limited indirect evidence in support of this for calmodulin. The levels of calmodulin in breast tumors appear higher than in normal tissue (O'Brian et al., 1989) and ER-negative tumors tend to express higher levels than ER-positive cells (Borner et al., 1987). Thus, it might be predicted that high concentrations of a calmodulin inhibitor would be required to growth inhibit ER-negative cells. The precise relevance of this association remains to be established.

It also must be clearly demonstrated that the concentrations at which nongenomic effects occur represent achievable intracellular Tamoxifen concentrations in tumors. Almost all of the nongenomic effects are observed at micromolar concentrations of Tamoxifen *in vitro*. The cell culture conditions used contain only low concentrations of serum, generally 10% or less, which will not reduce bioavailability to the same degree as occurs in blood. More compelling evidence could be gained from *in vivo* studies using either human tumor xenografts or chemically induced rodent mammary tumors. Until these various issues are resolved, the precise contribution of nongenomic effects to Tamoxifen's inhibitory effects will remain controversial.

Crossresistance

Cross resistance among antiestrogens. Crossresistance occurs frequently among drugs of the same structural class or that have a common mechanism/target. It is clear that most or all of the triphenylethylene antiestrogens and several non-steroidal compounds exhibit significant crossresistance (Clarke and Lippman, 1992). The structural and functional properties of the new steroidal antiestrogens (ICI 182,780, ICI 164,384) are sufficiently different from the non-steroidal antiestrogens that crossresistance cannot be presumed. For example, their interactions with ER, both in terms of effects on receptor dimerization (Fawell et al., 1990), recycling (Dauvois et al., 1992) and structure/function (McDonnell et al., 1995), are profoundly different from the triphenylethylenes.

We have addressed the potential for crossresistance by generating cellular models with resistance to 4-hydroxytamoxifen and ICI 182,780 (Brünner et al., 1993c; Brünner et al. 1993b) from hormone-independent, antiestrogen-responsive MCF-7 variants (Clarke et al., 1989b; Clarke et al., 1989c; Brünner et al., 1993a). Our preliminary data strongly suggest that cells acquiring resistance to a triphenylethylene may not exhibit crossresistance with the steroidal compounds (Brünner et al. 1993b). It is becoming apparent that this *in vitro* phenotype has predicted for the analogous clinical response pattern, since patients that have acquired resistance to Tamoxifen still exhibit responses to ICI 182,780 (Clarke et al., 1996b). In marked contrast, cells selected for resistance to the steroidal ICI 182,780 acquire crossresistance to Tamoxifen (Brünner et al. 1993b). There are many examples of schedule dependence in the efficacy of some cytotoxic chemotherapy regimes. However, such examples in endocrine therapy are less well described. Whether therapies based on combinations of antiestrogens are warranted remains to be established. Our data would suggest that the choice of schedule may be of critical importance when steroidal and non-steroidal antiestrogens are combined (Clarke et al., 1996b).

Gene networks. Tamoxifen can regulate the expression of several genes in the absence of estrogen. This could reflect differential effects on the two transcription activating domains present in the ER protein. One domain (TAF-1) appears to exhibit constitutive transcriptional regulatory activities when bound to DNA irrespective of ligand. The transcriptional activities of the other domain (TAF-2) are ligand dependent, and may only be activated when the receptor is occupied by estrogens (Danielian et al., 1992). This could provide a rational explanation for the partial agonism induced by the triphenylethylenes, since they could regulate transcription through TAF-1 but not TAF-2 (Danielian et al., 1992).

We have recently suggested that the ability of cells to acquire an estrogen-independent phenotype without concurrently acquiring antiestrogen resistance, and the lack of crossresistance between triphenylethylenes and steroidal antiestrogens, could reflect the differential regulation of interrelated and/or interdependent gene networks (Clarke and Brünner, 1995; Clarke et al., 1996b). The biophysical events regulating these gene networks could be explained by the conformational changes induced in the ER protein when occupied by different ligands. The physical properties of the ER protein appear associated with its ability to regulate reporter gene expression, and these properties are dependent upon the occupying ligand (McDonnell et al., 1995). The different protein conformations could explain how structurally diverse ligands could differentially regulate gene networks.

Resistance to one class of antiestrogens would not necessarily produce crossresistance to others if the regulated gene networks are interrelated but not interdependent. There may be several pathways that are concurrently influenced by the transcriptional activity of ER occupied by estrogen, but the end result of activation in terms of cell division may be the same. Thus, cells could switch from one pathway to another as these are selectively blocked by the action of different receptor-ligand complexes (Clarke et al., 1996b).

Reversal of Antiestrogen Resistance

Since Tamoxifen is an effective and nontoxic therapy for a significant number of breast cancer patients, a means to reverse resistance may induce additional/prolonged responses in patients. There is clear evidence from *in vitro* and *in vivo* studies that such approaches may be clinically feasible. Most of these approaches involve attempts to regulate the expression/function of ER, the primary target for Tamoxifen. These approaches primarily involve the interferons and to a lesser extent the retinoids.

Interferons as resistance modulators. Interferons generally fail to induce significant responses in breast cancer patients but can induce toxicity when administered as single agents or in combination chemotherapy regimens (Fentiman et al., 1987; Padmanabhan et al., 1985; Barreras et al., 1988; Pouillart et al., 1982). However, we (van den Berg et al., 1987) and others (Epstein et al., 1987; Porzsolt et al., 1989; Epstein et al., 1987; Goldstein et al., 1989; Kangas et al., 1985; Tiwari et al., 1991; Robinson et al., 1990) have demonstrated that interferons can potentiate the effects of antiestrogens in ER positive human breast cancer cells growing both *in vitro* and *in vivo*. Preliminary data from early clinical trials indicate that Tamoxifen can be safely combined with interferons in breast cancer patients (Miglietta et al., 1991; Tiwari et al., 1991). While somewhat sparse, there is now evidence that this may be a useful clinical strategy (Buzzi et al., 1992; Porzsolt et al., 1989; Recchia et al., 1990).

   Since the effects of antiestrogens are predominantly mediated through ER, the ability of interferons to potentiate these effects strongly suggests an effect on ER levels or function. Indeed, ER expression is induced by interferons in many cells, including ZR-75-1 (van den Berg et al., 1987) MCF-7 (Bezwoda and Meyer, 1990) and CG-5 human breast cancer cells (Sica et al., 1987), human breast tumor and uterine cell homogenates (Dimitrov et al., 1984), human endometrial adenocarcinomas (De Cicco et al., 1988), rabbit uterus (Dimitrov et al., 1984) and in MDBK cells (Zoon et al., 1986). Increased ER levels were observed in skin metastases of breast cancer patients treated with fibroblast interferon (Pouillart et al., 1982). While not universally observed (Goldstein et al., 1989; Porzsolt et al., 1989; Kerr et al., 1989), it seems likely that interferons could sensitize cells to antiestrogens by increasing ER expression.

The effects of interferons are mediated through interactions with their receptors, which have been demonstrated in several breast cancer models, including the ZR-75-1 (Martin et al., 1991), MCF-7 and Hs578T human breast cancer cell lines (Goldstein et al., 1989). TAM upregulates expression of interferon receptors in ZR-75-1 cells, while E2 reduces interferon receptor expression (Martin et al., 1991).

Retinoids as resistance modulators. The majority of ER positive human breast cancer cell lines express retinoic acid receptors (Lacroix et al., 1984; Marth et al., 1984; Swisshelm et al., 1994), and these cells generally appear more sensitive to the inhibitory effects of retinoids than ER-negative cells. Both estrogen and retinoid receptors are members of the same steroid receptor superfamily. Thus, there may be a beneficial interaction between antiestrogens and retinoids.

A number of investigators have described an additive ability of retinoids and tamoxifen to function as chemopreventive agents in chemically induced rodent mammary tumors (Ratko et al., 1989; McCormick and Moon, 1986; Teelmann and Bollag, 1988; Anzano et al., 1994). Similar interactions between ovariectomy and retinoids (McCormick et al., 1982) and between prolactin suppression and retinoid administration have been reported (Welsch et al., 1980). All-trans-retinoic acid and tamoxifen (Wetherall and Taylor, 1986; Fontana, 1987) produce an additive inhibition of MCF-7 and T47D cells. This may be drug specific, since the arotinoid RO 13-6298 does not produce such an interaction (Wetherall and Taylor, 1986), and may reflect a requirement for retinoid receptor selectivity. The ability of retinoic acid to increase ER expression in MCF-7 cells (Batra and Bengstonn, 1978) suggests that the mechanism of the interaction could be equivalent to that observed for the interferons and tamoxifen.

Conclusions

The precise mechanism(s) of resistance to Tamoxifen and the triphenylethylenes remains to be established. It seems likely that a preeminent mechanism of action may need to be established before the most important resistance mechanism(s) can be determined. It also is possible that no single mechanism is relevant, but that each tumor, or each subpopulation, will utilize a different resistance mechanisms (genomic and/or nongenomic) depending on the nature of the critical lesion that is produced by Tamoxifen. If this proves to be the case, it may be difficult to identify molecular biomarkers for response-resistance and to apply a rational approach for the generation of non-crossresistance strategies. While these remain viable possibilities, it seems most likely that the critical event(s) driving response and resistance to Tamoxifen are related to activities regulated through the ER signaling pathway(s). This would explain why so few ER-negative tumors respond to antiestrogens.

While a loss of ER expression may not be the primary resistance mechanism (Johnston et al., 1995), when it occurs this loss is associated with acquired resistance (Encarnacion et al., 1993). It appears that most tumors that acquire resistance in the clinic do so in the face of a continued expression of ER. With the exception of pharmacokinetic or receptor mutational events, the precise contribution of which remain to be established, this strongly implies a defect downstream of receptor-ligand interactions. This could involve modifications in the assembly/function of the ER-regulated transcription complex that drives different gene networks. If this hypothesis is correct, it may be possible to identify intermediate biomarkers that will predict for response/relapse. The earlier we could identify patients relapsing from Tamoxifen therapy, the better would be our chances of obtaining an effective intervention with another nontoxic antiestrogenic regimen. Such an approach could involve the use of a non-crossresistant antiestrogen therapy, e.g., ICI 182,780.

REFERENCES

Akimoto M, Ishii H, Nakajima Y, Iwasaki H (1986): Assesment of host immune response in breast cancer patients. *Cancer Detect Prev* 9:311-317

An T, Sood U, Pietruk T, Cummings G (1987): In situ quantitation of inflammatory mononuclear cells in ductal infiltrating breast carcinoma. *Am J Path* 128:52-60

Anzano MA, Byers SW, Smith JM, Peer CW, Mullen LT, Brown CC, Roberts AB, Sporn MB (1994): Prevention of breast cancer in the rat with 9-cis-retinoic acid as a single agent and in combination with Tamoxifen. *Cancer Res* 54:4614-4617

Aronica SM, Katzenellenbogen BS (1993): Stimulation of estrogen receptor-mediated transcription and alteration in the phosphorylation state of the rat uterine estrogen receptor by estrogen, cyclic adenosine monophosphate, and insulin-like growth factor-I. *Mol Endocrinol* 7:743-752

Arteaga CL, Kitten L, Coronado E, Jacobs S, Kull F, Osborne CK (1989): Blockade of the type-I somatomedin receptor inhibits growth of human breast cancer cells in athymic mice. *J Clin Invest* 84:1418-1423

Barreras L, Vogel CL, Koch G, Marcus SG (1988): Phase II trial of recombinant beta (IFN-Betaser) interferon in ythe treatment of metastatic breast cancer. *Invest New Drugs* 6:211-215

Bates SE, Davidson NE, Valverius EM, Dickson RB, Freter CE, Tam JP, Kudlow JE, Lippman ME, Salomon S (1988): Expression of transforming growth factor-alpha and its mRNA in human breast cancer: its regulation by estrogen and its possible functional significance. *Mol Endocrinol* 2:543-545

Batra S, Bengstonn B (1978): Effects of diethylstilbestrol and ovarian steroids on the contractile movements in rat uterine smooth muscle. *J Physiol* 276:329-342

Bezwoda WR, Meyer K (1990): Effect of alpha-interferon, 17beta-estradiol, and tamoxifen on estrogen receptor concentration and cell cycle kinetics of MCF-7 cells. *Cancer Res* 50:5387-5391

Birrell SN, Roder DM, Horsfall DJ, Bentel JM, Tilley WD (1995): Medroxyprogesterone acetate therapy in advanced breast cancer: the predictive value of androgen receptor expression. *J Clin Oncol* 13:1572-1577

Black MM, Zachrau RE, Hankey BF, Wesley M (1988): Skin window reactivity to autologous breast cancer. An index of prognostically significant cell-mediated immunity. *Cancer* 62:72-83

Bonilla F, Alvarez-Mon M, Merino F, de la Hera A (1988): IL-2 induces cytotoxic activity in lymphocytes from regional axillary nodes of breast cancer patients. *Cancer* 61:629-634

Borner C, Wyss R, Regazzi R, Eppenberger U, Fabbro D (1987): Immunological quantitation of phospholipid/Ca2+-dependent protein kinase of human mammary carcinoma cells: inverse relationship to estrogen receptors. *Int J Cancer* 40:344-348

Brandes LJ, Bogdanovic RP (1986): New evidence that the antiestrogen binding site may be a novel growth-promoting histamine receptor (?H3) which mediates the antiestrogenic and antiproliferative effects of tamoxifen. *Biochem Biophys Res Comm* 134:601-608

Brodie AMH, Santen RJ (1985): Aromatase in breast cancer and the role of aminogluthemide and other aromatase inhibitors. *CRC Crit Rev Oncol Hematol* 5:361-396

Brünner N, Boulay V, Fojo A, Freter C, Lippman ME, Clarke R (1993a): Acquisition of hormone-independent growth in MCF-7 cells is accompanied by increased expression of estrogen-regulated genes but without detectable DNA amplifications. *Cancer Res* 53:283-290

Brünner N, Boysen B, Kiilgaard TL, Frandsen TL, Jirus S, Clarke R (1993b):
    Resistance to 4OH-Tamoxifen does not confer resistance to the steroidal
    antiestrogen ICI 182,780 while acquired resistance to ICI 182,780
    results in cross resistance to 4OH-TAM. *Breast Cancer Res Treat*
    27:135(Abstract)

Brünner N, Frandsen TL, Holst-Hansen C, Bei M, Thompson EW, Wakeling
    AE, Lippman ME, Clarke R (1993c): MCF7/LCC2: A
    4-hydroxytamoxifen resistant human breast cancer variant which retains
    sensitivity to the steroidal antiestrogen ICI 182,780. *Cancer Res*
    53:3229-3232

Buzzi F, Brugia M, Rossi G, Giustini L, Scoponi C, Sica G (1992):
    Combination of beta-interferon and tamoxifen as a new way to
    overcome clinical resistance to tamoxifen in advanced breast cancer.
    Anticancer Res 12:869-872

Cabot MC, Zhang Z-C, Giuliano AE (1995): Tamoxifen elicits rapid
    transmembrane lipid signal responses in human breast cancer cells.
    Breast Cancer Res Treat 36:299-306

Catherino WH, Wolf DM, Jordan VC (1995): A naturally occuring estrogen
    receptor point mutation results in increased estrogenicity of a tamoxifen
    analog. *Mol Endocrinol* 9:1053-1063

Clarke R, Brünner N, Katz D, Glanz P, Dickson RB, Lippman ME, Kern F
    (1989a): The effects of a constitutive production of TGF-alpha on the
    growth of MCF-7 human breast cancer cells *in vitro* and *in vivo*. *Mol
    Endocrinol* 3:372-380

Clarke R, Brünner N, Katzenellenbogen BS, Thompson EW, Norman MJ, Koppi
    C, Paik S, Lippman ME, Dickson RB (1989b): Progression from
    hormone dependent to hormone independent growth in MCF-7 human
    breast cancer cells. *Proc Natl Acad Sci USA* 86:3649-3653

Clarke R, Brünner N, Thompson EW, Glanz P, Katz D, Dickson RB, Lippman
    ME (1989c): The inter-relationships between ovarian-independent
    growth, antiestrogen resistance and invasiveness in the malignant
    progression of human breast cancer. *J Endocrinol* 122:331-340

Clarke R, van den Berg HW, Murphy RF (1990): Tamoxifen and
    17beta-estradiol reduce the membrane fluidity of human breast cancer
    cells. *J Natl Cancer Inst* 82:1702-1705

Clarke R, Dickson RB, Lippman ME (1992): Hormonal aspects of breast
    cancer: growth factors, drugs and stromal interactions. *Crit Rev Oncol
    Hematol* 12:1-23

Clarke R, (1995): Human breast cancer cell line xenografts as models of breast
    cancer: the immunobiologies of recipient mice and the characteristics
    of several tumorigenic cell lines. *Breast Cancer Res Treat* (in press)

Clarke R, Hilakivi-Clarke LA, Cho E, James MR, Leonessa F (1996a): Estrogens, phytoestrogens and breast cancer. *Adv Exp Biol Med* (in press)

Clarke R, Skaar T, Leonessa F, Brankin B, James MR, Brünner N, Lippman ME (1996b): The acquisition of an antiestrogen resistant phenotype in breast cancer: the role of cellular and molecular mechanisms. *Adv Cancer Res* (in press)

Clarke R, Brünner N (1995): Cross resistance and molecular mechanisms in antiestrogen resistance. *Endocr Related Cancer* 2:59-72

Clarke R, Lippman ME (1992): Antiestrogens resistance: mechanisms and reversal. In: Drug Resistance in Oncology. Teicher BA ed. New York: Marcel Dekker, Inc, pp. 501-536

Cohen JHM, Danel L, Gordier G, Saez S, Revillard JP (1983): Sex steroid receptors in peripheral T cells: absence of androgen receptors and restriction of estrogen receptors to OKT 8 positive cells. *J Immunol* 131:2767-2771

Cole MP, Jones CTA, Todd IDH (1971): A new antioestrogenic agent in late breast cancer. An early clinical appraisal of ICI 46474. *Br J Cancer* 25:270-275

Colletta AA, Wakefield LM, Howell FV, van Roozendaal KEP, Danielpour D, Ebbs SR, Sporn MB, Baum M (1990): Anti-oestrogens induce the secretion of active transforming growth factor beta from human fetal fibroblasts. *Br J Cancer* 62:405-409

Contreras OO, Stoliar A (1988): Immunologic changes in human breast cancer. *Eur J Gynecol Oncol* 9:502-514

Custodio JBA, Almeida LM, Madeira VMC (1993a): The active metabolite hydroxytamoxifen of the anticancer drug tamoxifen induces structural changes in membranes. *Biochem Biophys Acta* 1153:308-314

Custodio JBA, Almeida LM, Madeira VMC (1993b): The anticancer drug tamoxifen induces changes in the physical properties of model and native membranes. *Biochim Biophys Acta Membranes* 123-129

Danel L, Souweine G, Monier JC, Saez S (1983): Specific estrogen binding sites in huma lymphoid cells and thymic cels. *J Steroid Biochem* 18:559-563

Daniel P, Gaskell SJ, Bishop H, Campbell C, Nicholson I (1981): Determination of tamoxifen and biologically active metabolites in human breast tumours and plasma. *Eur J Cancer Clin Oncol* 17:1183-1189

Danielian PS, White R, Lees JA, Parker MG (1992): Identification of a conserved region required for hormone dependent transcriptional activation by steroid hormone receptors. *EMBO J* 11:1025-1033

Dauvois S, Danielian PS, White R, Parker MG (1992): Antiestrogen ICI 164,384 reduces cellular estrogen receptor content by increasing its turnover. *Proc Natl Acad Sci USA* 89:4037-4041

De Cicco F, Sica G, Benedetto MT, Ciabattoni G, Rossiello F, Nicosia A, Lupi G, Iacopino F, Mancuso S, Dell'Acqua S (1988): *In vitro* effects of beta-interferon on steroid receptors and prostaglandin output in human endometrial adenocarcinoma. *J Steroid Biochem* 30:359-362

Dimitrov NY, Meyer CJ, Strander H, Einhorn S, Cantell K (1984): Interferon as a modifier of estrogen receptors. *Ann Clin Lab Sci* 14:32-39

Dotzlaw H, Alkhalaf M, Murphy LC (1992): Characterization of estrogen receptor variant mRNAs from human breast cancers. *Mol Endocrinol* 6:773-785

Duval D, Durant S, Homo-Delarche F (1983): Non-genomic effects of steroids. Interactions of steroid molecules with membrane structures and functions. *Biochim Biophys Acta* 737:409-442

Encarnacion CA, Ciocca DR, McGuire WL, Clark GM, Fuqua SA, Osborne CK (1993): Measurement of steroid hormone receptors in breast cancer patients on tamoxifen. *Breast Cancer Res Treat* 26:237-246

Epstein LB, Benz CC, Doty E (1987): Synergistic antiproliferative effect of interferon-alpha and tamoxifen on human breast cancer cells *in vitro*. *Clin Res* 35:196A

Etienne MC, Milano G, Fischel JL, Frenay M, Francois E, Formento JL, Gioanni J, Namer M (1989): Tamoxifen metabolism: pharmacokinetic and in vitro study. *Br J Cancer* 60:30-35

Farhat M, Abi-Younes S, Vargas R, Wolfe RM, Clarke R, Ramwell PW (1992): Vascular non-genomic effects of estrogen. In: Sex Steroids and the Cardiovascular System. Ramwell PW, Rubanyi G, Schillinger E eds. Berlin: Springer-Verlag, pp. 145-159

Fawell SE, White R, Hoare S, Sydenham M, Page M, Parker MG (1990): Inhibition of estrogen receptor-DNA binding by the "pure" antiestrogen ICI 164,384 appears to be mediated by impaired receptor dimerization. *Proc Natl Acad Sci USA* 87:6883-6887

Fentiman IS, Balkwill FR, Cuzick J, Hayward JL, Rubens RD (1987): A trial of human alpha interferon as an adjuvant agent in breast cancer after loco-regional recurrence. *Eur J Surg Oncol* 13:425-428

Fontana JA, (1987): Interaction of retinoids and tamoxifen on the inhibition of human mammary carcinoma cell proliferation. *Exp Cell Biol* 55:136-144

Fromson JM, Sharp DS (1974): The selective uptake of tamoxifen by human uterine tissue. *J Obstet Gynecol Br Commonwealth* 81:321

Fuqua SAW, Fitzgerald SG, Allred DC, Elledge RM, Nawaz Z, McDonnel D, O'Malley BW, Greene GL, McGuire WL (1992): Inhibition of estrogen receptor action by a naturally occurring variant in human breast tumors. *Cancer Res* 52:483-486

Goldstein D, Bushmeyer SM, Witt PL, Jordan VC, Borden EC (1989): Effects of type I and II interferons on cultured human breast cells: interactions with estrogen receptors and with tamoxifen. *Cancer Res* 49:2698-2702

Golinski P, Vesonder RF, Latus-Zietkiewicz D, Perkowski J (1988): Formation of fusarenone X, nivalenol, zearalenone, alpha-trans-zearalenol, -trans-zearalenol, and fusarin C by fusarium crookwellense. *Appl Environ Microbiol* 54:2147-2148

Gottardis MM, Wagner RJ, Borden EC, Jordan CV (1989): Differential ability of antiestrogens to stimulate breast cancer cell (MCF-7) growth *in vivo* and *in vitro*. *Cancer Res* 49:4765-4769

Greenberg DA, Carpenter CL, Messing RO (1987): Calcium channel antagonist properties of the antineoplastic antiestrogen tamoxifen in the PC12 neurosecretory cell line. *Cancer Res* 47:70-74

Hagler WM, Tyczkowska K, Hamilton PB (1984): Simultaneous occurrence of deoxynivalenol, zearalenone, and aflatoxin in 1982 scabby wheat from the Midwestern United States. *Appl Environ Microbiol* 47:151-154

Hanna N, Schneider M (1983): Enhancement of tumor metastases and suppression of natural killer cell activity by beta-estradiol treatment. *J Immunol* 130:974-980

Hardy JR, Judson IR, Sinnett HD, Ashley SE, Coombes RC, Ellin CL (1990): Combination of tamoxifen, aminoglutethimide, danazol and medroxyprogesterone acetate in advanced breast cancer. *Eur J Cancer* 26:824-827

Head JF, Elliott RL, McCoy JL (1993): Evaluation of lymphocyte immunity in breast cancer patients. *Breast Cancer Res Treat* 26:77-88

Herbst AL, Griffiths CT, Kistner RW (1964): Clomiphene citrate (NSC-35770) in disseminated mammary carcinoma. *Cancer Chemother Rep* 443:39-41

Horst HA, Horny HP (1987): Characterization and frequency distribution of lymphreticular infiltrates in axillary lymph node metastases of invasive ductal carcinoma of the breast. *Cancer*; 60 (12):3001-7 60:3001-7 1987

Huff KK, Knabbe C, Lindsey R, Kaufman D, Bronzert DA, Lippman ME, Dickson RB (1988): Multihormonal regulation of insulin-like growth factor-I-related protein in MCF-7 human breast cancer cells. *Mol Endocrinol* 2:200-208

James MR, Clarke R (1995): Role of steroid sulfatase in the promotion of breast tumors in MCF-7 human breast cancer cells. *Proc Endocr Soc* 658(Abstract)

Johnston SRD, Haynes BP, Smith IE, Jarman M, Sacks NPM, Ebbs SR, Dowsett M (1993): Acquired tamoxifen resistance in human breast cancer and reduced intra-tumoral drug concentration. *Lancet* 342:1521-1522

Johnston SRD, Saccanti-Jotti G, Smith IE, Newby J, Dowsett M (1995): Change in oestrogen receptor expression and function in tamoxifen-resistant breast cancer. *Endocr Related Cancer* 2:105-110

Kangas L, Nieminen A-L, Cantell K (1985): Additive and synergistic effects of a novel antiestrogen toremifene (Fc-1157a) and human interferons on estrogen responsive MCF-7 cells *in vitro. Med Biol* 63:187-190

Kaspar F, Klocker H, Denninger A, Cato AC (1993): A mutant androgen receptor from patients with Reifenstein syndrome: identification of the function of a conserved alanine residue in the D box of steroid receptors. *Mol Cell Biol* 13:7850-7858

Katzenellenbogen BS, Miller AM, Mullick A, Sheen YY (1985): Antiestrogen action in breast cancer cells: modulation of proliferation and protein synthesis, and interaction with estrogen receptors and additional antiestrogen binding sites. *Breast Cancer Res Treat* 5:231-243

Kayyali R, Marriott C, Wiseman H (1994): Tamoxifen decreases drug efflux from liposomes: relevance to its ability to reverse multidrug resistance in cancer cells?. *FEBS Lett* 344:221-224

Kellen JA, Wong ACH, Szalai JP, Gardner HA, Wood EM (1986): Characteristics of a tamoxifen-tolerant breast cancer cell subpopulation. *J Nutr Growth Cancer* 3:183-187

Kerr DJ, Pragnell IB, Sproul A, Cowan S, Murray T, George D, Leake R (1989): The cytostatic effects of alpha-interferon may be mediated by transforming growth factor-beta. *J Mol Endocrinol* 2:131-136

Kistner RW, Smith OW (1960): Observations on the use of a non-steroidal estrogen antagonist: Mer-25. *Surg Forum* 10:725-729

Knabbe C, Lippman ME, Wakefield LM, Flanders KC, Derynck R, Dickson RB (1987): Evidence that transforming growth factor-beta is a hormonally regulated negative growth factor in human breast cancer cells. *Cell* 48:417-428

Koehorst SGA, Cox JJ, Donker GH, da Silva SL, Burbach JPH, Thijssen JHH, Blankenstein MA (1994): Functional analysis of an alternatively spliced estrogen receptor lacking exon 4 isolated from MCF-7 breast cancer cells and meningiomas. *Mol Cell Endocrinol* 101:237-245

Kuiper-Goodman T, (1990): Uncertainties in the risk assessment of three mycotoxins: aflatoxin, ochratoxin, and zearalenone. *Can J Physiol Pharm* 68:1017-1024

Lacroix A, L'Heureux N, Bhat PV (1984): Cytoplasmic retinoic acid-binding protein in retinoic acid-resistant human breast cancer cell lines. *J Natl Cancer Inst* 73:793-800

Lam H-YP, (1984): Tamoxifen is a calmodulin antagonist in the activation of cAMP phosphodiesterase. *Biochem Biophys Res Comm* 118:27-32

Lenaz G, Curatola G, Mazzanti L, Parenti-Castelli G (1978): Biophysical studies on agents affecting the state of membrane lipids: biochemical and pharmacological implications. *Mol Cell Biochem* 22:3-32

Leonessa F, Jacobson M, Boyle B, Lippman J, McGarvey M, Clarke R (1994): The effect of tamoxifen on the multidrug resistant phenotype in human breast cancer cells: isobologram, drug accumulation and gp-170 binding studies. *Cancer Res* 54:441-447

Levy SM, Herberman RB, Whiteside T, Sanzo K (1990): Perceived social support and tumor estrogen/progesterone receptor status as predictors of natural killer cell activity in breast cancer patients. *Psychosom Med* 52:73-85

Lien EA, Solheim E, Lea OA, Lundgren S, Kvinnsland S, Ueland PM (1989): Distribution of 4-hydroxy-N-desmethyltamoxifen and their tamoxifen metabolites in human biological fluids during tamoxifen treatment. *Cancer Res* 49:2175-2183

Litherland S, Jackson IM (1988): Antioestrogens in the management of hormone-dependent cancer. *Cancer Treat Rev* 15:183-194

Lobaccaro JM, Lumbroso S, Belon C, Galtier-Dereure F, Bringer J, Lesimple T, Heron JF, Pujol H, Sultan C (1993a): Male breast cancer and the androgen receptor gene [letter]. *Nat Genet* 5:109-110

Lobaccaro JM, Lumbroso S, Belon C, Galtier-Dereure F, Bringer J, Lesimple T, Namer M, Cutuli BF, Pujol H, Sultan C (1993b): Androgen receptor gene mutation in male breast cancer. *Hum Mol Genet* 2:1799-1802

Luo Y, Yoshizawa T, Katayama T (1990): Comparative study on the natural occurrence of fusarium mycotoxins (trichothecenes and zearalenone) in corn and wheat from high- and low-risk areas for human esophageal cancer in China. *Appl Environ Microbiol* 56:3723-3726

Mandeville R, Ghali SS, Chausseau JP (1984): *In vitro* stimulation of NK activity by an estrogen antagonist (Tamoxifen). *Eur J Cancer Clin Oncol* 20:983-985

Marth C, Mayer I, Daxenbichler G (1984): Effect of retinoic acid and 4-hydroxytamoxifen on human breast cancer cell lines. *Biochem Pharmacol* 33:2217-2221

Martin HJ, McKibben BM, Lynch M, van den Berg HW (1991): Modulation by oestrogen and progestin/antiprogestin of alpha interferon receptor expression in human breast cancer cells. *Eur J Cancer* 27:143-146

Mayr U, Butsch A, Schneider S (1992): Validation of two *in vitro* test systems for estrogenic activities with zearalenone, phytoestrogens, and cereal extracts. *Toxicology* 74:135-149

McCormick DL, Mehta RG, Thompson CA, Dinger N, Caldwell JA, Moon RC (1982): Enhanced inhibition of mammary carcinogenesis by combined treatment with N-(4-hydroxyphenyl)retinamide and ovariectomy. *Cancer Res* 42:508-512

McCormick DL, Moon RC (1986): Retinoid-tamoxifen interaction in mammary cancer chemoprevention. *Carcinogenesis* 7:193-196

McDonnell DP, Clemm DL, Hermann T, Goldman ME, Pike JW (1995): Analysis of estrogen receptor function *in vitro* reveals three distinct classes of antiestrogens. *Mol Endocrinol* 9:659-669

Miglietta L, Repetto L, Gardin G, Amoroso D, Giudici S, Naso C, Merlini L, Queirolo P, Campora E, Pronzato P, Rosso R (1991): Tamoxifen and alpha interferon in advanced breast cancer. *J Chemother* 3:383-386

Miller AB, Bulbrook RD (1986): UICC multidisciplinary project on breast cancer: the epidemiology, aetiology and prevention of breast cancer. *Int J Cancer* 37:173-177

Morley P, Whitfield JF (1995): Effect of tamoxifen on carbachol-triggered intracellular calcium responses in chicken granulosa cells. *Cancer Res* 54:69-74

Murphy LC, Hilsenbeck SG, Dotzlaw H, Fuqua SAW (1995): Relationship of clone 4 estrogen receptor variant messenger RNA expression to some known prognostic variables in human breast cancer. *Clin Cancer Res* 1:155-159

Murphy LC, Dotzlaw H (1989): Variant estrogen receptor mRNA species in human breast cancer biopsy samples. *Mol Endocrinol* 3:687-693

Murphy LC, Sutherland RL (1985): Differential effects of tamoxifen and analogs with nonbasic side chains on cell proliferation *in vitro*. *Endocrinology* 116:1071-1078

Myers MJ, Peterson BH (1985): Estradiol indiced alterations in the immune system. I. Enhancement of IgM production. *Int J Immunopharmacol* 7:207-213

O'Brian CA, Liskamp RM, Solomon DH, Weinstein IB (1986): Triphenylethylenes: a new class of protein kinase C inhibitors. *J Natl Cancer Inst* 76:1243-1246

O'Brian CA, Housey GM, Weinstein IB (1988): Specific and direct binding of protein kinase C to an immobilized tamoxifen analogue. *Cancer Res* 48:3626-3629

O'Brian CA, Vogel VG, Singletary SE, Ward NE (1989): Elevated protein kinase C expression in human breast tumor biopsies relative to normal breast tissue. *Cancer Res* 49:3215-3217

Osborne CK, Coronado EB, Robinson JP (1987): Human breast cancer in athymic nude mice: cytostatic effects of long-term antiestrogen therapy. *Eur J Cancer Clin Oncol* 23:1189-1196

Osborne CK, Coronado EB, Allred DC, Wiebe V, DeGregorio M (1991): Acquired tamoxifen resistance: correlation with reduced breast tumor levels of tamoxifen and isomerization of trans-4-hydroxytamoxifen. *J Natl Cancer Inst* 83:1477-1482

Osborne CK, Wiebe VJ, McGuire WL, Ciocca DR, DeGregorio M (1992):
    Tamoxifen and the isomers of 4-hydroxytamoxifen in tamoxifen
    resistant tumors from breast cancer patients. *J Clin Oncol* 10:304-310

Padmanabhan N, Balkwill FR, Bodmer JG, Rubens RD (1985): Recombinant
    DNA human interferon alpha 2 in advanced breast cancer: a phase 2
    trial. *Br J Cancer* 51:55-60

Pasqualini JR, Nguyen B-L (1991): Estrone sulfatase activity and effect of
    antiestrogens on transformation of estrone sulfate in hormone-dependent
    vs independent human breast cancer cell lines. *Breast Cancer Res Treat*
    18:93-98

Pavlik EJ, Nelson K, Srinivasan S, Powell DE, Kenady DE, DePreist PD,
    Gallion HH, van Nagell JR (1992): Resistance to tamoxifen with
    persisting sensitivity to estrogen: possible mediation by excessive
    antiestrogen binding site activity. *Cancer Res* 52:4106-4112

Pollak M, Costantino J, Polychronakos C, Blauer S-A, Guyda H, Redmond C,
    Fisher B, Margolese R (1990): Effect of tamoxifen on serum
    insulinlike growth factor I levels in stage I breast cancer patients. *J
    Natl Cancer Inst* 82:1693-1697

Porzsolt F, Otto AM, Trauschel B, Buck C, Wawer AW, Schonenberger H
    (1989): Rationale for combining tamoxifen and interferon in the
    treatment of advanced breast cancer. *J Cancer Res Clin Oncol*
    115:465-469

Pouillart P, Palangie T, Jouve M, Garcie GE, Fridman WH, Magdalena H,
    Falcoff E, Billianus A (1982): Administration of fibroblast interferon
    to patients with advanced breast cancer: possible effects on skin
    metastasis and on hormone receptors. *Eur J Cancer Clin Oncol*
    18:929-935

Ramu A, Glaubiger D, Fuks Z (1984): Reversal of acquired resistance to
    doxorubicin in P388 murine leukemia cells by tamoxifen and other
    triparanol analogues. *Cancer Res* 44:4392-4395

Ratko TA, Detrisac CJ, Dinger NM, Thomas CF, Kelloff GJ, Moon RC (1989):
    Chemopreventative efficacy of a combined retinoid and tamoxifen
    treatment following surgical excision of a primary mammary cancer in
    female rats. *Cancer Res* 49:4472-4476

Ravdin PM, Fritz NF, Tormey DC, Jordan VC (1988): Endocrine status of
    premenopausal node-positive breast cancer patients following adjuvant
    chemotherapy and long-term tamoxifen. *Cancer Res* 48:1026-1029

Ravdin PM, Green S, Dorr TM, McGuire WL, Fabian C, Pugh RP, Carter RD,
    Rivkin SE, Borst JR, Belt RJ (1992): Prognostic significance of
    progesterone receptor levels in estrogen receptor-positive patients with
    metastatic breast cancer treated with tamoxifen: results of a prospective
    Southwest Oncology Group study. *J Clin Oncol* 10:1284-1291

Recchia F, Morgante A, Ercole C, Marchionni F, Rabitti G (1990): Differentiation induction and tamoxifen (TMX) therapy for stage IV breast cancer (BC). Preliminary report of a phase II study. *Proc Am Soc Clin Oncol* 9:abstr 193

Reed MJ, Owen AM, Lai LC, Coldham NG, Ghilchik MW, Shaikh NA, James VHT (1989): In situ oestrone synthesis in normal breast and breast tumour tissues: effect of treatment with 4-hydroxyandrostenedione. *Int J Cancer* 44:233-237

Robinson SP, Goldstein D, Witt PL, Borden EC, Jordan CV (1990): Inhibition of hormone-dependent and independent breast cancer cell growth *in vivo* and *in vitro* with the antiestrogen toremifene and recombinant human interferon-2alpha. *Breast Cancer Res Treat* 15:95-101

Schoental R, (1985): Trichothecenes, Zearalenone, and other carcinogenic metabolites of fusarium and related microfungi. *Adv Cancer Res* 45:217-290

Screpanti I, Santoni A, Gulino A, Herberman RB, Frati L (1987): Estrogen and antiestrogen modulation of mouse natural killer activity and large granular lymphocytes. *Cell Immunol* 106:191-202

Seaman WE, Blackman MA, Gindhart TD, Roubinian JR, Loeb JM, Talal N (1978): Beta-Estradiol reduces natural killer cells in mice. *J Immunol* 121:2193-2198

Seaman WE, Talal N (1980): The effect of 17beta-estradiol on natural killing in the mouse. In: Natural Cell-Mediated Immunity Against Tumors. Herberman RB ed. New York: Academic Press, pp. 765-777

Sica G, Natoli V, Stella C, Del Bianco S (1987): Effect of natural beta-interferon on cell proliferation and steroid receptor level in human breast cancer cells. *Cancer* 60:2419-2423

Stewart J, King RJB, Hayward JL, Rubens RD (1982): Estrogen and progesterone receptor: correlation of response rates, site and timing of receptor analysis. *Breast Cancer Res Treat* 2:243-250

Stewart T, Tsai S-CJ, Grayson H, Henderson R, Opelz G (1995): Incidence of de-novo breast cancer in women chronically immunosuppressed after organ transplantation. *Lancet* 346:796-798

Sthoeger ZM, Bentwich Z, Zinger H, Mozes E (1994): The beneficial effects of the estrogen antagonist, tamoxifen, on experimental systemic lupus erythematosus. *J Rheumatol* 21:2231-2238

Stimson WH (1980): Oestrogen and human T cell lymphocytes: presence of specific receptors n the T-suppressor/cytotoxic subset. *Scand J Immunol* 28:345-350

Strayer DR, Carter WA, Brodsky I (1986): Familial occurence of breast cancer is associated with reduced natural killer cytotoxicity. *Breast Cancer Res Treat* 7:187-192

Swisshelm K, Ryan K, Lee X, Tsou HC, Peacocke M, Sager R (1994): Down regulation of retinoic acid receptor beta in mammary carcinoma cell lines and its upregulation in senescing normal mammary epithelial cells. *Cell Growth Diff* 5:133-141

Szamel I, Hindy I, Vincze B, Eckhardt S, Kangas L, Hajba A (1994): Influence of toremifene on the endocrine regulation of breast cancer patients. *Eur J Cancer* 30A:154-158

Teelmann K, Bollag W (1988): Therapeutic effect of the arotinoid RO-15-0778 on chemically induced rat mammary carcinoma. *Eur J Cancer Clin Oncol* 24:1205-1209

Teodorczyk-Injeyan J, Cembryzynska M, Lalani S, Kellen JA (1993): Modulation of biological responses of normal human mononuclear cells by antiestrogens. *Anticancer Res* 13:279-284

Tiwari RK, Wong GY, Liu J, Miller D, Osborne MP (1991): Augmentation of cytotoxicity using combinations of interferons (types I and II), tumor necrosis factor-alpha, and tamoxifen in MCF-7 cells. *Cancer Lett* 61:45-52

Tsukada T, Inoue M, Tachibana S, Nakai Y, Takebe H (1994): An androgen receptor mutation causing androgen resistance in undervirilized male syndrome. *J Clin Endocrinol Metab* 79:1202-1207

Underwood JC, Giri DD, Rooney N, Lonsdale R (1987): Immunophenotype of the lymphoid cell infiltrates in breast carcinomas of low oestrogen receptor content. *Br J Cancer* 56:744-746

van den Berg HW, Leahey WJ, Lynch M, Clarke R, Nelson J (1987): Recombinant human interferon alpha increases oestrogen receptor expression in human breast cancer cells (ZR-75-1) and sensitises them to the anti-proliferative effects of tamoxifen. *Br J Cancer* 55:255-257

Verdeal K, Brown RR, Richardson T, Ryan DS (1980): Affinity of phytoestrogens for estradiol-binding proteins and effect of coumesterol on growth of 7,12-dimethylbenz(a)anthracene-induced rat mammary tumors. *J Natl Cancer Inst* 64:285-290

Wang Y, Miksicek RJ (1991): Identification of a dominant negative form of the human estrogen receptor. *Mol Endocrinol* 5:1707-1715

Welsch CW, Brown CK, Goodrich-Smith M, Chiusano J, Moon RC (1980): Synergistic effect of chronic prolactin suppression and retinoid treatment in the prophylaxis of N-methyl-N-nitrosourea-induced mammary tumorigenesis in female Sprague-Dawley rats. *Cancer Res* 40:3095-3098

Wetherall NT, Taylor CM (1986): The effects of retinoid treatment and antiestrogens on the growth of T47D human breast cancer cells. *Eur J Cancer Clin Oncol* 22:53-59

Wolf DM, Langan-Fahey SM, Parker CP, McCague R, Jordan VC (1993): Investigation of the mechanism of tamoxifen stimulated breast tumor growth; non-isomerizable analogues of tamoxifen and its metabolites. *J Natl Cancer Inst* 85:806-812

Yee D, Paik S, Lebovic GS, Marcus R, Favoni RE, Cullen KJ, Lippman ME, Rosen N (1989): Analysis of insulin-like growth factor-I gene expression in malignancy: evidence for a paracrine role in human breast cancer. *Mol Endocrinol* 3:509-517

Zoon K, Karasaki Y, zur Nedden DL, Hu R, Arnheiter H (1986): Modulation of epidermal growth factor receptors by human alpha interferon. *Proc Natl Acad Sci USA* 83:8226-8230

ACKNOWLEDGMENTS

This work was supported in part by grants NIH R01-CA58022 and the Cancer Research Foundation of America (R.Clarke), and NIH P30-CA51008 and NIH P50-CA58185 (Public Health Service) to R.Clarke/M.E.Lippman).

6. TAMOXIFEN AND MULTIDRUG RESISTANCE IN CANCER

J.A. Kellen

> *"Experience does not ever err, it is
> only your judgement that errs in
> promising itself results which are
> not caused by your experiments."*
> Leonardo da Vinci (c.1510)

So much has been said and written about the importance of multidrug resistance in cancer that it is hard to come up with an original introduction. Suffice to say that innate or acquired resistance to radiation and chemotherapy have become the major obstacle to successful cancer treatment. Notwithstanding the introduction of novel substances and our expanding understanding of the malignant process and its vulnerability, cancer cells are able to delve into their primordial resources and develop ingenious, multiple defence mechanisms which evolve, change with time, alternate and vary, depending on the host, tumour and treatment. The amazing ability of the cancer cell to adapt to an unfavourable environment is one of the inherent characteristics of malignancy, as well as phenotypic instability. It is probable that either small resistant cell subpopulations exist at any one time during the development of the tumour or that phenotypic alterations take place in response to the selective pressure of chemotherapy. Of course, both may proceed simultaneously and intertwine.

Once multidrug resistance was recognized as a major cause of treatment failure, ways and means have been sought to interfere with this apparently inexorable course of events. Since many specific and non-specific resistance mechanisms have been defined in great detail (Kellen, 1995), one would surmise that once the cause of a phenomenon is understood, recourse is not far away. So far, this has not been the case. The potential to eliminate or render harmless unwanted substances from a cell is ubiquitous and quite obviously a basic skill for any survival.Interference with these mechanisms is at best difficult, because of the necessity to inhibit physiological pathways which function normally or are prepared to function when need arises. Substances able to inhibit such pathways are either toxic themselves or, in order to achieve the desired effect, must be administered in heroic amounts. They are rarely specific for the tumour and will necessarily affect normal organs.

The regular and almost predictable appearance of drug resistance supports the search for a general strategy to prevent, overcome or at least delay resistance and restore or enhance sensitivity to the administered drug regime. This trend has been extensively reviewed (Kellen, 1994) and is still a very active field, judging by the number of papers published. A variety of compounds, many of them drugs currently in use for indications other than malignancy are being studied. Since they have few if any common characteristics and may inhibit entirely different resistance mechanisms, it is difficult to select promising candidates on theoretical grounds. Serendipity and empiricism have always played a helpful role. In brief, no single case of drug resistance in an individual patient can be generalized on its own merit and from a single perspective. Treatment success or failure will always be the outcome of an intricate interplay of forces, such as heterogeneity of the tumour itself as well as the genetic make-up, the immune responsiveness and the hormonal milieu of the host.

The list of substances studied in the wide context of resistance reversal is growing rapidly; this chapter must be restricted to antiestrogens (which of course, narrows the field considerably). This topic has been carefully reviewed (Clarke et al., 1992), is being exploited and remains a promising approach. Tamoxifen has been used in various settings; its generally excellent tolerance and minimum of side-effects makes it a popular adjuvant with few worries about toxicity in long term administration.

Of course, Tamoxifen must be evaluated as the sum of effects from itself and its metabolites. More than one mechanism of interference with more than one mechanism of resistance can be expected. Also, one must critically discern between *in vitro* and *in vivo* results; the former may raise much optimism leading to frustration with the latter. Data from animal models, while reproducible and showing some ressemblance with the human counterpart, can not be extrapolated without penalties either. Needless to say, once the big step into clinical application is made, selection, control and evaluation of suitable patients in statistically meaningful numbers becomes extremely difficult.

In very general terms, the apparently independent actions of Tamoxifen and its metabolites on tumours and drug resistance can be categorized as follows:

1) Facilitation for the chemotherapeutical agent to reach and enter the target cell by influx and efflux modification and/or possible competition (for ex. reversal of MDR phenotype).
2) Re-establishment of normal apoptotic pathways by interference with inhibitors of apoptosis.
3) Direct or indirect action on tumour cell multiplication including their accumulation in vulnerable phases of the cell cycle.
4) Enhancement of cytostatic action(s) and toxicity of drugs.
5) Synergistic effects with interferon(s) and the immune response.

This enumeration is tentative and certainly not complete, but it illustrates aptly the wide and colourful gamut of Tamoxifen actions. The mode of action exerted by Tamoxifen on multidrug resistance in a wide variety of tumours and clinical conditions can not be reduced to a single (and simple) denominator. While Tamoxifen undoubtedly reverses drug resistance in some, but not all resistant tumours and to some, but not all drugs, this effect is most impressive in situations where the mdr1 gene is overexpressed. Yet, simple competitive binding (the probable explanation for other "popular" chemosensitizers, such as Verapamil) or interference with the activity of the efflux pump system is not the direct cause of this phenomenon. In any case, Tamoxifen acts in a different way as other steroids (such as the synthetic progestine ORG 2058, estramustine, ZK112993 and Medroxyprogesterone-acetate) to name only a few (Huang Yang et al., 1994; Zibera et al., 1995; Leonessa et al., 1994). The action is independent of the receptor machinery.

REFERENCES

Clarke R, Dickson RB, Lippman ME (1992): Hormonal aspects of breast cancer. *Crit Rev Oncol/Hematol* 12:1-23

Huang Yang CP, Shen HJ, Horwitz SB (1994): Modulation of the Function of P-glycoprotein by Estramustine. *J Natl Cancer Inst* 86:723-725

Kellen JA (ed.) (1994): Reversal of Multidrug Resistance in Cancer. CRC Press, Boca Raton 1994

Kellen JA (ed.) (1995): Alternative Mechanisms of Multidrug Resistance in Cancer. Birkhäuser, Boston 1995

Leonessa F, Boyle B, Clarke R (1994): The antiprogestin ZK112993 increases the cytotoxic efficacy of vinblastine in multidrug resistant breast cancer. *Proc AACR* 35:352

Raderer M and Scheithauer W (1003): Clinical trails of agents that reverse multidrug resistance. A literature review. *Cancer* 72:3553-63

Zibera C, Gibelli N, Maestri L, Robustelli della Cuna G (1995): Medroxyprogesterone-Acetate Reverses the MDR Phenotype of the CG5-Doxorubicin Resistant Human Breast Cancer Cell Line. *Anticancer Res* 15:745-750

Sensitivity enhancement and delay of resistance development

While these two phenomena may be unrelated and result from entirely different mechanisms, their ultimate clinical effect is equally beneficial and desirable. Most of the observations on record are, however, in cell cultures. There is a definite indication that Platinum resistance (which again is not caused by a uniform mechanism) could be delayed or modulated by Tamoxifen. Some recent data are collated in Tab. 1.

The delay in the emergence of resistance to cisplatin may be restricted to some specific cell lines (such as the UM-SCC-10B squamous carcinoma or the MH ovarian carcinoma cells). The effect of Tamoxifen on cisplatin toxicity is neither specific nor universal and does not depend on interaction with estrogen receptors. It appears that Tamoxifen does not alter the cell cycle phase perturbation caused by cisplatin alone (McClay et al., 1993). A relatively small subset of patients with metastatic melanoma, initially treated with cisplatin until they demonstrated resistance, showed a favourable response when Tamoxifen was added (Mc Clay et al., 1993). Surprisingly, the sex of the patients and other endocrine parameters (such as menstrual status, age, etc.) were not taken into account in the evaluations; of course, the number of patients may become too small to allow any conclusions. Even if the steroid receptor status were unrelated to Tamoxifen action, levels of estrogens may hold the key to resistance modulation at least in some cancers. In human ovarian cancer cells (MH), resistant to cisplatinum, both clomiphene and tamoxifen alone or in combination markedly

Table 1. Enhancement of the cisplatinum effect by Tamoxifen

Tumour (model)	Characteristics	Effect	References
Melanoma cells	CisPt resistant	synergistic	Warso et al., 1995
Melanoma cells	-"-	delays develop. of resistance	McClay et al., 1993, 1994a
Squamous cell Ca	-"-	synergistic	Warso et al., 1995
Breast Ca, cells	-"- (ER neg.)	no effect	-"-
Head & Neck, Squamous cell Ca UM-SCC10B	-"-	delayed develop. of resistance	Nahata et al., 1995
Ovarian Ca human	-"-	synergistic	McClay et al., 1994b Kikuchi et al., 1992 & 1993
Ovarian Ca cells, A 2780	-"-	synergistic	De Vincenzo et al., 1994

enhanced the antiproliferative effect and uptake of cisplatinum (Kikuchi et al., 1993). Prospective clinical trials are underway to verify whether the addition of Tamoxifen to cisplatinum regimes improves clinical results.

REFERENCES

De Vincenzo R, Scambia G, Benedetti-Panici P, Bonnano G, Ferrandine G, Ercoli A, Isola G, Mancuso S (1994): Chemosensitizing Effect of Tamoxifen on Cisplatin Resistant A 2780 Ovarian Cancer Cells. *J Endocrin Invest* 17(Suppl 1):99

Kikuchi Y, Hirata J, Kita T, Tode T, Nagata I (1992): Enhancement of antitumor activity of cis-diaminedichlorplatinum (II) by antiestrogens. *Proc AACR* 33:483

Kikuchi Y Hirata J, Kita T, Imaizumi E, Tode T, Nagata I (1993): Enhancement of Antiproliferative Effect of cis-Diaminedichlorplatinum (II) by Clomiphene and Tamoxifen in Human Ovarian Cancer Cells. *Gyn Oncol* 49:365-372

McClay EF, McClay ME, Albright KD, Jones JA, Christen RD, Alacaraz J, Howell SB (1993): Tamoxifen Modulation of Cisplatin Resistance in Patients with Metastatic Melanoma. *Cancer* 72:1914-1918

Mc Clay EF, Albright KD, Jones JA, Christen RD, Howell SB (1994a): Tamoxifen Modulation of Cisplatin Sensitivity in Human Malignant Melanoma Cells. *Cancer Res* 53:1571-1576

Mc Clay EF, Albright KD, Jones JA, Christen RD, Howell SB (1994b): Tamoxifen delays the development of resistance to cisplatin in human melanoma and ovarian cancer cell lines. *Brit J Cancer* 70:449-452

Nakata B, Albright KD, Barton RM, Howell SB, Los G (1995): Synergistic interaction between cisplatin and tamoxifen delays the emergence of cisplatin resistance in head and neck cancer lines. *Cancer Chemother Pharmacol* 35:511-518

Pu YS, Hsieh TS, Tsai TC, Cheng AL, Hsieh CY, Su IJ, Lai MK (1995): Tamoxifen enhances the chemosensitivity of bladder carcinoma cells. *J Urol* 154:601-604

Warso MA, Menini P, Das Gupta TK (1995): Synergistic effect of tamoxifen on cisplatinum toxicity. *Proc AACR* 36:346

In vitro effect of Tamoxifen on multidrug resistance in cancer

The traditional approach when establishing the effect of resistance modulators follows a general line of thought: multidrug resistance in cancer is caused predominately by overexpression of mdr1, leading to elevated P-glycoprotein levels in the cell membrane. Decrease of P-gp, either by competitive binding or other mechanisms, leads to the increased cell content of the cytostatic drug(s) administered and therefore "reverses" resistance. The role of Tamoxifen as reverting agent is widely recognized, but there is no satisfactory explanation as to how this desirable effect is achieved. There is an indication that exposure to Tamoxifen *in vivo* decreased P-gp levels (Kellen et al., 1991; 1992). Hormonal regulation of P-gp activity has been described in various conditions, but not well understood (Plouzek and Yeh, 1995); in pregnancy, perhaps in answer to elevated levels of progestins, expression of the mdr1 gene increases in many organs (such as placenta, uterus, ovary, adrenal, kideny and colonic mucosa). On the other hand, increased expression of P-gp (in the rat liver, Smith et al., 1994) accelerates clearance of Tamoxifen and its metabolites.

The interaction between Tamoxifen and P-gp is not considered to be competitive. However, [^{3}H] tamoxifen aziridine, an electrophilic analog of Tamoxifen, does bind covalently and specifically to P-gp in multidrug resistant cells (Safa et al., 1994); Tamoxifen and it metabolites (N-desmethyltamoxifen and 4-hydroxytamoxifen) are potent inhibitors of this binding. Also, Tamoxifen was found to directly inhibit the binding of [3]azidopine to P-gp (Leonessa et al., 1994) as well as the uptake and metabolism of ethanolamine and choline in multidrug-resistant MCH-7 human breast carcinoma cells, inhibition of phosphatidylethanol amine (on which P-gp function depends) is an additional mechanism by which Tamoxifen may inhibit P-gp mediated drug efflux (Kiss and Crilly, 1995). Further proof of dependence of the Tamoxifen effect on reversal of drug resistance caused by P-gp is the observation that antiestrogens and their major metabolites act prinicipally on multidrug-resistant, P-gp positive cells (but not on intrinsically resistant, P-gp negative cells, Kirk et al., 1993).

In general, the effect on resistant tumour cell lines (for ex. in leukemia) differs between estrogens, Tamoxifen and pure antiestrogens (Zalcberg et al., 1993; Kirk et al., 1994) and differs in various cell lines. Thus, various human prostate cell lines resistant to Doxorubicin (DU-145 and LNCap) could be moderately sensitized by Tamoxifen by a non-mdr associated mechanism (Theyer et al., 1993). The partial reversal of Doxorubicin resistance in the drug resistant Chinese hamster ovary cell line appears to be the result of synergism between IFN-alpha and antiestrogens (Kang and Perry, 1993).

Some results obtained from studies with Tamoxifen as a resistance reversing agent are summarized in Table 2.

Table 2. In vitro effect of Tamoxifen on P-glycoprotein mediated multidrug resistance

Tumour (model)	Characteristics	Tamoxifen	References
(Review)	MDR	MDR reversal	Fine et al., 1992
Breast Ca (human) MCF-7^{ADR}	Receptor negative, Doxorubicin resist.	inhibition of mdr1 function	Leonessa et al., 1991 & 1994
Gastric Ca Colon Ca	Doxorubicin resist. -"-	increased intra-cellular drug concentration	Hotta et al., 1995
Leukemia CEM-VLB	-"-	-"-	Berman et al., 1991 & 1994
HL-60 RV	Vincristine resist.	-"- growth inhibit.	
Bladder Ca (human)	MDR	sensitization	Pu et al., 1995

REFERENCES

Berman E, Adams M, Duigou-Osternhof R, Godfrey L, Clarkson B, Andreef M (1991): Effect of Tamoxifen on Cell Lines Displaying the Multidrug Resistant Phenotype. *Blood* 77:818-825

Berman E, McBride M, Tong W (1994): Comparative Activity of Tamoxifen and N-Desmethyltamoxifen in Human Multidrug Resistant Leukemia Cell Lines. *Leukemia* 8:1191-1196

Fine RL, Sachs CW, Albers ME, Safa A, Rao US, Scarborough G, Burchette J, Jordan VC, Trump DL (1993): Inhibition of Multidrug Resistance in Human Cancer Cells by Tamoxifen: Laboratory to Clinical Studies. Proc Internatl Symp on Mechanism and New Approach to Drug Resist of Cancer Cells, Sapporo 1992, pp 323-332

Hotta T, Tanimura H, Yamane H, Iwahashi M, Tsunoda T, Tani M, Tamai M, Noguchi K, Mizobata S, Arii K, Terasawa H (1995): Adriamycin-resistance induced by P-glycoprotein is overcome by Tamoxifen and Cepharantin *in vitro*. *Proc AACR* 36:339

Kang Y and Perry RR (1993): Modulatory effects of tamoxifen and recombinant human alpha-interferon on doxorubicin resistance. *Cancer Res* 53:3040-3045

Kellen JA, Georges E, Ling V (1991): Decreased P-glycoprotein in a tamoxifen-tolerant breast carcinoma model. *Anticancer Res* 11:1243-1244

Kellen JA, Wong ACH, Mirakian A (1992): Immunohistochemical Determination of P-Glycoprotein in a Rat Mammary Tumour Treated with Tamoxifen. *In Vivo* 6:541-544

Kirk J, Houlbrook S, Stuart NS, Stratford IJ, Harris AL, Carmichael J (1993): Differential modulation of doxorubicin toxicity to multidrug and intrinsically drug resistant cell lines by anti-oestrogens and their major metabolites. *Brit J Cancer* 67:1189-1195

Kirk J, Syed SK, Harris AL, Jarman M, Roufogalis BD, Stratford IJ, Carmichael J (1994): Reversal of P-glycoprotein-mediated multidrug resistance by pure anti-oestrogens and novel tamoxifen derivatives. *Biochem Pharmacol* 48:277-285

Kiss Z and Crilly KS (1995): Tamoxifen inhibits uptake and metabolism of ethanolamine and choline in multidrug-resistant, but not in drug-sensitive, MCF-7 human breast carcinoma cells. *FEBS Let* 360:165-168

Leonessa F, Jacobson M, Boyle B, Lippman J, McGarvey M, Clarke R (1994): Effect of Tamoxifen on the Multidrug-resistant Phenotype in Human Breast Cancer Cells: Isobologram, Drug Accumulation, and M_r 170,000 Glycoprotein Binding Studies. *Cancer Res* 54:441-447

Plouzek CA and Yeh GC (1995): Hormonal regulation of P-glycoprotein expression in rat placental cells and rat tissues. *Proc AACR* 36:414

Safa AR, Roberts S, Agresti M, Fine RL (1994): Tamoxifen aziridine, a novel affinity probe for P-glycoprotein in multidrug resistant cells. *BBRC* 202:606-612

Smith LL, White I, Gant TW (1994): Increased clearance of tamoxifen and its metabolites in rat liver correlates with an increased expression of P-glycoprotein. Abstr. 33 Ann Meet Soc Toxicol, Dallas, pp 403

Theyer G, Schirmbock M, Thalhammer T, Sherwood ER, Baumgartner G, Hamilton G (1993): Role of the MDR-1-encoded multiple drug resistance phenotype in prostate cancer cell lines. *J Urol* 150:1544-1547

Zalcberg JR, Hu XF, Ching M, Wakeling A, Wall DM, Marschner IC, DeLuise M (1993): Differential effects of estrogen, tamoxifen and the pure antiestrogen ICI 182,780 in human drug-resistant luekemia cell lines. *Cancer Chemother Pharmacol* 33:123-129

In vivo effects of Tamoxifen on multidrug resistant tumours

Tamoxifen, by virtue of its relatively low toxicity and negligible side-effects, is currently one of the mainstays of long-term adjuvant cancer therapy. Together with its recognized potential to influence at least some multidrug resistance mechanisms, it is surprising how rarely it is part of chemotherapeutical protocols other than in breast cancer. Very little harm is to be expected even from random inclusion of Tamoxifen into therapy combinations and it is probable that the steroid receptor status of the tumour is irrelevant - which widens the selection of patients. It is true, eventually resistance to Tamoxifen will develop (apparently not caused by P-glycoprotein overexpression) but even a delay of drug resistance against cytostatics is a laudable goal and seems not to be correlated to resistance against Tamoxifen itself, which in turn does not close the door on second-line hormonal therapies (Dixon et al., 1992; Loenn et al., 1993).

The following table lists some more recent reports of *in vivo* effects of Tamoxifen; the table is not meant to be complete, but indicates a promising and perhaps undervalued trend.

Table 3. In vivo effects of Tamoxifen on MDR tumours

Tumour	Drug combination	Effect	Reference
Experimental:			
Rat mammary adenocarcinoma R3230AC	Tamoxifen only	P-gp decrease	Kellen et al., 1992
Clinical:			
Kidney Ca (metastat.)	Vinblastine, IFN	beneficial	Oudard et al., 1994
Kidney Ca	Chemotherapy, Cyclosporine	beneficial	Samuels et al., 1994a,b
Epithelial Ca	Vinblastine	beneficial	Trump et al., 1992
Lung Ca (small cell)	Chemotherapy, Verapamil	beneficial	Normandeau and Jones, 1990
Leukemia	Chemotherapy	beneficial	Berman et al., 1994

REFERENCES

Berman E, McBride M, Tong W (1994): Modulating multidrug resistance with tamoxifen in patients with advanced leukemia. *Ann Hematol* 68:A10

Dixon AR, Jackson L, Chan S, Haybittle J, Blameu RW (1992): A randomised trial of second-line hormone vs single agent chemotherapy in tamoxifen resistant advanced breast cancer. *Brit J Cancer* 66:402-404

Kellen JA, Wong AHC, Mirakian A (1992): Immunochemical determination of P-glycoprotein in a rat mammary tumour treated with tamoxifen. *In Vivo* 6:541-544

Loenn U, Loenn S, Stenkvist B (1993): Reduced occurrence of mdr-1 amplification in stage IV breast cancer patients treated with tamoxifen compared with other endocrine treatments. *Int J Cancer* 53:574-578

Normandeau R and Jones A (1990): Addition of verapamil and tamoxifen to the initial chemotherapy of small cell lung cancer. *Cancer* 65:1895-1902

Oudard S, Bouleuc C, Lotz JP, Lokiec F, Etienne MC, Milano G, Andre T, Gattegno B, Poupon MF, Izrael V (1994): Phase I-II study combining high dose tamoxifene as a modulator of multidrug resistance with vinblastine and alpha2b interferon in metastatic kidney carcinoma. *Proc Amer Soc Clin Oncol* 13:243

Samuels BL, Trump DL, Rosner G, Vogelsang NJ, Lyss AP, Shapiro CL, Schilsky RL (1994): Multidrug resistance modulation of renal cell carcinoma using cyclosporine A or tamoxifen. *Proc Amer Soc Clin Oncol* 13:252

Samuels BL, O'Brien SM, Vogelsang NJ, Bitran JD, Schilsky RL, Williams SF, Ratian MJ (1994): Phase I trial of double modulation of multidrug resistance with cyclosporine A and tamoxifen. *Proc Amer Soc Clin Oncol* 13:164

Trump DL, Smith DC, Ellis PG, Rogers MP, Schold SC, Winer EP, Panella TJ, Jordan VC, Fine RL (1992): High-dose oral tamoxifen, a potential multidrug-reversal agent: phase I trial in combination with vinblastine. *J Natl Cancer Inst* 84:1811-1816

Tamoxifen resistance

Prolonged exposure to Tamoxifen (which is routinely the case in postoperative maintenance treatment of breast cancer) may select for resistance to this drug. Cell cultures from the rat mammary adenocarcinoma R3230AC - a very popular experimental model because of its many similarities with the human counterpart - when exposed to gradually increasing Tamoxifen concentrations *in vitro*, become increasingly tolerant; prolonged treatment results in eventually unacceptable numbers of resistant cells. Toremifene, another triphenylethylene antiestrogen (Fc 1157a, FARMOS, Turku, Finland) induces resistance only at much higher levels; previous exposure to Tamoxifen results in some cross-resistance to Toremifene (Kellen et al., 1992).

The quest for more effective, "pure" antiestrogens is based on sound rationale: the currently used synthetic triphenylethylenes have a yin-yang effect, functioning both as estrogen agonists and antagonists and eventually induce resistance. There are apparent differences in the mode of action between these substances. While Tamoxifen promotes DNA binding but does not allow full transcriptional activation by the receptor, pure antiestrogens inhibit DNA binding by sterical interference with receptor dimerization (a dogmatic simplification which may be obsolete by the time this is published, Parker et al., 1991). So far, no consistent and dramatic improvement in clinical responses to novel antiestrogens has been reported; they also appear to induce resistance with time. *In vitro*, human breast cancer lines which had become resistant to pure antiestrogens were found to be sensitive to Tamoxifen (Lykkesfeldt et al., 1995). This, albeit solitary observation only helps to underscore the complexity and variability of resistance mechanisms.

On the other hand, overexpression of the mdr1 gene alone does not result in cross-resistance to endocrine therapies in breast cancer, including Tamoxifen (Clarke et al., 1991 & 1992). There is considerable intra- and intertumour variability, especially in breast cancer, as the result of phenotypic progressive changes in apparently independent parameters, such as estrogen-independent growth, antiestrogen resistance, and increased invasive potential (Clarke et al., 1989).

Two chapters in this book are devoted to different aspects of this important (and frustrating) feature of Tamoxifen treatment. The exact mechanism(s) as well as the causes for individual variations in the appearance of this phenomenon are not clear. One can safely assume that "classical" mdr1 amplification does not play a decisive role.

REFERENCES

Clarke R, Brunner N, Katzenellenbogen BS, Thompson EW, Glanz P, Katz D, Dickson RB, Lippman EM (1989): Relationships among antiestrogen resistance, ovarian-independent growth and invasiveness in human breast cancer. *Proc AACR* 30:206

Clarke R, Currier SJ, Kaplan O, Boulay V, Lovelace E, Pastan I, Gottesman MM, Dickson RB (1991): Role of MDR1 expression in the hormone responsiveness of MCF-7 human breast cancer cells. *Proc AACR* 32:366

Clarke R, Currier S, Kaplan O, Lovelace E, Boulay V, Gottesman MM, Dickson RB (1992): Effect of P-glycoprotein Expression on Sensitivity to Hormones in MCF-7 Human Breast Cancer Cell. *J Natl Cancer Inst* 84:1506-1512

Kellen JA, Georges E, Ling V, Dubsky M (1992): Toremifene Resistance in a Rat Tumour Model. *Anticancer Res* 12:1663-1666

Lykkesfeldt AE, Larsen SS, Briand P (1995): Human breast cancer cell lines resistant to pure anti-estrogens are sensitive to tamoxifen treatment. *Int J Cancer* 61:529-534

Parker MG, Arbuckle N, Danielian P, Emmas C, Fawell SE, White R (1991): Mechanism of action of estrogen receptor antagonists. Internatl Conf on Long-term Antihormonal Therapy for Breast Cancer. Lake Buena Vista, Florida 1991 (abstr)

Conclusions

In complex issues such as the modulation of multidrug resistance, there are multiple interpretations of how the effects come about. While there is no doubt that both *in vitro* and *in vivo* reversal of resistance can be achieved, there is the usual discrepancy between results obtained in cell cultures and in the clinic. It is well known that single and even confluent cancer cells, in a well-defined medium, constitute a clean, perfectly controlled model; it is also known that almost anything added or removed from such a medium will alter cell behaviour - much to the delight of researchers who get publishable data. Such models, while interesting and revealing, lack one major component which ultimately shapes the fate of the patient: the tumour-host interaction. The only useful and valid data, influencing therapeutic decisions and protocols, are results from trials which include resistance modifiers; they are still only few and often inconsistent. Persuading oncologists to include resistance modulators in large-scale trials (which would allow to evaluate the outcome from reasonable numbers of patients) is difficult and unpopular. There is some reluctance to add further substances to the drug burden and the move from a Petri dish to a live being is hesitant at best. Detailed and costly pre- and postoperative tests are mandatory to define, as close as possible, the predominant type of resistance in each individual. A case-by-case tailoring of the adjuvant therapy is probably necessary to optimize results.

All this has relegated combinations of chemotherapy with resistance modulators to anecdotal observations. To change this situation, for the ultimate benefit of the patient, requires wide acceptance of active, potent and otherwise inocuous substances, such as Tamoxifen, as an integrated tool in cancer therapy.

7. THE EFFECT OF TAMOXIFEN ON THE IMMUNE RESPONSE

Edward Baral, Eva Nagy, and Istvan Berczi

Introduction

The nonsteroidal anti-estrogenic agent, Tamoxifen (TX)[*], is widely applied for the treatment of breast carcinomas and of some other sex hormone dependent tumors (Patterson and Battersby, 1980). It is generally accepted that the mechanism of action of TX on these tumors is due to its antiestrogenic properties, which is exerted through its binding to of the estrogen receptor but without the growth promoting effect of estradiol (E2). For this reason, TX and related drugs (toremifene-TO, ethamoxytriphenol or MER25, and clomiphene) are referred to as nonsteroidal antiestrogens (Lerner and Jordan, 1990). Such nonsteroidal antiestrogenic agents are capable to inhibit the stimulatory effect of growth factors such as epidermal growth factor or insulin on human breast carcinoma cell lines in the complete absence of estrogens. A cytotoxic effect could also be observed when the antiestrogens were used at 4 micromole concentration or higher. The presence of the estrogen receptor was still necessary for these effects. Therefore, Rochefort (1987) suggested that these agents be named estrogen receptor targeted drugs, rather than antiestrogens. However, clinical observations revealed that TX is capable of inducing regression of some tumors that lack the classical receptor for E2 (Baum, 1985; Baral et al., 1987; Vogel, et al., 1987). This phenomenon could be explained by false negative receptor assay results. It is also possible that TX is capable of increasing host

---

[*]A list of abbreviations is given at the end of this chapter.

resistance against cancer by an estrogen receptor independent mechanism. Recent observations in our laboratory showed that TX, TO, some steroid hormones and their analogues prime a variety of murine and human tumor cells for cell mediated cytotoxicity. This sensitizing effect is not dependent on the classical estrogen receptor as receptor negative tumors are also sensitized. Our data also indicate that target cell sensitization is common to the biological effects of a variety of steroid hormones and thus it may be achieved through a variety of steroid receptors (unpublished).

The effect of Tamoxifen on the immune system

Tamoxifen has been studied in many laboratories for its possible influence on the immune system. Toremifene is the next in line in this respect and the other agents, which are of lesser clinical significance, have only been examined sporadically. Below, the studies on TX and TO will be discussed and studies on other agents will only be mentioned if they were done in comparison with TX or TO. The effect on primary lymphoid organs (bone marrow, thymus) and on mature lymphoid cells, mononuclear- and polymorphonuclear leukocytes and on immune function is surveyed here. A summary of this overview is given in Table 1.

Bone marrow. Normal human hemopoietic progenitor cells depleted of T cells and adherent cells were exposed *in vitro* to 5 micromole TX for 24 hrs. TX increased the growth of myeloid progenitors (CFU-GM) in 4 out of 10 experiments. When TX treated cells were subsequently exposed to doxorubicin, in 7 of 14 experiments there was a net increase in the number of surviving clonogenic cells when compared with cells exposed to doxorubicin alone. TX stimulated the growth of purified (CD34$^+$) progenitor cells, but did not increase the survival of these cells after exposure to doxorubicin. On the contrary, enhanced sensitivity was observed in 5 of 10 experiments (Woods et al., 1994).

The thymus. Steroid hormones in general and estradiol in particular have a suppressive effect on thymic function (Sakabe et al., 1994). TX antagonized the effect of E2 in the guinea pig thymus (Brandes et al., 1985).

Lymphocytes. B lymphocytes from human peripheral blood showed a diminished expression of the C'3 complement receptor after incubation with TX for 24 hrs (Baral et al., 1985). The pretreatment of T cells with therapeutically achievable concentrations of TX from human peripheral blood augmented the pokeweed mitogen (PWM) stimulated IgG but not IgM secretion by untreated autologous B cells. Cultures containing TX pretreated B cells and untreated T cells exhibited reduced secretion of both IgG and IgM (Baral et al., 1986). Paavonen and Andersson (1985)

Table 1. Immunodulation by tamoxifen and toremifene

Cell/tissue	Drug	Effect	Reference
Bone marrow	TX (*in vitro*)	Increased the growth of CFU-GM (human)	Woods et al., 1994
Thymus	TX (*in vivo*)	Antagonized the effect of estradiol (guinea pig)	Brandes et al., 1985
B lymphocytes	TX (*in vitro*)	Lipid A induced B cell mitogenesis is inhibited (rat)	Baral et al., 1989
	TX (*in vitro*)	Diminished expression of C'3 receptor; reduced IgG and IgM secretion (human)	Barel et al., 1985, 1986
	TX, FC1157a (*in vitro*)	PWM induced Ig secretion increased due to the inhibition of T suppressor cells (human)	Paavonen et al., 1985; Baral et al., 1986
	TX, TO, ICI 164,384 (*in vitro*)	PWM induced IgG and IgM secretion suppressed (human)	Teodorczyk-Injeyan et al., 1993
	TX (therapy)	Gradual fall in IgM levels (human)	Webster et al., 1979
	TX, TO (therapy)	Increased PFC response, decreased serum IgA, M, G levels (human)	Paavonen et al., 1991a, b
	TX (therapy)	C'3 receptor bearing cells decreased;	Joensuu et al., 1986;

Table 1, continued

T lymphocytes	TX (*in vitro*)	accelerated recovery from radiation induced lymphopenia (human)	Lukac et al., 1994
	TX (*in vitro*)	Inhibition of responses to PHA, Con A and PWM (rat)	Baral et al., 1989
	TX (*in vitro*)	Inhibition of the mixed lymphocyte reaction (rat)	Baral et al., 1991
	TX, FC1157a (*in vitro*)	Inhibited CD8[+] suppressor T cells (human)	Paavonen & Andersson 1985
	TX (*in vitro*)	Reversal of E2 mediated suppression of CD8[+] T suppressor cells (human)	Clerici et al., 1991
	TX, TO, ICI 164,384 (*in vitro*)	Suppressed mitogen-induced proliferation and L1-2 production; suppressed IL-2 receptor expression	Teodorczyk-Injeyan et al., 1993
	TO (*in vitro*)	Increased expression of progesterone receptors and Bcl 2 protein; decreased p53 expression (human)	Kellen, 1995
	TX (treatment)	Reduction of CD4[+] T cells and the proliferative response in AMLR (human)	Robinson et al., 1993

Table 1, continued

	TO (treatment)	Fewer CD4$^+$ helper T lymphocytes; increased response to Con A and PHA (human)	Valavaara et al., 1990
	TX (treatment)	SRBC receptor bearing (T) cells are decreased at 12 months (human)	Joensuuu et al., 1986
Phagocytes	TX (treatment)	Inhibition of E2 stimulated clearance of IgG coated erythrocytes from the circulation of guinea pigs	Maoz et al., 1985
	TX, TO ICI 164384 (in vitro)	Enhancement of LPS induced TNF-alphasecretion by normal human monocytes	Teodorczyk-Injeyan et al., 1993
	TX (in vitro)	Inhibition of giant cell formation by monocyts from breast cancer patients	Al-Sumidaie, 1988
	TX (in vitro)	Blockage of H_2O_2 production by human neutrophils	Troll & Lim, 1991
Antibody response	TX (in vitro)	Prevention of E2 mediated increase (human)	Clerici et al., 1991
	TX (treatment)	Inhibition of the antibody response, restored by additional PRL or GH treatment (rat)	Nagy & Berczi, 1986

Table 1, continued

	TX (treatment)	Inhibition of autoantibody and immune complex-mediated disease (Balb/c mice)	Sthoeger et al., 1994
	TX (treatment)	Decrease of serum immune complex levels in SLE patients at 4 months	Sturgess et al., 1984
Cell mediated immunity	TX (treatment)	Inhibition of contact sensitivity skin reaction, reversed by additional treatment with PRL or GH (rat)	Nagy & Berczi, 1986
	TX, TO (treatment)	High dose (50 mg/kg for 6 weeks) inhibited the activation of NK cells by IFN-gamma (NZB/NZW mouse)	Warri & Kangas, 1990
	TX (*in vitro*)	Inhibition of E2 induced NK activity (human)	Sarachi et al., 1988
	TX (treatment)	Increased NK activity after 1 month, decrease of NK activity after 1.5-2 yrs (human)	Sarachi et al., 1988
	TX (*in vitro*)	Enhancement of NK cytotoxicity (human)	Mandeville et al., 1984
	TX (*in vitro*)	Enhancement of tumor cell lysis by autologous killer cells (human)	Berczi & Vanky, 1987

Table 1, continued

Cell mediated immunity	TX, TO (*in vitro*)	Sensitization of ER⁻ target cells for NK, LAK and CTL mediated lysis (rat, mouse, human)	Berczi et al., 1992, Baral et al., 1994a,b, Baral et al., 1995a,c
	TX, TO (treatment)	Potentiation of immunotherapy of SL2-5 lymphoma in DBA2/J mice with IL-2 activated NK cells	Baral et al., 1995b
	TX, TO (treatment)	Potentiation of immunotherapy of P815 mastocytoma in DBA2 mice with LAK cells	Baral et al., 1995d
	TX, TO (treatment)	Potentiation of immunotherapy of P815 mastocytoma in DBA2 mice with CTL from tumor bearing animals	Nagy et al., 1995
		Potentiation of immunotherapy of H2712 mammary adenocarcinoma in C3H/HeJ mice with CTL from tumor bearing animals	Baral et al., (unpublished)
	TX (treatment)	Potentiation of the anti-metastatic effect of IL-2 against the MCA-106 sarcoma in C57B1/6 mice	Kim et al., 1990

found that TX and another antiestrogen, FC1157a, increased significantly the number of immunoglobulin secreting cells when added to 1-100 mM concentration of human lymphocytes stimulated with PWM. These concentrations of TX did not affect the proliferative response itself. The exposure of fractionated lymphocytes to TX revealed that the antiestrogens exerted their enhancing effect by inhibiting the suppressive function of CD8[+]cells. Teodorczyk-Injeyan and coworkers (1993) found that the exposure of human peripheral blood lymphocytes to TX, TO or to the pure antiestrogen, ICI 164,384 at 5 microgram/ml significantly suppressed the pokeweed mitogen induced IgG and IgM secretion.

In a randomized trial Webster et al. (1979) studied 72 patients with advanced breast cancer receiving chemotherapy and hormonal manipulation (ovariectomy and treatment with TX or androgens). A gradual decrease in IgM levels was observed as the study progressed. Lymphocyte DNA synthesis was decreased and the number of Ig secreting cells enhanced in unstimulated peripheral blood lymphocytes of patients with breast cancer, whereas PWM stimulated cultures showed a decreased Ig production.

TX or TO treatment of breast carcinoma patients increased the plaque forming cells (PFC) response and inhibited DNA synthesis by peripheral blood lymphocytes in more than half of the patients (Paavonen et al., 1991a). Serum immunoglobulin levels (IgA, IgM, IgG) were followed for up to 2 years in breast cancer patients undergoing TO therapy. Immunoglobulin levels decreased during the follow-up period in patients who responded to therapy and in those who did not (Paavonen et al., 1991b).

The treatment of human peripheral blood lymphocytes *in vitro* with TX, TO or ICI 164,384, at 2.5 and 5 microgram/ml concentrations, resulted in a suppression of mitogen induced proliferation, interleukin (IL)-2 production and IL-2 receptor-alpha expression (Teodorczyk-Injeyan, 1993). The exposure of normal human lymphocytes to TO (5 micromole/ml for 72 hrs) increased progesterone receptors and the expression of Bcl2 protein, whereas the expression of p53 was inhibited (Kellen, 1995).

Joensuu et al. (1986) studied 10 patients prior to, and 3, 6 and 12 months after, the initiation of TX treatment (20 mg twice daily). Complement receptor bearing cells decreased significantly at 6 months and those with receptors for sheep red blood cells (SRBC) (T lymphocytes) at 12 months after starting TX therapy. CD4[+], CD8[+], CD16[+] and B lymphocytes were decreased in breast carcinoma patients following radiotherapy. Recovery from this lymphopenia was accelerated if TX treatment was given after radiotherapy. Granulocyte phagocytosis was decreased in such TX treated patients (Lukac et al., 1994).

Tamoxifen at therapeutic concentrations suppressed significantly the proliferative response of rat spleen cells to phytohemagglutin (PHA), concanavalin A (Con A), PWM and to lipid A (LA), which is the active moiety of LPS (Baral et al., 1989). The mixed lymphocyte reaction conducted with spleen cells of Wistar-Furth and Fischer 344 rats was similarly suppressed (Baral et al., 1991). Estradiol did not have a consistent influence on lymphocyte mitogenesis or on the mixed lymphocyte reaction. The anti-proliferative effect of TX on rat spleen cells was compared with agents acting on protein kinase C (PKC), calmodulin (CM), and on calcium (Ca^{2+}). The PKC activator, phorbol 12-myristate 13-acetate (PMA), significantly inhibited the mitogenic response of PWM and Con A, had no effect on the response to PHA and enhanced markedly the response to LA. Chlorpromazine (CP), which is a PKC inhibitor, had no significant influence on mitogenesis. The calmodulin inhibitor, R24571, tended to enhance the PHA response and had no effect on the responses to other mitogens. The Ca^{2+} ionophore, A23187 was mitogenic on its own, enhanced significantly the LA response and tended to inhibit the responses to PWM, Con A and PHA. TX inhibited significantly the response to PWM, Con A, PHA, and LA, but had no influence on the mitogenic response to A23187. Therefore, none of these agents mimicked the general antiproliferative effect of TX on mitogen-stimulated lymphocytes. When TX was applied jointly with the mitogens, and the PKC, CM or Ca^{2+} modulating agents, the overall response was lowered by TX, but the pattern was identical to those obtained without TX. The intracellular Ca^{2+} chelating agent, TMB-8, the Ca^{2+} channel blocking agents, verapamil (VE) and nifedipine, and the extracellular Ca^{2+} chelating agent, EGTA, were strong inhibitors of mitogenesis and synergized with TX. Excess Ca^{2+} placed into the culture medium antagonized the inhibitory effect of TX on T lymphocyte mitogenesis, but had no influence on the inhibitory effect of this drug on B cell proliferation. Additional experiments revealed that treatment of spleen cells with TX led to an elevation of cytoplasmic free Ca^{2+} as measured by the fluorescent dye, fura-2. When Con A stimulated cells were treated with TX, the mitogen-induced increase of cytoplasmic Ca^{2+} was further elevated by the drug. Neither E2 nor verapamil caused similar alterations of Ca^{2+} in normal or Con A treated rat spleen cells.

Treatment of spleen cells with TX, E2 or VE for 4 hrs prior to Con A stimulation had no influence on the extent of mitogen induced Ca^{2+} elevation (unpublished).

The antibody response. The addition of E2 ($2x10^{-9}$-10^{-5} M final concentrations) augmented significantly the antigen-antigen-specific antibody response *in vitro*. This augmentation could be prevented by the incubation of the lymphoid cells with 10^{-6}-10^{-8} M TX prior to culture. The augmentation of the immune response was due to the inhibition of $CD8^{+}T$ suppressor cells by E2, which was reversed by TX (Clerici et al., 1991).

Treatment of rats with (1 mg s.c./150-175 g rat/day) TX during immunization with SRBC significantly inhibited the antibody response, which could be reversed by additional treatment with either prolactin (PRL) or growth hormone (GH) (Nagy and Berczi, 1986). Balb/c female mice were immunized with the human monoclonal anti-DNA antibody bearing the 16/6 idiotype. Six weeks following immunization when high levels of autoantibodies were demonstrated, the mice were treated with TX (200-800 microgram/mouse twice a week) up to 8 months. TX had no influence on autoantibody production under these conditions, but normal numbers of white blood cells and thrombocytes were observed in treated mice, whereas the untreated groups had significant leukopenia and thrombocytopenia. Moreover, the treated animals lacked proteinuria and immune complex deposits in the kidneys which were present in untreated animals. Delayed TX treatment starting a year following immunization also demonstrated a beneficial therapeutic effect (Sthoeger et al., 1994). Eleven female patients with stable systemic lupus erythematosus (SLE) were treated with TX in a double blind crossover trial. No patient improved on TX and 2 deteriorated. However, serum levels of immune complexes fell 4 months after treatment (Sturgess et al., 1984). A role for estrogens in the development or exacerbation of SLE has been suggested by many studies. Recently, three cases have been reported where otherwise healthy women received ovulation inducing agents and subsequently developed full blown SLE (Ben-Chetrit and Ben-Chetrit, 1994).

No consistent immunological changes could be observed in breast cancer patients treated with TX (20 mg, twice daily) for 3, 6 or 12 months. T lymphocytes (erythrocyte rosette forming cells), B lymphocytes (surface Ig^{+} cells) and responses to PHA and Con A were studied. The expression of complement receptors (erythrocyte-antibody-complement rosette forming cells) was decreased significantly at 6 months and active erythrocyte rosette forming cells (T cells) at 12 months after starting TX (Joensuu et al., 1986). Immune functions were determined before the start of TO treatment and at 3, 6 and 12 months in 12 postmenopausal women with advanced estrogen receptor-positive breast cancer. No significant changes in T cell subsets or NK cell cytotoxicity were observed in comparison with controls during the treatment period. However, during TO treatment, the patients had fewer CD4[+] cells (helper T lymphocyte) than did controls. In cancer patients the number of B cells prior to treatment was higher than in controls, which decreased to control levels during the first month of TO treatment and remained within the normal range. A stimulatory effect on lymphocyte responses to PHA and Con A was observed during the first month of treatment which stabilized at a higher level thereafter (Valavaara et al., 1990).

Cell mediated immunity. Treatment of rats with TX inhibits the development of contact sensitivity skin reactions in a dose dependent manner. Additional treatment with either prolactin or growth hormone reversed the immunosuppressive effect of TX (Nagy and Berczi, 1986). The antiproliferative effect of TX in the mixed lymphocyte reaction *in vitro* (Baral et al., 1991) also indicates that the induction of cell mediated immunity is suppressed by TX.

The effect of TX on natural killer cells has been studied in several laboratories. Treatment of NZB/NZW mice with TX or TO for 6 weeks did not influence the activity of natural killer (NK) cells. Moreover, low doses (0.1 and 10 mg/kg) did not interfere with the *in vivo* activation of NK cells by interferon-alpha (IFNalpha), but high doses (50 mg/kg for 6 weeks) were inhibitory (Warri and Kangas, 1990). In 21 patients with bilateral breast cancer, a significant increase in NK activity was found in comparison with controls and a significant decrease in CD4[+] T cells. The proliferative response of T lymphocytes in the autologous mixed lymphocyte reaction (AMLR) was in the normal range. Lymphocytes derived from 10 bilateral breast carcinoma patients during TX treatment was significantly reduced when compared to the pretreatment period and was at the level of controls. TX treated patients also showed a reduction in the proportion of CD4[+] T cells and in the proliferative response in AMLR (Robinson et al., 1993). Estradiol enhanced the NK activity of large granular lymphocytes obtained from normal subjects which could be antagonized by TX treatment (Sorachi et al., 1993). Rotstein et al. (1988) studied 23 breast cancer patients treated with TX for 1.5-2 years. A significant lower NK activity was found against K562 target cells. In contrast, Berry et al. (1987) found in 17 post-menopausal breast carcinoma patients treated with TX for one month that NK activity was significantly increased.

That TX is capable of enhancing cell mediated cytotoxicity *in vitro* was first suggested by Mandeville et al. (1984) who performed NK mediated cytotoxicity assays with human peripheral blood lymphocytes using the K562 erythroleukemic cell line as target. When TX was present during the assay, significant enhancement of cytotoxicity was observed by TX from 8 different donors, 10^{-7} and 10^{-8} M concentrations being effective. TX had no cytotoxic effect on the K562 target cells. An additive effect in the augmentation of cytotoxicity was observed when the cells were exposed simultaneously to human leukocyte interferon and TX.

Peripheral blood lymphocytes were isolated from 20 patients, 18 with various types of carcinomas and 2 with malignant mesenchymal tumors. Autologous tumor cells and the K562 cell line were used as targets in the ^{51}Cr release assay. Aliquots of the lymphocytes were preincubated for 15 h with various concentrations of TX (50, 100, 200, 400 ng/ml), washed and examined for target cell destruction. Untreated peripheral blood lymphocytes of 4 patients lysed autologous tumor cells. After TX treatment, lymphocytes from eight patients lysed autologous targets. TX induced autotumor lysis in lymphocytes of 6 patients, enhanced cytotoxicity in 1, and inhibited existing cytotoxicity in 2. The optimal concentration for enhancing cytotoxicity was 200 ng/ml in 5 cases, 400 ng/ml in 2 cases, and 50 ng/ml in 1 case. High density small lymphocytes which showed specific cytotoxicity for autologous tumor cells, but did not kill K562 targets, were also studied. TX induced autotumor lysis in one of 5 cases (Baral and Vanky, 1987).

We also studied the effect of E2 and TX on NK cell activity from rat spleen cells using the YAC-1 murine lymphoma as target. TX enhanced and E2 inhibited cell killing if placed into cultures for the duration (5 h) of the cytotoxic reaction. In this system E2 interfered with the enhancing effect of TX if applied jointly. Pretreatment of the target cells with TX led to highly significant enhancement of cytotoxicity. E2 also enhanced target cell killing but less effectively. When target cells were treated with TX + E2 the level of cytotoxicity was comparable to the one obtained with TX alone. These effects on target cells were detectable at pharmacological (1 micromole) and physiological (1 nM) E2 and equimolar TX concentrations. Pretreatment of effector spleen cells with TX enhanced their cytotoxic potential in some combinations but was inhibitory in others. Pharmacological levels of estradiol inhibited effector cells when applied alone, or in combination with TX. Highly significant enhancements of target cell destruction occurred if both target and effector cells were pretreated with TX. Estradiol treatment of both cell types resulted in slight enhancement or no effect on cytotoxicity. Similar results were obtained when the spleen cells were pretreated with IL-2 for 48 h. In this case the treatment of both the targets and effectors with TX and E2 for 4 h led to superior cytotoxicity compared to that achieved by TX treatment alone. Sensitization required the active metabolic participation of target cells, and the killer cell mediated release of the nuclear label, ^{3}H-thymidine was significantly increased from TX treated cells. These results indicate that TX primed the target cells for apoptosis. Both E2 and TX changed the kinetics of ^{3}H-thymidine incorporation by YAC-1 cells, but the cells were capable of growing in the presence of drug concentrations (1 micromole) used in the cytotoxicity experiments. YAC-1 cells have no measurable E2 receptors, and are weakly positive for progesterone receptors (Baral et al., 1995a).

We also conducted *in vitro* cytotoxicity experiments with the SL2-5 lymphoma of DBA2/J mice using interleukin-2 activated syngeneic NK cells as effectors. Both TX and TO enhanced signficantly the susceptibility of the SL2-5 lymphoma to lysis by IL-2 activated NK cells *in vitro*. The effect of TX and TO (10 mg/kg/day/animal in feed) on the immunotherapy of SL2-5 lymphoma with syngeneic IL-2 activated NK cells was also investigated in DBA2 mice. Treatment was initiated when the subcutaneous tumors reached 5 mm in diameter. Both TX and TO potentiated significantly the tumor regression and cure rate when compared to groups receiving NK therapy alone (Fig. 1) (Baral et al., 1995b).

The effect of TX and E2 was examined on IL-2 activated killer (LAK) cell-mediated cytotoxicity using spleen cells of Fisher 344 rats as the source of effectors and the P815 murine mastocytoma cells as targets. Treatment of the target cells with either TX or E2 for 4 or 18 h rendered them highly sensitive to LAK cell mediated lysis. TX was more effective in this regard than was E2. When joint treatment was applied, cytotoxicity remained at the level of TX treatment. The cytotoxic potential of IL-2 primed LAK cells was also modified by TX and E2 but to a lesser extent. Enhancement and inhibition of cytotoxic potential could be observed in certain experimental designs. When drug-treated target and effector cells were combined, a high cytotoxicity characteristic of sensitized target cells was observed in most experiments. Evidence of synergism and of inhibition of cytotoxicity was also seen in some of these

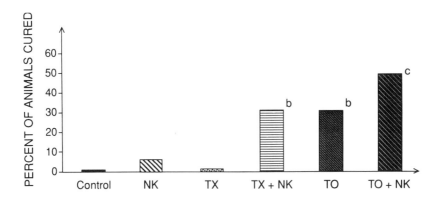

Figure 1. Potentiation by TX or TO of the therapeutic effect of IL-2 activated NK cells on the SL2-5 lymphoma in DBA/2 mice. DBA2/J mice received 10^7 SL2-5 tumor cells s.c. (LD_{100}). Therapy was initiated when the tumors reached 0.5 cm in diameter by feeding the relevant groups with either TX or TO (10 mg/kg/day). Treated and control mice were injected 2 days later with 50×10^7 IL-2 activated NK cells i.p., which was repeated 3 times, 6 days apart. Cumulative cure rates are shown in the figure from 4 different experiments with a total of 16 mice in each group. Control animals succumbed to the tumor by day 42 in all experiments. Retarded tumor growth was observed in all treated groups. Only the animals showing complete tumor regression and long term tumor free survival are included in the figure as animals cured. The cured animals have been challenged with a lethal dose of tumor cells 205-360 days after the initial tumor inoculum. Six of 15 animals so treated resisted the lethal inoculum and tumor growth was inhibited in the rest. All the 5 controls succumbed to this tumor dose by day 35.
Statistics (t test): Control group compared to treated groups, b = $P < 0.01$; c = $P < 0.005$

experiments. Target cells could be sensitized for LAK cell mediated destruction by physiological concentration (1 nM) of E2 and equimolar concentrations of TX. Neither E2 nor TX exerted a direct cytotoxic effect on P815 cells. Cytosol preparations of P815 cells had no measurable receptors for E2 or progesterone (Baral et al., 1995c).

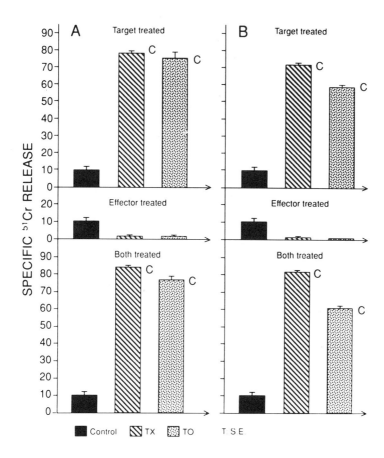

Figure 2. TX and TO potentiate the IL-2 activated killer (LAK) cell mediated lysis of P815 mastocytoma cells. <u>Panel A:</u> TX was used at 1 micromole and TO at 5 micromole concentrations. <u>Panel B:</u> Both TX and TO were used at 100 nM concentration.

Statistics (t test): Control compared to TX or TO treated cells, c = P<0.001

Tamoxifen and TO enhanced the lysis of P815 mastocytoma cells *in vitro* by syngeneic DBA2 spleen cells that had been activated by human recombinant IL-2 for 6 days (LAK cells) (Fig. 2). Similarly, enhanced tumor suppression occurred when TX or TO treated P815 cells were mixed with LAK cells and injected s.c. to normal DBA2 recipients. Tumor suppression could be increased further by the treatment of such recipients orally by TX or TO and by the repeated injections of LAK cells to the tumor site. The treatment of animals bearing subcutaneous tumors of 5 mm in diameter orally with TX or TO (10 mg/kg/day/animal) or with LAK cells i.p. resulted in tumor suppression. When the drug treatment was combined with LAK cells, tumor suppression was more pronounced and complete tumor regression was induced in a significant number of the animals so treated. The mice cured by combination LAK cell therapy have been rechallenged with a lethal tumor dose (LD_{100}) 312-334 days after the original tumor inoculum. Five of the 9 animals so treated were tumor free at 355-418 days, whereas in the remaining 4 tumor growth was retarded in comparison with the controls. All controls died by day 29. These experiments indicate that the immunotherapeutic effect of LAK cells can be significantly amplified by joint treatment with the antiestrogens, TX or TO and that immunological memory is also generated by such treatment (Baral et al., 1995d).

The effect of E2 and TX was studied on the lytic activity of cytotoxic T lymphocytes (CTL) generated in mixed cultures of rat spleen cells, using female Fisher 344 cells as responders and female Wistar rat cells as stimulators. Con A stimulated Wistar lymphoblasts were used as target cells. CTL harvested on day 5 exerted 16-25 % cytotoxicity when used at 1:12 - 1:50 target:effector cell ratios. Day 6 CTL had no cytotoxic activity. Treatment of target cells with either TX or E2, or both, at 1 micromole concentrations for 4 h prior to cytotoxicity testing raised the target cell killing to 100 %. Highly significant enhancement of cytotoxicity was observed also when the drugs were used at 100-, 10-, or 1 nM concentrations. Treatment of effector cells under similar conditions led to inhibition of cytotoxicity at 1 micromole concentration, some enhancement at 100 nM and no effect at 10 and 1 nM. When treated target and effector cells were combined, the amplification of target cell lysis was similar in magnitude to tests with treated targets only (Baral et al., 1994). These results illustrate that CTL mediated cytotoxicity is amplified by physiological concentrations (1 nM) of E2 and equimolar concentrations of TX. Even the highest concentration (1 micromole) of TX tested can be obtained during cancer therapy (Patterson and Battersby, 1980).

Killer cells capable of lysing P815 mastocytoma cells have been detected in the spleens of tumor bearing DBA2/J mice 12-14 days after tumor inoculation. The lysis of tumor cells by these effector spleen cells could be significantly increased if the target cells were pretreated for four hrs with TX (1 micromole) or TO (5 micromole). Similar treatments of

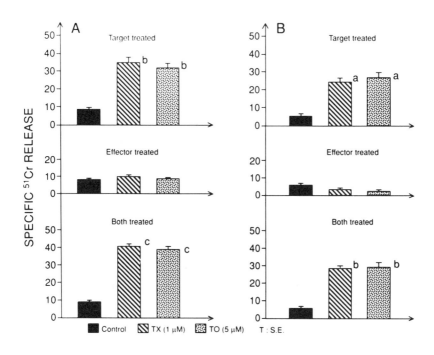

Figure 3. TX and TO potentiate the cytotoxic effect of spleen cells from P815 tumor bearing animals against P815 target cells. Panel A: Effector cells were obtained from spleens of mice bearing P815 mastocytoma for 12 days. Panel B: Effector cells were obtained from mice bearing P815 tumors for 14 days. *Statistics* (t test): Control compared to TX or TO treated cells, a = P<0.05; b = P<0.01; c = P<0.001

the effector cells had no effect (Fig. 3). The oral treatment of animals bearing 5 mm subcutaneous tumors with TX or TO suppressed tumor growth significantly. Similarly, the transfer of killer cells from spleens of tumor bearing mice produced tumor suppression in the recipients. When the tumor bearing animals were treated orally with TX or TO and with killer cells i.p., a stronger tumor suppression was induced than with either treatment alone, and complete cure has been achieved in a significant number of animals (Fig. 4A) (Nagy et al., 1995).

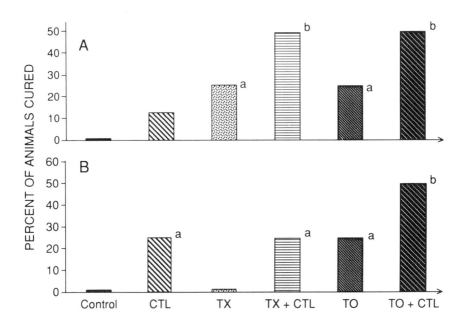

Figure 4. Potentiation by TX or TO of the therapeutic effect of CTL cells on the P815 mastocytoma in DBA/2J mice (A) and on the H2712 mammary carcinoma in C3H/HeJ mice (B). <u>Panel A:</u> P815 tumor cells were given to DBA2/J mice 10^4 cells s.c. Therapy of animals bearing 0.5 cm subcutaneous tumors was initiated by oral treatment of TX or TO (10 mg/kg/day) and 2 days later with 50 x 10^4 spleen cells i.p. from tumor bearing animals that had CTL activity. This treatment was repeated 2 times, 4 days apart. The results shown in the panel were obtained in 2 experiments and represent 8 animals/group. Termination at 28 days. <u>Panel B:</u> The design of this experiment is identical to that of Panel A, except that the H2712 mammary carcinoma was injected to C3H/HeJ mice (10^6 cells s.c.) followed by TX or TO treatment orally and treatment with 25 x 10^6 spleen cells from tumor bearing animals i.p. 3 times, 6 days apart. The results are the mean of two experiments representing 8 animals per group. Control animals died at 32 days.
Statistics (t test): Control group compared to treated groups, a = $P<0.05$; c = $P<0.01$

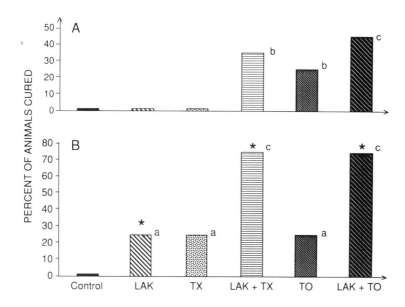

Figure 5. Potentiation by TX or TO of the therapeutic effect of LAK cells and LAK + CTL on the P815 mastocytoma in DBA/2J mice. <u>Panel A:</u> DBA2/J mice received 10^4 P815 cells s.c. Oral treatment with TX or TO (10 mg/kg/day in feed) was initiated when the tumors were 0.5 cm in diameter. Two days later 25 x 10^4 LAK cells were injected i.p. which was repeated 2 times, 4 days apart. Control animals succumbed to tumor by day 32. The results presented in the figure were calculated from 5 experiments, representing 20 mice/group. <u>Panel B:</u> These experiments were identical to the one presented on Panel A except that 50 x 10^4 LAK cells were injected i.p. 4 times, 4 days apart, which was combined with spleen cell treatment from tumor bearing animals that contained CTL (indicated in the figure with an asterisk only) (50 x 10^4 spleen cells i.p.) 4 times, commencing 2 days after the first LAK treatment and given alternately with LAK cells, 4 days apart. All controls died by day 34. The results in the figure represent 2 experiments with 8 animals/group.
Statistics (t test): Control group compared to treated groups, a = P<0.05; b = P<0.01; c = P<0.001

The combination immunotherapy of this tumor with TX or TO and killer cells could further be improved when syngeneic LAK cells and CTL from tumor bearing animals were given alternately 2 days apart for a total of 8 injections (Fig. 5). Killer cells could also be isolated from C3H/HeJ mice bearing the H2712 mammary adenocarcinoma. The treatment of tumor bearing animals (5 mm diameter s.c. tumors) with TX or TO orally (10 mg/kg/day/animal) and with spleen cells from tumor bearing animals i.p. 3 times 6 days apart, resulted in the cure of 25-50% of the animals where all the untreated controls succumbed to cancer (Fig. 4B) (unpublished results).

Tumor cells and lymphoid cells were isolated from the ascites fluid of patients with ovarian cancer using a discontinuous Ficoll-Hypaque density gradient (75-100%). Tumor-associated lymphocytes (TAL) were then cultured in the presence of autologous tumor cells (TAL:tumor ratio 10:1) in RPMI-1640 medium supplemented with human recombinant IL-2 (100 Cetus units/ml). The cytotoxic activity of TAL derived cells was measured on days 0, 6 and 14. No cytotoxicity was observed against the autologous tumor at the time of separation, but all the lymphoid cells became cytotoxic by day 6 which increased by day 14. A significant enhancement of cytotoxicity occurred in 5 of 13 patients so examined on day 6 and in 8 of 13 patients on day 14 when the autologous tumor cells were treated with TO (Fig. 6) (unpublished). TX also enhanced tumor lysis under these conditions, but less efficiently.

These results indicate that immune cytolysis mediated by NK, LAK, or CTL effector cells is amplified by TX and, to a lesser extent, E2. This amplification is due to the sensitization of the target cells to lysis, whereas the treatment of effector cells by either of these agents is usually, but not always, inhibitory. When drug-treated target and effector cells are combined for cytotoxic reactions, the rule is enhanced cytotoxicity for TX and TO without exception, and usually for E2. This is also true when the cells are treated jointly with both TX and E2. None of the target cells (Yac-1, P815, Nb2, H2712) studied so far expressed conventional estrogen receptors, yet physiological concentrations of E2 sensitized these cells for immune cytolysis. Comparable concentrations of TX were also effective. Clearly, the concentrations of antiestrogens used are nontoxic. According to our latest observations, the sensitizing effect is dependent on active nucleic acid and protein synthesis as pretreatment of the target cells with actinomycin D or cycloheximide, interferes with subsequent sensitization. The lytic reaction triggered in

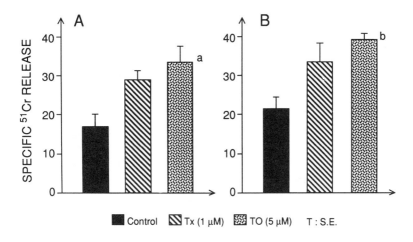

Figure 6. Enhancement by TX or TO of the cytotoxic activity of tumor-derived lymphocytes on autologous ovarian carcinoma cells. Panel A: Tumor associated lymphocytes (TAL) were activated with human recombinant interleukin-2 for 6 days in culture. Panel B: TAL were activated for 14 days. Only those data are represented where TX or TO showed a significant sensitizing effect on target cells. Panel A has been derived from 5 experiments conducted with cells from 5 different patients. In Panel B the results from 3 additional patients, that became significant on day 14, have been included, for a total of 8 patients. *Statistics* (T test): Control compared to TX or TO treated targets, a $= P < 0.05$; b $= P < 0.01$

sensitized target cells by NK, LAK or CTL effectors involves nuclear breakdown, suggesting that apoptosis is the mechanism of cell death.

Screpanti et al. (1991) also observed that estradiol enhances the natural killer cell susceptibility of human breast cancer cells. Treatment of the MCF-7 cell line with 50 nM estradiol for 24 h increased significantly the susceptibility of these cells to lysis by IL-2 activated or non-activated human peripheral blood lymphocytes. This increase in susceptibility reached the maximum after 3 days and was maintained throughout 10 days of treatment. A monoclonal antibody specific for CD16 abrogated completely the cytotoxic activity of effector cells against MCF-7 and K562 indicating that NK-type cells were involved. Estradiol had no effect on the susceptibility of the estrogen receptor negative breast cancer cell line, BT-20, to NK cell mediated lysis.

Albertini and coworkers (1992) studied the susceptibility of breast cancer cell lines to lysis by LAK cells after treatment with E2 and TX. The estrogen receptor positive (ER^+), MCF-7, and the ER^-, MDA-MB-231 cell lines were used as targets. MCF-7 cells stimulated with E2 were more susceptible to lysis by LAK cells than the corresponding TX treated cells or controls. Treatment with E2 or TX had no effect on the susceptibility of MDA-MB231 cells for lysis.

Our results suggest that treatment of tumor bearing hosts with TX could enhance host defence by amplifying the cell mediated killing of tumor cells. Indeed, it has been observed by Kim and coworkers (1990) that TX potentiates *in vivo* the anti-metastatic activity of IL-2 in C57BL/6 mice. The weakly immunogenic fibrosarcoma MCA-106 was injected i.v. and some of the animals received 50,000 units of IL-2 twice a day i.p. on days 3-12. Some IL-2 treated and non-treated mice also received 2 micromole/ml of TX in the drinking water which was supplied ad libitum leading to an average daily intake of 10 micromole/mouse/day TX. At termination of the experiment on day 18 the number of pulmonary tumor nodules were reduced by 66% in the IL-2 treated group, by 32% in the TX treated group, and by 95% in the IL-2 plus TX treated animals.

Phagocytic cells. E2, estriol, and a structural estrogen analogue with minimal estrogenic activity, 1,3,5(10)-estratrien-3,16ß-diol, enhanced the clearance of IgG coated erythrocytes from the circulation of guinea pigs, which could be partially inhibited by TX. On the other hand, estradiol in physiological concentrations increased the number of monocyte colonies developed from peripheral blood leukocytes of male and female donors and TX did not inhibit this effect (Maoz et al., 1985). We observed that TX upregulated the production of TNFalpha and downregulated IL-1 production in lipid A stimulated rat peritoneal macrophages (unpublished).

The LPS induced secretion of tumor necrosis factor-alpha (TNFalpha) by normal human monocytes was enhanced by TX, TO and ICI 164,384. This was true for all TX and ICI exposed and for about 30% of TO exposed cultures (Teodorczyk-Injeyan et al., 1993).

The incubation of peripheral blood monocytes from patients with breast cancer under agarose for 6 days at 37°C in 5% CO_2 resulted in giant cell formation. This reaction was significantly inhibited if TX was placed into the culture medium. Furthermore, the incubation of monocytes from mastectomy patients treated with TX for 3 months, showed a significant reduction in the number of giant cells compared to the samples tested before the commencement of treatment (Al-Sumidaie,

1988). TX blocked completely the tumor promoter-induced H_2O_2 production by human neutrophils in a dose dependent fashion (Troll and Lim, 1991).

Inflammation and host defense. A case of autoimmune progesterone dermatitis did not respond to estrogen, but marked improvement occurred after TX treatment (Stephens et al., 1989). The occurrence of purpuric vasculitis has been described during TX therapy. Withdrawal of TX resulted in complete clearing of the lesions. Histological examination suggested that the vasculitis was immune complex mediated.

Clark et al. (1991) reported the treatment of retroperitoneal fibrosis with TX, which has subsequently been confirmed (Benson and Baum, 1993; Spillane and Whitman, 1995). Retroperitoneal fibrosis is the result of fibroblast proliferation and collagen deposition. Benson and Baum suggested that TX treatment increases the secretion of TGF-ß by the fibroblasts and immune cells present in the inflammatory mass which in turn inhibits the inflammatory process.

The resistance of B10 mice against malaria (caused by *Plasmodium chabaudi*) was decreased by testosterone and more effectively by E2. The immunosuppressive effect of E2 could be prevented by TX or clomifene treatment. The immunosuppressive effect of testosterone but not of E2 could be adaptively transferred to syngeneic mice by spleen T cells (Benten et al., 1993).

The endocrine effects of antiestrogens

Oral administration of TX (20 mg/day) to 6 women volunteers for 5 or 10 days during the follicular phase of their cycle caused no change in either the overall length of the cycle or the time of occurrence of mid-cycle gonadotrophin surge. LH, FSH, and progesterone changed little during the control and test cycles. Estradiol levels increased 2 to 8-fold during the test cycle. Deceleration was most pronounced at the time of mid-cycle and midluteal hormone phase. There was a significant decrease in plasma prolactin levels in mid-cycle, but not during the remainder of the cycle (Groom and Griffiths, 1976). Forty-five postmenopausal women with recurrent breast cancer were treated with TX, 20 mg twice daily. Estradiol concentrations rose steadily in patients whose tumors did not respond to treatment. TX treatment did not change PRL concentrations when its serum level was within normal range, but reduced significantly concentrations in hyperprolactinemic patients within 2 weeks in those whose cancer responded well and by 6 weeks in those who showed no remission. In patients with normal PRL values, the PRL response to thyrotrophin releasing hormone (TRH) was significantly higher in cases without remission than in those who responded to treatment. Patients with hyperprolactinemia showed a reduced response to TRH challenge which was about half the control values and the response occurred faster in those who were successfully treated (Willis et al., 1977). Serum concentrations of E2, progesterone, testosterone, FSH, LH, PRL, GH, and sex hormone binding globulin (SHBG) were monitored in 30 patients on oral TO therapy, one half receiving 60 mg and the other half 300 mg daily. The above parameters were measured prior to treatment and at the second, sixth, eighth and twelfth weeks of treatment. The secretion of E2 decreased during TO therapy with 60 mg and 300 mg doses. PRL was significantly suppressed. SHBG increased significantly at both doses, testosterone was decreased as a consequence of elevated SHBG. The TRH induced PRL release was also suppressed in both groups of patients. The other hormones measured were not significantly altered and there was no significant difference in the hormonal effects of the two doses (Szamel et al., 1994).

The type I growth hormone receptor (GHR_1) was recently shown to be liver specific and is present at a higher level in females. In male rats, estradiol induced GHR_1, whereas in females ovariectomy and TX reduced the expression of this receptor. The induction of GHR_1 by E2 was GH dependent and it is diminished in GH deficient dwarf rats and absent in Hypox rats. Corticosterone also reduced the E2-induced increase in GHR_1 even though it had no effect alone (Gabrielsson et al., 1995).

Postmenopausal breast cancer patients treated with long term TX therapy showed normal levels of insulin-like growth factor I (IGF-I) and insulin-like growth factor binding protein-III (IGFBP-III), whereas IGFBP-I was significantly increased. Insulin levels were normal. During the treatment, serum IGF-I decreased at 6 months and began to increase at 12 months and IGFBP-I increased at 6 months and remained elevated at 12 months (Lahti et al., 1994).

The growth of two TX-resistant variants (RR-3 and AL-1) of the MCF-7 human breast carcinoma cell line was stimulated both by estradiol and TX, but not by ICI 164,384, a pure antiestrogen. TX-stimulated cell proliferation was dependent on IGF-I (Wiseman et al., 1993). In rats, the uterotrophic action of TX is mediated at least in part by IGF-I. In contrast, ICI 182780 reduces IGF-I gene expression and uterine weight. At the same time both estradiol and TX suppress the IGFBP-III gene expression to less than one third of control values, whereas oophorectomy and ICI 182780 both increase IGFBP-III expression. Therefore, the uterotrophic activity of chronic E2 and TX treatment may be the consequence of both the inhibition of uterine IGFBP-III and the stimulation of uterine IGF-I production (Huynh and Pollack, 1993, 1994).

Estradiol and TX acted as partial T_3 agonists on GH induction in rats. On the other hand, E2 and TX antagonized the induction of somatic growth by T_3. The feedback inhibition of TSH release and the induction of PRL by T_3 was not influenced by E2 or TX. TX mimicked the effects of E2 in antagonizing T_3, but acted as an antiestrogen in other responses (Dipippo et al., 1995).

Discussion

It is clear from this brief overview that all the organs and cells of the immune system are affected by tamoxifen. One study suggests that bone marrow function may be stimulated by TX. This finding is supported by the observation that TX therapy accelerates the recovery of patients from radiation-induced lymphopenia. TX appears to antagonize the inhibitory effect of estradiol on the thymus (Berczi and Asa, 1996). The proliferative response of B lymphocytes to mitogens and the expression of the C'3 receptor are inhibited *in vitro* by TX. The effect of immunoglobulin secretion is variable. It is implied that TX has a direct inhibitory effect on Ig secretion by B cells, but the activity of suppressor T cells inhibiting Ig secretion is also abolished by TX which may lead to a net increase of secreted Ig in culture. Tamoxifen inhibited the antibody response in rats, which could be reversed by additional treatment with either PRL or GH. TX also inhibited the development of autoantibody and immune complex mediated disease in mice and decreased serum immune complex levels in SLE patients after 4 months of treatment. Decreased serum immunoglobulin levels were observed in patients after long term TX therapy.

The mitogenic response of T lymphocytes is inhibited by TX, as is the mixed lymphocyte reaction *in vitro*, and the production of IL-2. Some investigators found that TX has an inhibitory effect on suppressor T lymphocytes, whereas others described that the inhibitory effect of E2 on suppressor T cells was antagonized by TX. Long term TX treatment of patients resulted in the reduction of CD4$^+$ helper T cells and of the proliferative response in the autologous mixed lymphocyte reaction. Long term treatment with TO similarly reduced CD4$^+$T lymphocytes, but the response of lymphocytes from such patients to Con A and PHA was increased (see: Table 1).

The development of contact sensitivity skin reactions was also inhibited by TX treatment in rats, which could be reversed by additional treatment with either PRL or GH. High doses (50 mg/kg for 6 weeks) of either TX or TO given to mice inhibited the activation of NK cells by a single dose of interferon-alpha. The stimulatory effect of E2 on the NK activity of human lymphocytes *in vitro* was also antagonized by TX. Increased NK activity was found in patients one month after the initiation of TX treatment, whereas a decrease was observed after 1.5-2 years of treatment (Table 1).

The original observation of Mandeville et al. (1984) that TX is capable of enhancing the lysis of target cells by NK cells *in vitro* has been confirmed in our laboratory and we discovered that the enhancing effect is due to the sensitization of target cells to killer cell mediated lysis (Berczi et al., 1992; Baral et al., 1994, 1995b). Sensitization took place when estrogen receptor negative target cells were treated with TX, TO or E2. Therefore, this effect was not dependent on classical estrogen receptors, but rather, a different receptor is implied by the similar effects of E2 and TX/TO on the targets used by us. Natural killer, lymphokine activated killer, and cytotoxic T lymphocytes recovered from tumor bearing animals, were all suitable effector cells for the enhanced killing of TX/TO-treated targets. However, it was obligatory to have a cytotoxic effector cell capable of killing the target in order to take advantage of the sensitizing effect of these agents. TX or TO were not cytotoxic for target cells. The target cells could be grown in culture media containing the maximum concentrations of TX (1 micromole) and TO (5 micromole) that were used in our *in vitro* experiments. The treated cells also formed tumors when injected to animals, though their oncogenic potential has been decreased. The sensitizing effect of TX and TO could be prevented by metabolic inhibitors (actinomycin-D and cycloheximide) and the sensitized cells showed an accelerated release of the nuclear label ^{3}H-thymidine into the culture medium (Baral et al., 1994, 1995a). Taken together, these results indicate that the antiestrogens, TX and TO, activate metabolic pathways in the target cell, which lead to priming for killer cell induced apoptosis. In recent years, it has been established that cytotoxic T lymphocytes can induce target cell lysis, either by signaling the cell to commit suicide or by the release of cytolysins which initiate the lytic process through a membrane attack mechanism. The suicide signal is delivered by membrane bound TNF through the Fas membrane receptor on the target cell (Suda et al., 1993; Takahashi et al., 1994; Ramsdell et al., 1994). Whether or not the mTNF-Fas pathway is facilitated by TX and TO remains to be established.

Tamoxifen also exerts an inhibitory effect on phagocytic cells and on inflammation. However, the secretion of TNFalpha from lipopolysaccharide (LPS)-activated macrophages is enhanced by TX and by the pure anti-estrogen ICI164,384 and, to a lesser extent, by TO (Table 1). As TNFalpha is known to induce tumor regression, this may also contribute to the potentiation of cancer immunotherapy by antiestrogens.

The enhancement of target cell destruction by various killer cells after treatment with TX or TO made it possible to design effective protocols for the immunotherapy of lethal cancer in mice with NK, LAK and CTL effectors, combined with oral TX or TO treatment. Moreover, a remarkable inhibition of tumor growth was observed in animals treated orally with TX, and especially with TO alone. It is probable that this is the result of increased sensitivity of the tumor in treated animals to killer cells, such as NK and CTL, that are present in the tumor bearing animal (Berczi, 1972, 1983; Berczi et al., 1973; Berczi and Sehon, 1979; Wang et al., 1980).

We found that normal murine spleen cells in which the NK activity was stimulated by recombinant human IL-2 for 2 days could be used for the immunotherapy of lethal cancer in syngeneic recipients in combination with oral TX or TO treatment with good results. Therefore, the use of IL-2 stimulated NK cells instead of LAK cells, which require at least 6 days of IL-2 treatment in conjunction with TX or TO, may be a simple and economical approach to antiestrogen facilitated immunotherapy of NK sensitive tumors in man.

The enhancement of NK activity by low doses of IL-2 treatment for 24-48 hrs has also been observed in other laboratories (Magazachi et al., 1988; Sarin et al., 1989). Ferguson and McDonald (1985) observed that the treatment of NK cells with estrogen suppressed cytolysis *in vitro* in a dose dependent manner. We made an identical observation; however, we also found that TX is capable of antagonizing the suppressive effect of estradiol on NK cells (Baral et al., 1995a).

The treatment of mice with estradiol stimulated NK cell activity for the first 30 days, which was followed by suppressed activity (Screpanti et al, 1987). *In vitro* physiological concentrations of ß-estradiol, progesterone, and testosterone had little effect on the level of NK cytotoxicity, whereas high concentrations (1-10 micromole/ml) inhibited cytotoxicity (Sulke et al.,1985).

On the basis of our results, it is clear that estradiol has a dual effect on NK cell mediated cytotoxicity. It sensitizes the targets for cytolysis which is not dependent on the presence of classical estrogen receptors. At the same time it inhibits the cytotoxic activity of the effector cells, which is likely to be dependent on classical estrogen receptors and can be antagonized by TX (Baral et al., 1995a). Therefore, it is conceivable that *in vivo* TX and TO do not only act through the sensitization of the tumor to immune cytolysis, but also, especially in female hosts, these drugs might counteract the inhibitory effect of estrogens on NK cells.

Screpanti and coworkers (1991) also observed that NK cell susceptibility of human breast cancer cells is enhanced by estradiol. Treatment of the estrogen receptor positive MCF-7 cells for 24 hrs or more with estradiol increased their sensitivity to lysis by non-activated or IL-2-activated peripheral blood lymphocytes. The ER- breast cancer line (BP20) did not change its NK susceptibility after estradiol treatment. A similar increase in susceptibility was observed if the target cell was transfected with the v-Ha-*ras* oncogene. This observation concurs with our findings that E2 is capable of sensitizing tumor targets for NK cell mediated lysis. However, we did not observe the requirement for the presence of estrogen receptor in the cells we used in our experiments (Baral et al., 1994 , 1995a). Nevertheless, the observation of Screpanti et al. (1991) that not all cells can be sensitized to cell mediated lysis has been confirmed by our observations with ovarian carcinoma cells using autologous killer cells (unpublished).

Lymphokine activated killer cells are cytotoxic for a wide spectrum of tumor cells. LAK cells have been demonstrated to suppress tumor growth in animals and also in some patients (Rosenberg, 1987). Nevertheless, the immunotherapy of human cancer with such cells remains experimental with poor predictability of the outcome. The therapeutic effect of LAK cells on the P815 mastocytoma could be enhanced by additional treatment with either TX or TO.

Albertini and coworkers (1992) found that human LAK cells killed the estrogen receptor positive MCF-7 breast carcinoma target cells more efficiently after stimulation with estradiol for 6 days. Treatment of the receptor negative MBA-MD-231 cells with estradiol did not influence its lysis by LAK cells. Treatment of both cell lines with TX in an identical manner had no effect on target cell lysis. These results caution that some tumors may not be sensitized to LAK mediated lysis by TX treatment.

Cytotoxic T lymphocytes present in the spleen of mice bearing the P815 mastocytoma, or the H2712 mammary adenocarcinoma had a therapeutic effect when transformed into syngeneic hosts bearing progressing tumors. Additional treatment with TX or TO amplified this therapeutic effect, indicating that it is possible to increase the killing potential of CTL from tumor bearing animals by these drugs. This supports further the hypothesis that the suppression of tumor growth by TX or TO treatment alone is due to the sensitizing effect of these drugs on tumor cells towards endogenous killer cells. Killer cells are frequently detectable in tumor bearing animals and in cancer patients, and may be present in the tumor tissue itself (Berczi, 1972, 1983; Berczi et al., 1973; Berczi and Sehon, 1979; Wang et al., 1980). Killer cells recovered from tumor bearing hosts are capable of lysing the tumor target *in vitro*, yet they are incapable of rejecting the same cancer *in vivo* (Berczi et al., 1973; Berczi and Sehon, 1977; Berczi, 1983). In tumor bearing hosts, the emergence of more than one kind of killer cells can be demonstrated, which invariably fade away during tumor progression (Wang et al., 1980). One may suggest on the basis of available information that TX and TO, in addition to sensitizing tumor cells to cell mediated destruction, also delay or even prevent the switching of the immune response from cell mediated reactions, which are protective, to humoral antibody responses, which are known to enhance tumor growth, rather than to protect the host (Berczi, 1972).

In many of our *in vitro* experiments and in all of the *in vivo* experiments, TO was more effective in sensitizing tumor cells and potentiating immunotherapy when compared to TX. This was true even when tumor cells were treated with TX and TO *in vitro* mixed with NK cells and injected s.c. to animals. Given the fact that the chemical structure of these two agents is very similar and that their action on the estrogen receptor is virtually identical, this difference in their ability to sensitize target cells was unexpected and cannot be explained at this time.

Preliminary experiments with ascites from patients with ovarian carcinoma revealed that after separation, the tumor associated lymphocytes could be activated for cytotoxicity by recombinant human IL-2 treatment in all the 13 patients so examined. The treatment of the tumor cells with TX or TO did induce significant elevations in target cell destruction, TO being more effective in this respect than was TX. After the activation of killer cells by IL-2 for 14 days, TO treatment of target cells induced significant increase in cytotoxicity in 8 of 13 patients. However, it is also indicated that in addition to the properties of the target cell the length of activation of the killer cell also contributes to the manifestation of enhanced target cell lysis after TO treatment. The reason for this phenomenon is not understood at the present time.

Based on the information available to date, a rational protocol for the combination immunotherapy of cancer may be designed as follows: (i) Test in *in vitro* cytotoxic assay whether or not killer cells are present in the patient against the autologous tumor cells and if the cancer of the patient can be sensitized by TX/TO for killer cell induced lysis. If killer cells are found, initiate therapy by giving toremifene orally. An optimal dose for this purpose has not been established yet. Therefore, the usual dose used in the therapy of estrogen receptor positive tumors is recommended. We suggest the use of TO because it is consistently more efficient in target cell sensitization and also in combination immunotherapy experiments in all the systems examined so far by us. (ii) If killer cells are not present in the patient, one may consider the induction of killer cells by the surgical removal of the tumor, vaccination, treatment with interleukin-2, interleukin-12, interferon-alpha, macrophage-granulocyte colony stimulating factor, etc. Again, it is necessary to test for the presence of effective killer cells in the patient before initiating cancer therapy. The experiments of Kim et al. (1990) and our preliminary observations indicate that interleukin-2 treatment can be given jointly with TX or TO treatment with the end result of potentiating the anti-tumor effect of IL-2. (iii) The third approach for combination immunotherapy is to activate killer cells (e.g. IL-2 activated NK, LAK and CTL cells) from the patient according to established methodology, reinfuse the killer cells to the donor in sufficient numbers (10^9-10^{11}) (Rosenberg et al., 1987) and apply oral treatment with TO at the same time. The killer cells may be given repeatedly to patients while maintaining anti-estrogen therapy continuously. The combination of more than one kind of killer cell (e.g. LAK and CTL) can also be used to good advantage according to our animal experiments. During such combination therapy, it is advisable to monitor the presence of killer cells in the patient and try to boost, induce or replenish, if significant decrease is detected.

The cytotoxic action of TX on the ER^+ human breast carcinoma cell line, MCF-7, was augmented, when the treatment was combined with TNFalpha (Tiwari et al., 1991). In MCF-7 cells which were relatively resistant to TX or TNF, cytotoxicity increased significantly if TX was combined with either TNF or IFN, or when the two cytokines were combined (Matsuo, 1992). These observations raise the possibility that combination therapy of cancer with TX and cytokines could be advantageous.

In addition to the estrogen receptor, tamoxifen is known to act on protein kinase C (Su et al., 1985; O'Brien et al., 1988), on calmodulin (Lam, 1984), on intracellular histamine receptors (Brandes and LaBella, 1992), on membrane associated antiestrogen binding sites (Biswas and Vonderhaar, 1989), on plasma membrane glycoprotein (P-gp) (Kellen et al., 1992; Kirk et al., 1994; Safa et al., 1994). We found that the modulation of PKC and calmodulin activity influenced the response of rat spleen cells to mitogens differently than did TX. Only Ca^{2+} antagonist agents had a general inhibition of lymphocyte proliferation similarly to TX. The anti-proliferative effect of TX was partially reversed by the increase of Ca^{2+} in the culture medium when T cell mitogens were used, but not when the B lymphocyte stimulant, lipid A, was applied. TX induced Ca^{2+} influx to spleen cells. However, pretreatment of spleen cells with TX for 4 hrs did not alter the Ca^{2+} influx induced by Con A, yet cell proliferation in response to this mitogen was significantly inhibited. On the other hand, the direct mitogenic effect of the Ca^{2+} ionophore, A23187, on spleen cells could not be influenced by TX. The calmodulin inhibitor, R24571, reversed significantly in most experiments the inhibition of spleen cell proliferation in response to PWM and Con A, but not to PHA, all of which are T cell mitogens. Therefore, calmodulin may be involved in the generation of the inhibitory signal by TX, at least in these cases (unpublished).

Among lymphocytes, only the $CD8^+$ subset of T cells (suppressor/killer T cells) has classical estrogen receptors, whereas the $CD4^+$ subset and B lymphocytes are negative. The Nb2 rat lymphoma cell line also lacks classical estrogen receptors as described by Biswas and Vonderhaar (1989), which was confirmed by us (Baral et al., 1994). These authors also found that estrogens were without effect on Nb2 cells, whereas antiestrogens, such as TX and nafoxidine, inhibited the growth stimulatory effect of PRL at concentrations as low as 10^{-10} M. The growth inhibition could be partially reversed by the increase of PRL concentrations. Estrogen-noncompetitive membrane binding sites were detected in Nb2 cells by these authors, which were specific for antiestrogens (average kD for TX 3.1×10^{-10} M). The treatment of Nb2 cells with antiestrogens inhibited lactogenic hormone binding to membrane receptors. The order of affinities of the anti-estrogens to this binding site was: TX > nafoxidine > 2-(4-tert-butyl-phenoxy)ethyl diethylamine hydrochloride > LY117018, which paralleled the order of their potencies as growth and lactogenic binding inhibitors.

Additional studies revealed that the antiestrogen binding site was physically associated with the PRL receptor. The authors suggested that the binding of TX to this site inhibits the binding of lactogens to the PRL receptor and the subsequent growth and differentiation in target tissues (Das et al., 1993). The findings by Vonderhaar and co-workers are compatible with our observation in rats that the immunosuppressive effect of TX could be reversed by additional PRL treatment (Nagy and Berczi, 1986). TX also antagonized the growth promoting effect of IL-6 on the human breast carcinoma cell line, MCF-7 (Speirs et al., 1993).

Glucocorticoids and sex hormones have long been known to induce thymic involution. This is now known to be due to the promotion of apoptosis in thymocytes. These steroid hormones have an overall inhibitory effect on immune reactions. The possible exception to this is estradiol which is suppressive for cell mediated immune reactions, but may promote antibody formation, at least in some situations (Berczi and Asa, 1996). Current evidence suggests that TX has an overall suppressive effect on immune reactions which indicates that in this case it behaves as an estradiol agonist rather than an antagonist. Therefore, the findings that TX is capable of regulating lymphocyte mitogenesis in a reversible manner may bear relevance to the hormonal regulation of lymphocyte threshold for proliferative signals and to the long recognized role of hormones in the pathogenesis of autoimmune disease (Berczi et al., 1993).

Even though estradiol has no influence on the proliferation of Nb2 lymphoma cells, physiological concentrations of E2 sensitize these cells for lysis by CTL, which is similar to the effect of TX. This sensitizing process requires active metabolic participation which leads to priming the target cell for accelerated nuclear breakdown after the cytotoxic insult. TX had a similar sensitizing effect on Con A-stimulated rat spleen cells used as targets for CTL (Baral et al., 1994). Therefore, estradiol at physiological concentrations and TX at equimolar concentrations are capable of priming Nb2 cells and normal rat spleen cells for killer cell mediated apoptosis. The receptor for apoptotic signaling is a membrane-bound protein called Fas, which belongs to the nerve growth factor-tumor necrosis factor receptor family. The ligand for Fas is a type II transmembrane protein that belongs to the TNF family (Suda et al., 1993). Apoptosis plays a major role in the maintenance of immune homeostasis and self tolerance. The strong potentiating effect of estradiol and tamoxifen on apoptotic signaling by killer cells indicates that steroid hormones play a major role in the maintenance of normal immune functions (Takahashi et al., 1994; Ramsdell et al., 1994).

At this stage it is not known whether or not the anti-proliferative effect and the priming effect of target cells for apoptosis by TX are distinct or related phenomena. The absence of the anti-proliferative effect of estradiol on Nb2 cells and its ability to prime these cells for killer cell mediated apoptosis suggests that these are different phenomena. Spleen cells have to be activated first by concanavalin A for 3 days in order to make them suitable as target cells for CTL. This observation suggests that apoptotic signaling of small lymphocytes by killer cells is not possible. Indeed, there is abundant evidence in the literature that cells are primed for apoptosis during mitogenic activation, and it will depend on the succeeding signals whether or not the cell will undergo mitosis or apoptosis. If the additional growth factors necessary for mitosis are not available, apoptosis will follow, whereas stimulation of the cell with the appropriate growth factor is capable of preventing apoptotic death (Arends and Wyllie, 1991).

The major pathways by which tamoxifen affects immune reactions are summarized in Figure 7. As is shown, TX and related antiestrogens have a direct effect on the immune system and on target cells for cell mediated cytolysis. In addition, these drugs also interact with the neuroendocrine system and modulate the secretion of imunoregulatory hormones, their receptors, and binding proteins.

Conclusions

Tamoxifen has an antiproliferative effect on lymphocytes and inhibits the induction of humoral and cell mediated immune reactions. It is also inhibitory for suppressor T lymphocytes which under certain situations could lead to enhanced immunoglobulin secretion in response to mitogens. TX antagonizes the stimulatory effect of E2 on phagocytosis, inhibits giant cell formation by monocytes and blocks the H_2O_2 production by human neutrophils. However, the LPS induced production of TNFalpha by normal human monocytes and by rat peritoneal cells is enhanced by TX treatment.

The inhibitory effect of E2 on natural killer cells is antagonized by TX. NK, LAK and CTL effector cells are capable of target cell lysis after treatment with 1 micromole TX or 5 micromoles TO, which are the concentrations commonly achievable during cancer therapy. Both TX

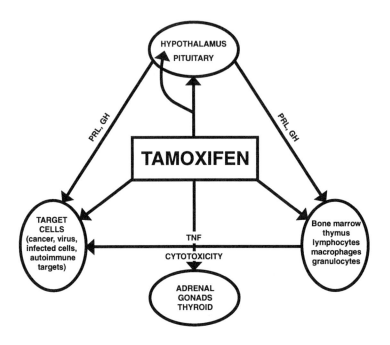

Figure 7. Major pathways of immunomodulation by nonsteroidal antiestrogens. Tamoxifen exerts an overall suppressive effect on the immune system which is mediated by the estrogen receptor and in all probability, 2 additional receptors, one mediating the antiproliferative effect and the other the priming of target cells for cell mediated lysis. The production of TNF by monocytes is enhanced by TX. TX antagonizes the suppressive effect of E2 on NK cells and in general has little, if any, effect on killer cells, whereas it boosts cell mediated immune cytolysis by priming the target cells for programmed cell death. TX decreases the serum levels of PRL and IGF-I and also antagonizes their effect at the cellular level, and thus interferes with these immunostimulatory hormones. The evidence available to date suggests that TO affects the immune system by similar mechanisms. Current evidence suggests that the amplifying effect of TX and TO on the effector phase of cytotoxic immune reactions against tumor cells will be useful for the immunotherapy of cancer.

and TO enhanced the cell mediated destruction (e.g. by NK, LAK or CTL effectors) of several estrogen receptor negative tumor cells *in vivo*, which lead to the cure and long term survival of a significant proportion (50-75%) of the animals harboring lethal cancer.

Killer and suppressor cells (CD8$^+$T lymphocytes) and NK cells express classical estrogen receptors and TX or TO may act on these receptors as antiestrogens. However, the antiproliferative effect of TX on lymphocytes is independent of classical estrogen receptor and of estrogen action. Current evidence indicates that the sensitizing effect of TX and TO on estrogen receptor negative target cells for cell mediated lysis is mediated by yet another receptor on which estradiol has a similar effect to that of TX and TO. This receptor is present in Con A activated lymphocytes, in the Nb2 rat lymphoma, in the Yac-1 and SL2-5 murine lymphomas, in the P815 murine mastocytoma, in the K562 human erythroid leukemia cell line, and in the majority of human ovarian carcinoma cells.

TX and TO decrease serum PRL, GH and IGF-I levels, influence the expression of hormone receptors and their binding proteins, which also affect the immune system. TX induced immunosuppression in rats could be reversed by treatment with either GH or PRL, suggesting that these hormones are effective antagonists of TX induced immunosuppression. TX also antagonizes the stimulatory effect of PRL on lymphoid cells.

The potentiation of cell mediated tumor destruction by TX and TO in tumor bearing animals indicates that these drugs can be used for the combination immunotherapy of cancer. The prerequisite for such therapy is the availability of killer cells capable of lysing the tumor cells in question and the susceptibility of the tumor target to sensitization. Both of these parameters can be monitored by laboratory testing.

Abbreviations

A23187, Ca2$^+$ionophore; AMLR, autologous mixed lymphocyte reaction; Bcl 2, survival gene; C'3, complement receptor; CD, cluster designation; CFU-GM, granulocyte-macrophage colony forming unit; CM, calmodulin; CP, chlorpromazine; CTL, cytotoxic T lymphocyte; E2, estrogen; ER, estrogen receptor; FC1157a, antiestrogen; FSH, follicle stimulating hormone; GH, growth hormone; GHR, growth hormone receptor; H2712, murine mammary carcinoma; ICI 164,384, pure antiestrogen; IFNalpha, interferon-alpha; IGF, insulin-like growth factor; IGFBP, insulin-like growth factor binding protein; K562, human erythromyeloid leukemia cell line; LAK, lymphokine activated killer; LH, luteinizing hormone; LPS, lipopolysaccharide; LY 117018, antiestrogen; MBA-MD-231, MCF-7, human breast carcinoma cell lines; MER-25, ethamoxytriphenol-antiestrogen; Nb2, rat lymphoma; NK, natural killer; P53, tumor suppressor gene; PFC, plaque forming cells; PGP, plasma membrane glycoprotein; PHA, phytohemagglutinin; PKC, protein kinase C; PMA, phorbol 12-myristate 13-acetate; PRL, prolactin; PWM, pokeweed mitogen; R24571, calmodulin inhibitor; SHBG, sex hormone binding globulin; SRBC, sheep red blood cells; TAL, tumor associated lymphocytes; TNFalpha, tumor necrosis factor-alpha; TO, toremifene; TRH, thyrotropin releasing hormone; TSH, thyroid stimulating hormone; TX, tamoxifen.

REFERENCES

Albertini MR, Gibson DFC, Robinson SP, Howard SP, Tans KJ, Lindstrom MJ, Robinson RR, Tormey DC, Jordan VC and Sondel PM (1992): Influence of estradiol and tamoxifen on susceptibility of human breast cancer cell lines to lysis by lymphokine-activated killer cells. *J Immunother* 11:30-39

Al-Sumidaie AM (1988): The effect of tamoxifen and medroxyprogesterone on giant cell formation by monocytes from patients with breast cancer. *J Cancer Res Clin Oncol* 114:399

Arends MJ and Wyllie AH (1991): Apoptosis: Mechanisms and roles in Pathology. *Int Rev Exp Pathol* 32:223-254

Baral E and Vanky F (1987): Effect of tamoxifen on the cell-mediated autotumor lysis. *J Clin Lab Immunol* 22:97

Baral E, Blomgren H, Rotstein S and Virving L (1985): Antiestrogen effects on human blood lymphocyte subpopulations in vitro. *J Clin Lab Immunol* 17:33

Baral E, Blomgren H, Wasserman J, Rotstein S and von Stedingk LV (1986): Effect of tamoxifen on pokeweed mitogen stimulated immunoglobulin secretion in vitro. *J Clin Lab Immunol* 21:137

Baral E, Glas U, Rutqvist LE and Skoog L (1987): Adjuvant therapy in postmenopausal patients with operable breast cancer. In: Fundamental problems in breast cancer, Paterson AHG and Lees AW, eds. Martinus Nijhoff.

Baral E, Kwok S and Berczi I (1989): Suppression of lymphocyte mitogenesis by tamoxifen. *Immunopharmacology* 18:57-62

Baral E, Kwok S and Berczi I (1991): The influence of estradiol and tamoxifen on the mixed lymphocyte reaction in rats. *Immunopharmacology* 21:191-198

Baral E, Nagy E and Berczi I (1994): Target cells are sensitized for cytotoxic T lymphocyte mediated destruction by estradiol and tamoxifen. *Int J Cancer* 58:64-68

Baral E, Nagy E and Berczi I (1995a): Enhancement of natural killer cell mediated cytotoxicity by tamoxifen. *Cancer* 75:591-599

Baral E, Nagy E, Kangas L and Berczi I (1995b): Immunotherapy of the SL2-5 murine lymphoma with natural killer cells and tamoxifen or toremifene. Submitted to *Cancer*

Baral E, Nagy E and Berczi I (1995c): The modulation of lymphokine activated killer cell mediated cytotoxicity by estradiol and tamoxifen. *Int J Cancer* (accepted)

Baral E, Nagy E, Kangas L and Berczi I (1995d): Anti-estrogens enhance the therapeutic effect of lymphokine activated killer cells on the P815 murine mastocytoma. Submitted to *Int J Cancer*

Baum M (1985): Nolvadex Adjuvant Trial Organisation: Controlled trial of tamoxifen as single adjuvant agent in management of early breast cancer; analysis at six years. *Lancet* 1:836

Ben-Chetrit A and Ben-Chetrit E (1994): Systemic lupus erythematosus induced by ovulation induction treatment. *Arthritis Rheum* 37:1614-1617

Benson JR and Baum M (1993): Tamoxifen for retroperitoneal fibrosis (letter). *Lancet* 341:836

Benten WPM, Wunderlich F, Herrmann R and Kühn-Velten WN (1993): Testosterone-induced compared with oestradiol-induced immunosuppression against Plasmodium chabaudi malaria. *J Endocrinol* 139:487-494

Berczi I (1972): Studies in tumor immunology. Ph.D. thesis, The University of Manitoba

Berczi I (1983): Cancer Immunology - Quo Vadis? An overview. *J Exp Clin Cancer Res* 2:135-144

Berczi I and Asa S (1996): Endocrine-immune interaction. In: Functional Endocrine Pathology, 2nd edition, Kovacs K and Asa S, eds. Boston, MA: Blackwell Scientific Publishers (in press)

Berczi I and Sehon AH (1977): Tumor inhibition by effector cells cultured from progressing sarcomas. *Immunol Commun* 6:617-632

Berczi I and Sehon AH (1979): Effector and suppressor lymphoid cells in tumor bearing guinea pigs. *Int J Cancer* 23:274-282

Berczi I, Strausbach P, Sehon AH (1973): Rejection of tumor cells in vitro. *Science* 180:1289-1291

Berczi I, Nagy E, Baral E (1992): The amplification of cell-mediated cytolysis by estradiol and tamoxifen. 8th International Congress of Immunology, August 23-28, 1992, Budapest, Hungary

Berczi I, Baragar FD, Chalmers IM, Keystone EC, Nagy E and Warrington RJ (1993): Hormones in self tolerance and autoimmunity: a role in the pathogenesis of rheumatoid arthritis? *Autoimmunity* 16:45-56

Berry J, Green BJ and Matheson DS (1987): Modulation of natural killer cell activity by tamoxifen in stage I post-menopausal breast cancer. *Eur J Cancer Clin Oncol* 23:517

Biswas R and Vonderhaar BK (1989): Antiestrogen inhibition of prolactin-induced growth of the Nb2 rat lymphoma cell line. *Cancer Res* 49:6295-6299

Brandes LJ and LaBella FS (1992): Histamine and calcium are independently regulated intracellular mediators of lymphocyte mitogenesis. *Biochem Biophys Res Commun* 182:786-793

Brandes LJ, MacDonald LM and Bogdanovic RP (1985): Evidence that the antiestrogen binding site is a histamine-like receptor. *Biochem Biophys Res Commun* 126:905

Clark CP, Vanderpool D and Preskitt JT (1991): The response of retroperitoneal fibrosis to tamoxifen. *Surgery* 109:502-506

Clerici E, Bergamasco E, Ferrario E and Villa ML (1991): Influence of sex steroids on the antigen-specific primary antibody response in vitro. *J Clin Lab Immunol* 34:71-78

Das RB, Biswas R and Vonderhaar BK (1993): Characteristics of a membrane-associated antilactogen binding site for tamoxifen. *Mol Cell Endocrinol* 98:1-8

Dipippo VA, Lindsay R and Powers CA (1995): Estradiol and tamoxifen interactions with thyroid hormone in the ovariectomized-thyroidectomized rat. *Endocrinology* 136:1020-1033

Ferguson MM and McDonald FG (1985): Oestrogen as an inhibitor of human NK cell cytolysis. *FEBS Lett* 191:145-8

Gabrielsson BG, Carmignac DF, Flavell DM and Robinson ICAF (1995): Steroid regulation of growth hormone (GH) receptor and GH-binding protein messenger ribonucleic acids in the rat. *Endocrinology* 136:209-217

Groom GV and Griffiths K (1976): Effect of the anti-oestrogen tamoxifen on plasma levels of luteinizing hormone, follicle-stimulating hormone, prolactin, oestradiol and progesterone in normal pre-menopausal women. *J Endocr* 70:421-428

Huynh HT and Pollak M (1993): Insulin-like growth factor I gene expression in the uterus is stimulated by tamoxifen and inhibited by the pure antiestrogen ICI 182780. *Cancer Res* 53:5585-5588

Huynh P and Pollak M (1994): Uterotrophic actions of estradiol and tamoxifen are associated with inhibition of uterine insulin-like growth factor binding protein 3 gene expression. *Cancer Res* 54:3115-3119

Joensuu H, Toivanen A and Nordman E (1986): Effect of tamoxifen on immune functions. *Cancer Treat Rep* 70:381-382

Kellen JA (1995): The effect of toremifene on lymphocyte gene product expression. AACR Abstract 514

Kellen JA, Wong ACH and Mirakian A (1992): Immunohistochemical determination of P-glycoprotein in a rat mammary tumour treated with tamoxifen. *In Vivo* 6:541-544

Kim B, Warnaka P and Konrad C (1990): Tamoxifen potentiates in vivo antitumor activity of interleukin-2. *Surgery* 108:139

Kirk J, Syed SK, Harris AL, Jarman M, Roufogalis BD, Stratford KJ and Carmichael J (1994): Reversal of P-glycoprotein-mediated multidrug resistance by pure anti-oestrogens and novel tamoxifen derivatives. *Biochem Pharmacol* 48:277-285

Lahti EI, Knip M and Laatikainen TJ (1994): Plasma insulin-like growth factor I and its binding proteins 1 and 3 in postmenopausal patients with breast cancer receiving long term tamoxifen. *Cancer* 74:618-624

Lam HYP (1984): Tamoxifen is a calmodulin antagonist in the activation of cAMP phosphodiesterase. *Biochem Biophys Res Commun* 118:27-32

Lerner LJ and Jordan VC (1990): Development of antiestrogens and their use in breast cancer: eighth Cain memorial award lecture. *Cancer Res* 50:4177

Lukac J, Kusic Z, Kordic D, Koncar M and Bolanca A (1994): Natural killer cell activity, phagocytosis, and number of peripheral blood cells in breast cancer patients treated with tamoxifen. *Breast Cancer Res Treat* 29:279-285

Maghazachi AA, Vujanovic NL, Herberman RB and Miserodt JC (1988): Lymphokine activated killer cells in rats. IV. Developmental relationships among large agranular lymphocytes, large granular lymphocytes and lymphokine activated killer cells. *J Immunol* 140:2846-2852

Mandeville R, Ghalli SS and Chausseau J-P (1984): In vitro stimulation of human NK activity by an estrogen antagonist (tamoxifen). *Eur J Cancer Clin Oncol* 20:983

Maoz H, Kaiser N, Halimi M, Barak V, Haimovitz A, Weinstein D, Simon A, Yagel S, Biran S and Treves AJ (1985): The effect of estradiol on human myelomonocytic cells. 1. Enhancement of colony formation. *J Reprod Immunol* 7:325

Matsuo S, Takano S, Yamashita J and Ogawa M (1992): Synergistic cytotoxic effects of tumor necrosis factor, interferon-gamma and tamoxifen on breast cancer cell lines. *Anticancer Res* 12:1575-1580

Nagy E and Berczi I (1986): Immunomodulation by tamoxifen and pergolide. *Immunopharmacology* 12:145

Nagy E, Baral E, Kangas L and Berczi I (1995): Anti-estrogens potentiate the immunotherapeutic effect of cytotoxic T lymphocytes on the P815 murine mastocytoma. Submitted to *Int J Cancer*

O'Brian CA, Housey GM and Weinstein IB (1988): Specific and direct binding of protein kinase C to an immobilized tamoxifen analogue. *Cancer Res* 48:3626-3629

Patterson JS and Battersby LA (1980): Tamoxifen: an overview of recent studies in the field of oncology. *Cancer Treat Rep* 64:775

Paavonen T (1994): Hormonal regulation of immune responses. *Ann Med* 26:255-258

Paavonen T and Andersson LC (1985): The oestrogen antagonists, tamoxifen and FC-1157a, display oestrogen like effects on human lymphocyte functions in vitro. *Clin Exp Immunol* 61:467-474

Paavonen T, Aronen H, Pyrhönen S, Hajba A and Andersson LC (1991a): The effects of anti-estrogen therapy on lymphocyte functions in breast cancer patients. *APMIS* 99:163-170

Paavonen T, Aronen H, Pyrhönen S, Hajba A and Andersson LC (1991b): The effect of toremifene therapy on serum immunoglobulin levels in breast cancer. *APMIS* 99:849-853

Ramsdell F, Seaman MS, Miller RE, Tough TW, Alderson MR and Lynch DH (1994): gld/gld mice are unable to express a functional ligand for Fas. *Eur J Immunol* 24:928-933

Robinson E, Rubin D, Mekori T, Segal R and Pollack S (1993): In vivo modulation of natural killer cell activity by tamoxifen in patients with bilateral primary breast cancer. *Cancer Immunol Immunother* 37:209-212

Rochefort H (1987): Nonsteroidal antiestrogens are estrogen-receptor-targeted growth inhibitors that can act in the absence of estrogens. *Hormone Res* 28:196

Rosenberg SA, Lotze MT, Muul LM, Chang AE, Avis FP, Leitman S, et al. (1987): A progress report on the treatment of 157 patients with advanced cancer using lymphokine activated killer cells and interleukin 2 or high-dose interleukin 2 alone. *New Engl J Med* 316:889-897

Rotstein S, Blomgren H, Petrini B, Wasserman J and Von Stedingk LV (1988): Influence of adjuvant tamoxifen on blood lymphocytes. *Breast Cancer Res Treat* 12:75

Safa AR, Roberts S, Agresti M and Fine RL (1994): Tamoxifen aziridine, a novel affinity probe for P-glycoprotein in multidrug resistant cells. *Biochem Biophys Res Comm* 202:606-612

Sakabe K, Kawashima I, Urano R, Seiki K and Itoh T (1994): Effects of sex steroids on the proliferation of thymic epithelial cells in a culture model: a role of protein kinase C. *Immunol Cell Biol* 72:193-199

Sarin A, Adler WH and Saxena RK (1989): Lack of optimal activation of natural killer levels by interleukin-2 in rat spleen cells: evidence of suppression. *Cell Immunol* 122:548-554

Screpanti I, Santoni A, Gulino A, Herberman RB and Frati L (1987): Estrogen and antiestrogen modulation of the levels of mouse natural killer activity and large granular lymphocytes. *Cell Immunol* 106:191-202

Screpanti I, Felli MP, Toniato E, Meco D, Martinotti S, Frati L, Santoni A and Gulino A (1991): Enhancement of natural killer-cell susceptibility of human breast-cancer cells by estradiol and v-Ha-ras oncogene. *Int J Cancer* 47:445

Sorachi K, Kumagai S, Sugita M, Yodoi J and Imura H (1993): Enhancing effect of 17ß-estradiol on human NK cell activity. *Immunol Lett* 36:31-36

Speirs V, Adams EF and White MC (1993): The anti-estrogen tamoxifen blocks the stimulatory effects of interleukin-6 on 17 beta-hydroxysteroid dehydrogenase activity in MCF-7 cells. *J Steroid Biochem Mol Biol* 46:605-611

Spillane RM and Whitman GJ (1995): Treatment of retroperitoneal fibrosis with tamoxifen (letter). *AJR* 164:515-516

Stephens CJM, Wojnarowska FT and Wilkinson JD (1989): Autoimmune progesterone dermatitis responding to Tamoxifen. *Brit J Dermatol* 121:135

Sthoeger ZM, Bentwich ZVI, Zinger H, Mozes E (1994): The beneficial effect of the estrogen antagonist, tamoxifen, on experimental systemic lupus erythematosus. *J Rheumatol* 21:2231-2238

Sturgess AD, Evans DTP, Mackay IR and Riglar A (1984): Effects of the oestrogen antagonist tamoxifen on disease indices in systemic lupus erythematosus. *J Clin Lab Immunol* 13:11-14

Su HD, Mazzei GJ, Vogler WR and Kuo JF (1985): Effect of tamoxifen, a nonsteroidal antiestrogen, on phospholipid/calcium-dependent protein kinase and phosphorylation of its endogenous substrate proteins from the rat brain and ovary. *Biochem Pharmacol* 34:3649-3653

Suda T, Takahashi T, Golstein P and Nagata S (1993): Molecular cloning and expression of the Fas ligand, a novel member of the tumor necrosis factor family. *Cell* 75:1169-1178

Sulke AN, Jones DB and Wood PJ (1985): Hormonal modulation of human natural killer cell activity in vitro. *J Reprod Immunol* 7:105-10

Szamel I, Hindy I, Vincze B, Eckhardt S, Kangas L and Hajba A (1994): Influence of toremifene on the endocrine regulation in breast cancer patients. *Eur J Cancer* 30A:154-158

Takahashi T, Tanaka M, Brannan CI, Jenkins NA, Copeland NG, Suda T and Nagata S (1994): Generalized lymphoproliferative disease in mice, caused by a point mutation in the Fas ligand. *Cell* 76:969-976

Teodorczyk-Injeyan J, Cembrzynska-Nowak M, Lalani S and Kellen JA (1993): Modulation of biological responses of normal human mononuclear cells by antiestrogens. *Anticancer Res* 13:279-283

Tiwari RK, Wong GY, Liu J, Miller D and Osborne MP (1991): Augmentation of cytotoxicity using combinations of interferons (types I and II), tumor necrosis factor-alpha, and tamoxifen in MCF-7 cells. *Cancer Lett* 61:45-52

Troll W and Lim JS (1991): Tamoxifen suppresses tumor promoter-induced hydrogen peroxide in human neutrophils. *Proc Am Assn Cancer Res* 32:149 (Abstract #891)

Valavaara R, Tuominen J and Toivanen A (1990): The immunological status of breast cancer patients during treatment with a new antiestrogen, toremifene. *Cancer Immunol Immunother* 31:381-386

Vogel CL, East DR, Voigt W and Thomsen S (1987): Response to tamoxifen in estrogen receptor-poor metastatic breast cancer. *Cancer* 60:1184

Wang KC, Berczi I, Hoffman EG and Sehon AH (1980): Effector and enhancing lymphoid cells in plasmacytoma bearing mice. II. Dynamic changes during tumor progression. *Int J Cancer* 25:493-501

Wärri A and Kangas L (1990): Effect of toremifene on the activity of NK-cells in NZB/NZW mice. *J Steroid Biochem* 36:207-209

Webster DJT, Richardson G, Baum M, Priestman T and Hughes LE (1979): Effect of treatment on the immunological status of women with advanced breast cancer. *Brit J Cancer* 39:676

Willis KJ, London DR, Ward HWC, Butt WR, Lynch SS and Rudd BT (1977): Recurrent breast cancer treated with the antioestrogen tamoxifen: correlation between hormonal changes and clinical course. *Brit Med J* 1:425-428

Wiseman LR, Johnson MD, Wakeling AE, Lykkesfeldt AE, May FEB and Westley BR (1993): Type I IGF receptor and acquired tamoxifen resistance in oestrogen-responsive human breast cancer cells. *Eur J Cancer* 29A:2256-2264

Woods KE, Grant S, Yanovich S and Gewirtz DA (1994): Variable effects of tamoxifen on human hematopoietic progenitor cell growth and sensitivity to doxorubicin. *Cancer Chemother Pharmacol* 33:509-514

ACKNOWLEDGEMENTS

The work discussed in this chapter has been supported in part by the Manitoba Cancer Treatment and Research Foundation, the Seller's Foundation, the Manitoba Health Research Foundation, the Manitoba Health Services Foundation, and Orion-Pharmos Corporation of Finland. The authors are indebted to Mrs. Jean Sylwester for her devoted work on this manuscript.

8. CELLULAR EFFECTS OF EARLY EXPOSURE TO TAMOXIFEN

Taisen Iguchi and Yasuhiko Ohta

Historically, Tamoxifen has been synthesized as an antiestrogen by Harper and Walpole (1966). However, this substance showed some estrogenic effects when examined in laboratory animals: a complete estrogen agonist in the chick oviduct (Sutherland et al., 1977), a partial agonist with antiestrogenic activity in the immature and ovariectomized rat (Harper and Walpole, 1967; Jordan and Koerner, 1976), and a full agonist in the immature and ovariectomized adult mouse (Harper and Walpole, 1966; Terenius 1971; Jordan et al., 1978; Chou et al., 1992). Two-dimensional electrophoresis revealed that proteins from the vagina of postpuberty Tamoxifen-exposed ovariectomized adult mice showed the same behavior as in those from the vagina of postpubertally estrogen-exposed mice, suggesting that Tamoxifen acts as an estrogen agonist (Takamatsu et al., 1992). Tamoxifen can inhibit the estradiol-stimulated increased in uterine wet weight (Harper and Walpole, 1967), however it simultaneously induced hypertrophy of uterine luminal epithelial cells (Kang et al., 1975) and progesterone receptor (PR) synthesis (Dix and Jordan, 1980; Jordan and Gosden, 1982) in rats. Since some human breast tumors are directly dependent on estrogen for growth, Tamoxifen was tested clinically for breast cancer therapy and proved to be at least as effective as other endocrine therapies (Cole et al., 1971; Baum et al., 1995).

The study of permanent changes in target organs induced by early exposure of sex hormones during a critical period of development began with experiments on the neonatal mouse treated with estrogen by Takasugi et al. (1962). The vaginal epithelium of mice exposed to 17ß-estradiol showed persistent proliferation and cornification, which were not abolished by removal of adrenals and hypophysis following ovariectomy (Takasugi, 1963). This persistent vaginal cornification was thus estrogen-independent and could be induced not only by estrogen but by aromatizable or non-aromatizable androgens only when the treatment was started within 3 days after birth, indicating the presence of a critical period. The vaginal epithelium showing estrogen-independent persistent proliferation and cornification resulted in cancerous lesions (for reviews, Bern et al, 1976; Takasugi, 1976). Neonatal estrogen or androgen exposure in male mice induces persistent suppression of spermatogenesis and atrophy of seminal vesicles and prostates (Ohta and Takasugi, 1974). Effects of perinatal exposure to sex hormones on the reproductive system of female and male animals have been reviewed by Bern (1992a,b), Takasugi (1979), Forsberg (1979), Herbst and Bern (1981), Arai et al. (1983), Newbold and McLachlan (1988), Mori and Nagasawa (1988), Kincl (1990), and Iguchi and Bern (1995). In addition, various abnormalities have been demonstrated in rats and mice exposed neonatally to Tamoxifen (Iguchi, 1992). This review deals with studies including an update of permanent effects on genital and nongenital organs from perinatal exposure to Tamoxifen, with special consideration of the cellular basis for the changes observed.

Genital abnormalities induced by perinatal exposure to Tamoxifen female rat

In female Sprague-Dawley rats, neonatal and prepubertal exposure to 10 microgram/day Tamoxifen inhibited the formation of uterine glands (Branham et al., 1985, 1988a,b). In prepubertal rats, 5 daily exposures to hydroxytamoxifen (1-100 microgram) and Tamoxifen (10 and 100 microgram) beginning at 20 days of age induced glandular epithelial hypertrophy up to 2 fold in size compared to controls (Branham et al., 1993a). Also, luminal epithelial spheres (LES) appeared in the culture of 11-day-old rat uterine epithelial and stromal cells. Estrogen is beneficial to the formation and maintenance of LES, however LES formation was inhibited by exposure of uteri to 10 microgram Tamoxifen for 5 days from the day of birth. Tamoxifen exposure affected the normal differentiation of both luminal epithelium and stroma, since neither tissue supported the formation of LES when the exposed tissues were combined with normal tissues.

Döhler et al., (1986) demonstrated that perinatal exposure to Tamoxifen (from 16 days of pregnancy to delivery, 200 microgram/day to mothers, and 10 microgram/day to neonates for 10 days) induced permanent anovulatory sterility in rats. Ohta et al. (1989) also showed that 5 daily administrations of 100 or 200 microgram Tamoxifen/day in neonatal life induced sterility characterized by acyclicity of estrus and anovulation in female rats similar to rats and mice exposed neonatally to Tamoxifen (Chamness et al., 1979; Forsberg, 1985; Taguchi and Nishizuka, 1985; Iguchi et al., 1986a, 1988a). Ovaries of these rats exhibited persistent vaginal mucification and contained various maturation stages of follicles but no corpora lutea. This is in contrast to the findings of Chamness et al. (1979) and Iguchi et al. (1986a) who demonstrated that Tamoxifen-exposed rats and mice showing continued vaginal diestrus had atrophic ovaries with small follicles and degenerated oocytes; the vagina was lined by atrophic epithelium without mucus. The vagina of Tamoxifen-exposed rats ovariectomized at ages of 10 and 60 days failed to respond to estrogen-priming, showing no estrous smears (Ohta et al., 1989). Therefore, continued vaginal diestrus in neonatally Tamoxifen-exposed rats may be explained by changed sensitivity of the ovary to gonadotropin and/or of the vagina to sex hormones. The endometrium of neonatally Tamoxifen-exposed rats had a reduced capacity for proliferation and transformation into deciduoma, in response to intraluminal oil instillation as compared with that of controls (Ohta et al., 1989). These findings suggest that the effect of Tamoxifen administered in neonatal life is primarily due to the sustained, low uterine responsiveness to the deciduogenic stimuli. Ohta (1982, 1985) has demonstrated that endogenous estrogen is not needed for the capacity of the uterus to form deciduoma within 10 days after birth. It is likely that in neonatally Tamoxifen-exposed rats, the lowered uterine responsiveness to the deciduogenic stimulus does not result from the action of estrogen but from that of the estrogen agonist on the developing uterus (Ohta, 1995).

Female guinea pigs

In guinea pigs exposed prenatally to Tamoxifen (5 mg/kg/day) for 12 days from approximately the 50th day of pregnancy and neonatally to 100 microgram Tamoxifen for 2-12 days, enhancement of synthetic and secretory activities in the uterine epithelium was similar to those induced by estrogen as demonstrated by electron microscopy, (Pasqualini and

Lecerf, 1986). In newborn guinea pigs exposed to Tamoxifen together with estradiol, similar effects on growth of uterus were stronger than in the animals exposed to Tamoxifen or estradiol alone (Pasqualini et al., 1986a). Tamoxifen stimulated the fetal and newborn guinea pig vagina, resulting in an increase in DNA content, wet weight and PR expression (Nguyen et al., 1986). When a combination of Tamoxifen and progesterone was given to neonatal guinea pigs, progesterone blocked the Tamoxifen-induced production of PR (Pasqualini et al., 1986b). N-Desmethyltamoxifen and 4-hydroxytamoxifen are more effective than cis-tamoxifen on growth and PR induction in the uterus and vagina of newborn guinea pigs (Lecerf et al., 1988). These findings indicate that Tamoxifen may act as an estrogen agonist on the uterus and vagina of guinea pigs during the perinatal period.

Female mice

In female C57BL/Tw mice given daily injections of 2, 20 or 100 microgram Tamoxifen starting with the day of birth, uteri were examined at 35 and 150 days of age (Iguchi et al., 1986a). Uterine hypoplasia was found in neonatally Tamoxifen-exposed mice as previously observed in similarly treated NMRI mice (Taguchi and Nishizuka, 1985). Uterine metaplasia and myometrial disorganization have been reported as major uterine abnormalities of mice exposed perinatally to estrogen (Newbold and McLachlan, 1982; Ostrander et al., 1985; Iguchi et al., 1986b,e, 1987b). In contrast, no uterine metaplasia was found in neonatally Tamoxifen-exposed mice, although the number of uterine glands significantly decreased in Tamoxifen-exposed mice, similar to Tamoxifen-exposed rats (Branham et al., 1985). Prenatal DES exposure (2 mg from Day 15 to 18 of gestation) also caused a retardation of uterine gland genesis and reduced the number of glands in mouse uteri (Iguchi and Takasugi, 1987). Vaginal hypoplasia and hypospadias were common abnormalities in 150-day-old Tamoxifen-exposed mice. Vaginal adenosis was encountered in 35-day-old mice exposed neonatally to 20 or 100 microgram Tamoxifen/day, but not permanent vaginal epithelial proliferation (Iguchi et al., 1986a). These results indicate that Tamoxifen has little permanent effect on the vaginal epithelium of neonatal mice.

In ovaries of Tamoxifen-exposed mice, luteinization was never observed (Forsberg, 1985; Taguchi and Nishizuka, 1985). Ovaries of Tamoxifen-exposed 150-day-old mice contained small follicles whose oocytes frequently underwent degeneration. Frequency of oocyte death

(14, 77 and 89%) rose with increase in Tamoxifen dose (2, 20 and 100 microgram) given to the neonates (Iguchi et al., 1986a). Follicular growth was markedly suppressed in ovaries of Tamoxifen-exposed mice, being similar to the ovary of hypophysectomized rats (cf. Selye et al., 1933). In addition, responsiveness of ovaries to prepubertally injected gonadotropin (hCG) was strikingly reduced in Tamoxifen-exposed mice (Iguchi et al., 1986a). These findings imply that the hypothalamo-hypophysio-ovarian system was impaired by neonatal Tamoxifen exposure comparable to neonatal estrogen exposure (Takasugi, 1976; Gorski et al., 1977). We found that specific binding of follicle-stimulating hormone to ovaries of 40-day-old C57BL mice exposed neonatally to 5 microgram DES and 100 microgram Tamoxifen for 5 days from the day of birth to be significantly lower than that in the controls (Iguchi, 1992).

Extensive adenosis-like lesions have been reported in 2- to 6-month-old NMRI mice exposed neonatally to Tamoxifen (Forsberg, 1985; Taguchi and Nishizuka, 1985) as reported in human females exposed prenatally to DES (Herbst et al., 1971; Herbst and Bern, 1981) and perinatally DES-exposed mice (Forsberg, 1969, 1979; Plapinger and Bern, 1979; Iguchi et al., 1986b, 1988a). Only small lesions were observed in the vaginal fornix of 35-day-old C57BL mice exposed neonatally to 20 or 100 microgram Tamoxifen/day (Iguchi et al., 1986a); however, extensive lesions were seen in the upper vaginal region of 35-day-old ICR mice exposed neonatally to 2-200 microgram Tamoxifen/day (22-100%), reflecting a probable strain difference (Iguchi et al., 1989b). Adenosis-like lesions were found in the cervical and upper vaginal regions derived from the Müllerian duct, especially in the common cervical canal and the vaginal fornix, but not in the lower vagina derived from the urogenital sinus; this result is in accordance with observations in prenatally DES-exposed mice (Iguchi et al., 1986b,c).

In neonatally Tamoxifen-exposed (200 microgram/day) mice, uteri were heavier and the epithelial cells were taller than in the controls, at 5 to 20 days of age. The uteri of Tamoxifen-exposed mice at 35 days had a significantly taller columnar epithelium and a smaller number of glands than the controls (Iguchi et al., 1989b). These findings suggest that neonatal Tamoxifen acts as an estrogen agonist on the uterovaginal epithelium and uterine glands. Uteri of mice exposed neonatally to Tamoxifen showed a reduced number of glands, a disorganization of the circular musculature and lowered responsiveness to estradiol given prepubertally (Iguchi et al., 1989b). Nascent uterine glands in intact mice appeared at 5-7 days (Plapinger, 1982; Iguchi and Takasaugi, 1987), however, in neonatally Tamoxifen-exposed mice, uterine epithelium began to invaginate at 5 days and formed nascent glands at 10 days (Iguchi et al., 1989b), suggesting a delay in the commencement of gland formation as reported in both neonatally Tamoxifen-exposed rats and prenatally DES-exposed mice (Branham et al., 1985; Iguchi and Takasugi, 1987).

In mice exposed neonatally to Tamoxifen, the organization of the stroma and the circular musculature was disrupted at ages of 5 and 10-15 days in ICR and C57BL strains, respectively (Iguchi et al., 1986a, 1989b). Neonatal Tamoxifen exposure induced changes in the density and distribution of types I and III collagen, fibronectin and laminin (Iguchi et al., 1989b). Irisawa and Iguchi (1990) found that type I collagen and fibronectin were absent from the uterine stroma of the edematous region, while laminin disappeared from the tunica muscularis in neonatally Tamoxifen-exposed, 15-day-old C57BL mice. Thus the suppression of gland formation and the lowered responsiveness to estrogen may result from changes in extracellular matrix proteins, and the increase in uterine weight in Tamoxifen-exposed mice during the prepubertal period is due to edema of the stroma. Tamoxifen induced a high incidence of polyovular follicles (Irisawa and Iguchi, 1990).

Tamoxifen (100 microgram/day) injections starting within 5 days after birth caused a high incidence of polyovular follicles in the ovary and aplasia of the tunica muscularis in the uterus at 60 days. Tamoxifen exposure starting within 7 postnatal days also induced atrophy of the uterine luminal epithelium. In mice given Tamoxifen within 3 days after birth, the vagina had a thinner epithelium than that in the controls (Irisawa and Iguchi, 1990). These findings suggest that the postnatal limit of the critical period for Tamoxifen induction of female genital abnormalities is within 3-7 days after birth.

Female human feti

The potential estrogenicity and teratogenicity of Tamoxifen were examined in 54 genital tracts isolated from 4- to 19-week-old human female fetuses and grown for 1 to 2 months in untreated athymic nude mice or host mice exposed to Tamoxifen or to DES (Cunha et al., 1987). Proliferation and maturation of the squamous vaginal epithelium were observed in specimens treated with these agents only when the feti were maintained to a gestational age equivalent to 16 weeks or more. The number of their endometrial and cervical glands was 87% of the control specimens maintained to a gestational age equivalent to 13 weeks or more in untreated hosts. By contrast, Tamoxifen-exposed specimens showed a 44% reduction of the glands seen in the control specimens. The developing uterus of untreated controls was separated into stroma and myometrium, whereas in Tamoxifen-exposed specimens, condensation and separation of the mesenchyme were greatly impaired. The oviduct was also affected by Tamoxifen, resulting in hyperplasia and disorganization of its epithelium. These findings emphasize the unrecognized estrogenicity and potential teratogenicity of Tamoxifen on the developing human genital tract, indicating the need for caution to prevent inadvertent exposure of the developing fetus to antiestrogens (see, Heel et al., 1978). This needs particular attention in view of the ongoing preventive administration of Tamoxifen in healthy women.

Male mice

In C57BL male mice given 5 daily injections of 2, 20 and 100 microgram Tamoxifen starting within 24 h after birth, weights of testes, gubernacula, seminal vesicles and epididymides were significantly lower in Tamoxifen-exposed (20 and 100 microgram/day) mice than in the controls at 160 days (Iguchi and Hirokawa, 1986). One of 10 Tamoxifen-exposed (2 microgram/day) mice possessed testes with extended intertubular spaces largely occupied by proliferated fibroblasts and showed a low spermatogenic index. In 13 mice given 20 microgram Tamoxifen, the mean spermatogenic index (67%) was lower than in the controls (88%). One mouse had testes lacking spermatids and spermatozoa; two mice had testes showing proliferation of fibroblasts in the intertubular spaces. In half of the 100 microgram Tamoxifen-exposed mice, spermatogenic indices were lowered (0-35%), whereas in the other half, the indices remained unaffected. In all mice exposed neonatally to Tamoxifen, coloidal secretion in the lumina of the seminal vesicles was reduced in amounts correlated with the dose, suggesting a reduced androgen secretion.

Taguchi (1987) has demonstrated genital abnormalities including testicular hypoplasia, suppression of spermatogenesis, intraabdominal testes, epididymal cysts and squamous metaplasia of seminal vesicles in 8-month-old NMRI/Tg male mice given 3 daily injections of 20 microgram Tamoxifen from the day of birth. Five daily injections of 100 microgram Tamoxifen from the day of birth resulted in a decrease in spermatogenic index (22%) in 60-day-old C57BL mice (Irisawa et al., 1990).

In C57BL mice exposed to 100 microgram Tamoxifen/day for 5 days beginning at various early postnatal ages (0=day of birth 3, 5, 7 and 10 days), the spermatogenic index, diameter of seminiferous tubules and Leydig cell nuclei were significantly less than in controls at 60 days (Irisawa et al., 1990). In mice given Tamoxifen starting at 0 and 3 days, 70% had testes with spermatogenic indices lower than 25%. Epithelial cell height in the epididymis and seminal vesicles of mice given Tamoxifen starting at 0 and 3 days was significantly lower than those in controls. The postnatal limit of the critical period for Tamoxifen-induced male genital organ dysfunction is 3 days after birth (Irisawa et al., 1990).

Abnormalities in os penis induced by neonatal exposure to Tamoxifen

The os penis of adult rats and mice is divided into two regions: the proximal segment is composed of bone with hyaline cartilage containing type II collagen at its proximal end, and the distal segment is composed of fibrocartilage having type I collagen (Glucksmann and Cherry, 1972). Hyaline cartilage, bone marrow and trabeculae formed in the proximal segment of control mice at 5 days were lacking in mice exposed neonatally to 100 microgram/day Tamoxifen for 5 days at ages of 10 and 30 days. The size of the proximal segment in neonatally Tamoxifen-exposed mice at 10-60 days was significantly smaller than that in age-matched controls (Iguchi et al., 1990b). The distal segment of the os penis developed into fibrocartilage by 30 days in the controls, whereas such cartilage was undetectable in mice exposed to Tamoxifen at 30 days neonatally (Iguchi et al., 1990b). Growth and ossification of the distal segment were also delayed in mice exposed neonatally to the antiandrogen, cyproterone acetate (Glucksmann et al., 1976), and castration within 4 days after birth inhibited the growth and ossification (Howard, 1959; Glucksmann et al., 1976). These results suggest that the growth and formation of fibrocartilage in the distal segment of the penis are caused by androgens present at birth.

In 60-day-old mice given Tamoxifen injections starting within 5 days, hyaline cartilage was undetectable in the proximal segment. In mice exposed to Tamoxifen starting at 7 or 10 days, hyaline cartilage was formed at 60 days; however, the size of the proximal segment was significantlly smaller than in controls (Iguchi et al., 1990b). These results indicate that Tamoxifen has a specific effect on suppression of hyaline cartilage in os penis, and that there is a critical period for the suppression of cartilage formation by Tamoxifen.

Spines on the glans penis skin begin to form in both control and neonatally Tamoxifen-exposed mice between 5 and 10 days of age, but the density was lower in neonatally Tamoxifen-exposed mice from 10 to 60 days than in the controls (Iguchi et al., 1990b). The epidermis of the glans penis and the prepuce began to separate at 10 days in the controls. In neonatally Tamoxifen-exposed mice, however, even at 60 days they remained unseparated. Spine formation was significantly suppressed by Tamoxifen exposure starting within 5 days but not by nafoxidine and clomiphene (Iguchi et al., 1990b), suggesting that Tamoxifen has a specific inhibitory effect on penal spine formation.

Nongenital abnormalities induced by perinatal exposure to Tamoxifen

Sexually dimorphic brain nuclei. The volume of the sexually dimorphic nucleus in the preoptic area (SDN-POA) of the rat brain is several-fold-larger in adult males than in adult females (Gorski et al., 1978; Jacobson et al., 1981; Döhler et al., 1982, 1984a). A single injection of Tamoxifen (Döhler et al., 1984b) permanently reduced the SDN-POA volume in male rats but not in female rats. Perinatal Tamoxifen exposure resulted in permanent anovulatory sterility without influencing SDN-POA in female rats (Döhler et al., 1986). Tamoxifen exposure did not alter serum levels of testosterone in male rats during the perinatal period, but inhibited the development of SDN-POA. The development of SDN-POA is primarily under estrogenic control and Tamoxifen acts as an estrogen antagonist on this structure.

Mouse pelvis. Sexual dimorphism of the pelvis has been described in mice (Gardner, 1936; Iguchi et al., 1989a; Uesugi et al., 1992a,b, 1993). Iguchi et al. (1986a) demonstrated that neonatal Tamoxifen exposure caused a long-lasting inhibition of pubic bone calcification, suggesting that the elastic and cartilaginous nature of the symphysis region persevered into adulthood. Neonatally Tamoxifen-exposed mice showed a hernia of urinary bladder with or without descent of the caecum through the subpubic space. Mice exposed to Tamoxifen starting at 0 to 10 days had significantly longer pubic ligaments than did the corresponding controls. However, mice exposed neonatally to clomiphene and nafoxidine show normal pubic bones.

In 120-day-old female mice exposed neonatally to 100 microgram Tamoxifen, the total area of the pelvis, and the individual areas of the ilium, ischium and pubis were significantly smaller than in the controls. There was no difference in length of the ischium between Tamoxifen-exposed and control mice of both sexes. However, lengths of ilium and pubis, and widths of ilium, pubis and ischium in Tamoxifen-exposed male and female mice were significantly smaller than in the respective controls. These results suggest that neonatal Tamoxifen exposure retards the growth of ilium and os pubis in mice (Uesugi et al., 1993). Neonatal exposure to Tamoxifen also altered the developmental pattern of the pelvis and femur, which contained lower concentrations of calcium and phosphorus than controls (Iguchi et al., 1995).

In 15-day-old neonatally Tamoxifen-exposed mice, the osteoclastic surface, the number of osteoclasts per unit area, and the number of nuclei per osteoclast were significantly smaller than those in the controls. The ratio of ossified area to pubic bone was significantly larger (Uesugi et al., 1993). These findings indicate that neonatal Tamoxifen suppressed osteoclastic activity. Inhibition of ossification persisted in the junction of pubis and ischium of a pelvis transplanted under the kidney capsule after *in vitro* Tamoxifen exposure (Uesugi et al., 1993). Further studies are needed to clarify alterations of gene expression of bone matrix proteins and alkaline phosphatase (Turner et al., 1990) in the innominate bone of mice exposed neonatally to Tamoxifen.

Estrogen is required to maintain bone density and prevent osteoporosis (Takano-Yamamoto and Rodan, 1990). Tamoxifen is an antiestrogen but there appears to be a target site specificity to its action (Jordan, 1990). Tamoxifen has an estrogen-like effect upon bone in ovariectomized adult rats (Turner et al., 1987, 1988, 1994); although it inhibits estrogen-stimulated increase in ovariectomized rat uterine wet weight, it has an additive estrogenic effect on bone density in rats (Jordan et al., 1987). Fentiman et al. (1989) reported that Tamoxifen administration (10 or 20 mg/day) for periods of 3-6 months did not influence spinal or femoral bone density, osteocalcin, alkaline phosphatase and electrolytes in humans.

Molecular changes in reproductive tracts by Tamoxifen

The growth stimulatory effect of estrogen on the uterus involves regulation of expression of immediate early responses genes, *jun* and *fos* protooncogenes, whose products control the cell cycle (Loose-Mitchell et al., 1988; Hyder et al., 1992; Chiapetta et al., 1992; Cicatiello et al., 1992; Weisz and Bresciani, 1988; Weisz and Rosales, 1990; Weisz et al.,

1990; Webb et al., 1991; Iguchi et al., 1995; Kamiya et al., 1995). The molecular events that mediate transcription of estrogen-regulated genes include binding of estrogen to the estrogen receptor (ER), activation of the receptor-ligand complex, binding of the receptor to ER elements on the chromatin and transactivation of factors that initiate gene transcription (for review, Carson-Jurica et al., 1990).

In mice, uterine epithelial cells (Korach et al., 1988; Yamashita et al., 1989; Bigsby et al., 1990; Greco et al., 1991; Sato et al., 1992), seminal vesicles and prostate (Sato et al., 1994a) have no ER, at least for 5 postnatal days. A single injection of estrogen on the day of birth induced ER protein expression (Yamashita et al., 1990; Sato et al., 1992), and a single injection of 100 microgram Tamoxifen at 0 day also induced ER protein expression in mouse uterine epithelial cells within 24 h thereafter (Sato et al., 1994b), and 5 daily injections of 5 microgram DES induced ER in seminal vesicles and prostate (Sato et al., 1994a). ER mRNA expression of uterine stromal cells and epithelial cells in newborn mice increased after 4 h and 8 h, respectively, after a single injection of Tamoxifen on day 0. In the ovariectomized adult mice, a single injection of 100 microgram Tamoxifen increased both ER mRNA expression and mitotic rates in uterine and vaginal epithelial cells 12 h and 24 h after the injection (Sato et al., 1994b).

In immature ovariectomized Sprague-Dawley rat, 1 mg/kg Tamoxifen increased c-fos mRNA expression ca. 20-fold in 8 h, which is comparable in magnitude to that produced by 40 microgram/kg estradiol. c-fos mRNA induction is observed at doses of 0.1-10 mg/kg Tamoxifen. The induction of c-fos mRNA by both estradiol and Tamoxifen is blocked by medroxyprogesterone acetate. Tamoxifen also increased uterine levels of c-jun, jun-B and c-myc mRNAs (Kirkland et al., 1993). In ovariectomized adult rat uterus, 1 mg/kg Tamoxifen induced elevation of c-fos mRNA 2.4- to 6.2-fold 6 to 24 h after Tamoxifen injection. Tamoxifen also induced marked elevation of jun-B mRNA by ca. 10-fold in 24 h. Only a slight induction of c-jun and jun-D expression occurred by 12 h after Tamoxifen treatment (Nephew et al., 1993). In the ovariectomized adult mouse uterus, 100 microgram Tamoxifen increased ER, c-jun and c-fos mRNAs 1, 3 and 3 h after the injection, respectively (Nishimura et al., 1992). These results indicate that Tamoxifen acts in $vivo$ as an estrogen agonist, activating expression of cellular oncogenes in normal uterine tissue in rats and mice.

In humans, Tamoxifen showed a down-regulation of growth factors (Jordan, 1993) such as insulin-like growth factor I (Colletti et al., 1989;

Pollak et al., 1990) and transforming growth factor-alpha (Noguchi et al., 1993), and oncogenes such as c-*erb*B-2 and c-*myc* (Le Roy et al., 1991) in patients with breast cancer. The estrogenic and uterine stimulatory effects of Tamoxifen are a safety concern in long term Tamoxifen therapy (Jordan, 1992). Recent clinical trials demonstrated an increased incidence in uterine cancer in patients receiving long term Tamoxifen therapy (Fornander et al., 1989; Malfetano, 1990; Anderson et al., 1991; DeMuylder et al., 1991; Gal et al., 1991; Ismail, 1994; Neven et al., 1994). Estrogenic activity of Tamoxifen has been reported in human endometrial carcinoma cells in culture (Anzai et al., 1989; Gong et al., 1992). In addition, human endometrial carcinoma displays enhanced growth in athymic nude mice treated with Tamoxifen (Satyaswaroop et al., 1984; Clark and Satyaswaroop, 1985; Gottardis et al., 1990). Studies using nude mice transplanted with both breast tumour and endometrial carcinoma cells demonstrated that while Tamoxifen controlled estrogen-stimulated growth of the breast tumor, endometrial tumor growth was enhanced by Tamoxifen (Gottardis et al., 1988). In human endometrial carcinoma grown in nude mice, Tamoxifen stimulated c-*fos* and c-*jun* expression in a similar pattern but to a lesser degree than estradiol (Sakakibara et al., 1992). Thus, in addition to mammary cells, endometrial cells also appear to be a primary target for Tamoxifen.

Conclusions

Tamoxifen increases uterine weight, protein and DNA in ovariectomized adult mice, and neonatal exposure to Tamoxifen induces infertility by modification of the hypothalamo-hypophysio-ovarian axis, vaginal adenosis, uterine hypoplasia, ovarian dysgenesis, polyovular follicles in female mice, reduction of decidual response in rat uterus to an artifical stimulus, and persistent suppression of spermatogenesis and atrophy of seminal vesicle, epididymis and gubernaculum in male mice. In addition to these abnormalities in reproductive organs, neonatal exposure to Tamoxifen affects the development of bones such as pelvis, femur and os penis (Iguchi, 1992).

During long term adjuvant Tamoxifen therapy, levels of Tamoxifen and its metabolites are high and tissues will be saturated with antiestrogens. Even if Tamoxifen were stopped in a patient immediately after discovery of her pregnancy, the long plasma half-life at steady state would result in the drug being present for at least 6 weeks (Furr and Jordan, 1984; Jordan, 1990). A fetus could thus be exposed to the drug throughout the first trimester. Therefore, as suggested by Jordan and Murphy (1990), the present authors strongly suggest that Tamoxifen should not be taken during an ambiguous period of pregnancy as well as the obvious period.

The prenatal and neonatal mouse models continue to provide information of possible occurrence of genital abnormalities in human offspring exposed to Tamoxifen and related compounds. In further studies, however, as indicated in this review, attention should be paid to non-genital organs as well as genital organs exposed to Tamoxifen during fetal and early postnatal development in mammals including humans.

ACKNOWLEDGMENTS

The author wishes to thank Emeritus Professor Noboru Takasugi, Yokohama City University for his continuous encouragement, valuable advice and critical reading of this review. Some studies described herein were supported by a Grant-in-Aid from the Ministry of Education, Science and Culture of Japan, a grant from the Kihara Foundation for Scientific research and a grant in Support of the Promotion of Research at Yokohama City University.

REFERENCES

Anderson M, Storm H and Mouridsen HT (1991): Incidence of new primary cancers after adjuvant tamoxifen therapy and radiotherapy for early cancer. *J Natl Cancer Inst* 83:1013-1017

Anzai Y, Holinka CF, Hirouki K Na Gurpide E (1989): Stimulatory effects of 4-hydroxytamoxifen on proliferation of human endometrial adenocarcinoma cells (Ishikawa line). *Cancer Res* 49:2362-2365

Arai Y, Mori T, Suzuki Y and Bern HA (1983): Long-term effects of perinatal exposure to sex steroids and diethystilbestrol on the reproductive system of male mammals. *Int Rev Cytol* 84:235-268

Baum M, Brinkley DM, Dossett JA, McPherson K, Patterson JS, Rubens RD, Smiddy FG, Stoll BA, Wilson A, Richards D and Ellis SH (1985): Controlled trial of tamoxifen as single adjuvant agent in management of early breast cancer. *Lancet* 1:836-840

Bern HA (1992a): Diethylstilbestrol (DES) syndrome: present status of animal and human studies. In: *Hormonal Carcinogenesis*. Li, J, Nandi S, Li SA, eds. Springer-Verlag, New York, pp 1-8

Bigsby RM, Aixin L, Luo K and Cunha GR (1990): Strain differences in the ontogeny of estrogen receptors in murine uterine epithelium. *Endocrinology* 126:2592-2596

Branham WS, Lyn-Cook BD, Andrews A and Sheehan DM (1993b): Growth of separated and recombined neonatal rat uterine luminal epithelium and stroma on extracellular matrix: Effects of in vivo tamoxifen exposure. *In Vitro Cell Dev Biol* 29A:408-414

Branham WS, Sheehan DM, Zehr DR, Medlock KL, Nelson CJ and Ridlon E (1985): Inhibition of rat uterine gland genesis by tamoxifen. *Endocrinology* 117:2238-2248

Branham WS, Zehr DR, Chen JJ and Sheehan DM (1988a): Postnatal uterine development in the rat: Estrogen and antiestrogen effects on luminal epithelium. *Teratology* 38:29-36

Branham WS, Zehr DR, Chen JJ and Sheehan DM (1988b): Alterations in developing rat uterine cell populations after neonatal exposure to estrogens and antiestrogens. *Teratology* 38:271-279

Branham WS, Zehr DR and Sheehan D (1993a): Differential sensitivity of rat uterine growth and epithelium hypertrophy to estrogens and antiestrogens. *Proc Soc Exp Biol Med* 203:297-303

Carson-Jurica MA, Schrader WT and O'Malley BW (1990): Steroid receptor family: structure and functions. *Endocr Rev* 11:201-220

Chamness GC, Bannayan GA, Landry Jr LA, Scheridan PJ and McGuire WL (1979): Abnormal reproductive development in rats after neonatally administered anti-estrogen (tamoxifen). *Biol Reprod* 21:1087-1090

Chiappetta C, Kirkland JL, Loose-Mitchell DS, Murphy L and Stancel GM (1992): Estrogen regulates expression of the *jun* family of protooncogenes in the uterus. *J Steroid Biochem Mol Biol* 41:113-123

Chou Y-C, Iguchi T and Bern HA (1992): Effects of antiestrogens on adult and neonatal mouse reproductive organs. *Reprod Toxicol* 6:439-446

Cicatiello L, Ambrosino C, Coletta B, Scalona M, Sica V, Bresciani F and Weisz A (1992): Transcriptional activation of *jun* and actin genes by estrogen during mitogenic stimulation of rat uterine cells. *J Steroid Biochem Mol Biol* 41:523-528

Clark LL and Satyaswaroop PG (1985): Photoaffinity labeling of the progesterone receptor from human endometrial carcinoma. *Cancer Res* 45:5417-5420

Cole MP, Jones CTA and Todd IDH (1971): A new anti-oestrogenic agent in late breast cancer. *Br J Cancer* 25:270-275

Colletti RB, Roberts JD, Devlin JT and Copeland KC (1989): Effect of tamoxifen on plasma insulin-like growth factor I in patients with breast cancer. *Cancer Res* 49:1882-1884

Cunha GR, Taguchi O, Nishizuka Y and Robboy SJ (1987): Teratogenic effects of clomiphene, tamoxifen and diethylstilbestrol on the developing human femal genital tract. *Hum Pathol* 18:1132-1143

DeMuylder X, Neven P, DeSomer M, VanBelle Y, Vanderick G and DeMuylder E (1991): Endometrial lesions in patients undergoing tamoxifen therapy. *Int J Gynaecol Obstet* 36:127-130

Dix CJ and Jordan VC (1980): Modulation of rat uterine steroid hormone receptors by estrogen and antiestrogen. *Endocrinology* 107:2011-2020

Döhler K-D, Coquelin A, Davis F, Hines M, Shryne JE and Gorski RA (1984a): Pre- and postnatal influence of testosterone propionate and diethystilbestrol on differentiation of the sexually dimorphic nucleus of the preoptic area in male and female rats. *Brain Res* 302:291-295

Döhler K-D, Coquelin A, Davis F, Hines M, Shryne JE, Sickmöller PM, Jarzab B and Gorski RA (1986): Pre- and postnatal influence of an estrogen antagonist and an androgen antagonist on differentiation of sexually dimorphic nucleus of the preoptic areas in male and female rats. *Neuroendocrinology* 42:443-448

Döhler K-D, Hines M, Coquelin A, Davis F, Shryne JE and Gorski RA (1982): Pre- and postnatal influence of diethylstilbestrol on differentiation of the sexually dimorphic nucleus in the preoptic area of the female rat brain. *Neuroendocr Lett* 4:361-365

Döhler K-D, Srivastava SS, Shryne JE, Jarzab B, Sipos A and Gorski RA (1984b): Differentiation of the sexually dimorphic nucleus in the preoptic area of rat brain is inhibited by postnatal treatment with an estrogen antagonist. *Neuroendocrinology* 38:297-301

Fentiman IS, Caleffi M, Rodin A, Murby B and Fogelman I (1989): Bone mineral content of women receiving tamoxifen for mastalgia. *Br J Cancer* 60:262-264

Fornander T, Rutqvist LE, Cedermark BV, Glas U, Mattson A, Silversward JD, Skoog L, Somell A, Theve T, Wilking N, Askergren J and Hjolmar ML (1989): Adjuvant tamoxifen in early breast cancer: occurrence of new primary cancers. *Lancet* 1:117-119

Forsberg J-G (1969): The development of atypical epithelium in the mouse uterine cervix and vaginal fornix after neonatal oestradiol treatment. *Br J Exp Pathol* 50:187-195

Forsberg J-G (1979): Development mechanism of estrogen-induced irreversible changes in the mouse cervicovaginal epithelium. *Natl Cancer Inst Monogr* 51:41-50

Forsberg J-G (1985): Treatment with different antiestrogens in the neonatal period and effects in the cervicovaginal epithelium and ovaries of adult mice: A comparison to estrogen-induced changes. *Biol Reprod* 32:427-441

Furr BJA and Jordan VC (1984): The pharmacology and clinical uses of tamoxifen. *Pharmac Ther* 25:127-205

Gal D, Kopel S, Bashevkin M, Lebowitcz L, Lev R and Tancer ML (1991):
    Oncogenic potential of tamoxifen on endometria of postmenopausal
    women with breast cancer - preliminary report. *Gynecol Oncol* 42:120-
    123

Gardner WU (1936): Sexual dimorphism of the pelvis of the mouse, the effect
    of estrogenic hormones upon the pelvis and upon the development of
    scrotal hernias. *Am J Anat* 59:459-483

Herbst AL and Bern HE (eds) (1981):   Developmental Effects of
    Diethylstilbestrol (DES) in Pregnancy. New York, Thieme-Stratton, pp
    203

Herbst AL, Ulfelder H and Poskanzer DC (1971):   Adenocarcinoma of the
    vagina: association of maternal stilbestrol therapy with tumor appearance
    in young women. *New Engl J Med* 284:878-881

Howard E (1959):   A complementary action of corticosterone and
    dehydropiandrosterone on the mouse adrenal, with observations on the
    reactivity of reproductive tract structures to dehydroepiadrosterone and 11-
    hydroxy-androstenedione. *Endocrinology* 65:785-801

Hyder SM, Stancel GM, Nawaz Z, McDonnell DP and Loose-Mitchell DM
    (1992): Identification of an estrogen response element in the 3'-flanking
    region of the murine c-*fos* protooncogene. *J Biol Chem* 267:18047-18054

Iguchi T (1992):   Cellular effects of early exposure to sex hormones and
    antihormones. *Int Rev Cytol* 139:1-57

Iguchi T and Bern HA (1995): Transgenerational effects: intrauterine exposure
    to diethylstilbestrol (DES) in humans and the neonatal mouse model. In:
    Comments on Toxicology, A Soto ed., Gordon and Breach (in press)

Iguchi T, Fukazawa Y and Bern HA (1995):   Effects of sex hormones on
    oncogene expression in vagina and on development of sexual dimorphism
    of pelvis and anococcygeus muscle in the mouse. *Environment Health
    Perspect* (in press)

Iguchi T and Hirokawa (1986): Changes in male genital organs of mice exposed
    neonatally to tamoxifen. *Proc Japan Acad* 62B:157-160

Iguchi T, Hirokawa M and Takasugi N (1986a):   Occurence of genital tract
    abnormalities and bladder hernia in female mice exposed neonatally to
    tamoxifen. *Toxicology* 42:1-11

Iguchi T, Irisawa S, Fukazawa Y, Uesugi Y and Takasugi N (1989a):
    Permanent chondrification in the pelvis and occurence of hernias in mice
    treated neonatally with tamoxifen. *Reprod Toxicol* 2:127-134

Iguchi T, Irisawa S, Uesugi Y, Kusunoki S and Takasugi N (1990b): Abnormal
    development of the os penis in male mice treated neonatally with
    tamoxifen. *Acta Anat* 139:201-208

Iguchi T, Ostrander PL, Mills KT and Bern HA (1987b): Ovary-independent
    and ovary-dependent uterine squamous metaplasia in mice induced by
    neonatal exposure to diethylstilbestrol. *Med Sci Res* 15:489-490

Iguchi T, Ostrander PL, Mills KT and Bern HA (1988b): Vaginal abnormalities in ovariectomized BALB/cCrgl mice after neonatal exposure to different doses of diethylstilbestrol. *Cancer Lett* 43:207-214

Iguchi T, Takase M and Takasugi N (1986b): Development of vaginal adenosis-like lesions and uterine epithelial stratification in mice exposed perinatally to diethylstilbestrol. *Proc Soc Exp Biol Med* 181:59-65

Iguchi T, Takase M and Takasugi N (1986c): Persistent anovulation in the ovary of mice treated with human chorionic gonadotropin starting at different early postnatal ages. *IRCS Med Sci* 14:187-188

Iguchi T, and Takasugi N (1987): Postnatal development of uterine abnormalities in mice exposed to DES in utero. *Biol Neonate* 52:97-103

Iguchi T, Takei T, Takase M and Takasugi N (1986e): Estrogen participation in induction of cervicovaginal adenosis-like lesions in immature mice exposed prenatally to diethylstilbestrol. *Acta Anat* 127:110-114

Iguchi T, Todoroki R, Yamaguchi S and Takasugi N (1989b): Changes in the uterus and vagina of mice treated neonatally with antiestrogens. *Acta Anat* 136:146-154

Irisawa S and Iguchi T (1990): Critical period of induction by tamoxifen of genital organ abnormalities in female mice. *In Vivo* 4:175-180

Irisawa S, Iguchi T and Takasugi N (1990): Critical period of induction by tamoxifen of genital organ abnormalities in male mice. *Zool Sci* 6:541-545

Ismail SM (1994): Pathology of endometrium treated with tamoxifen. *J Clin Pathol* 47:827-833

Jacobson CD, Csernus VJ, Shryne JE and Gorski RA (1981): The influence of gonadectomy, androgen exposure, or a gonadal graft in the neonatal rat on the volume of the sexually dimorphic nucleus of the preoptic area. *J Neurosci* 1:1142-1147

Jordan VC (1990): Long-term adjuvant tamoxifen therapy for breast cancer. *Breast Cancer Res Treat* 15:125-136

Jordan VC (1992): The role of tamoxifen in the treatment and prevention of breast cancer. *Curr Problems Cancer* 16:134-176

Jordan VC (1993): Growth factor regulation by tamoxifen is demonstrated in patients with breast cancer. *Cancer* 72:1-2

Jordan VC, Dix CJ, Naylor KE, Prestwich G and Rowsby L (1978): Non-steroidal antiestrogens: Their biological effects and potential mechanisms of action. *J Toxicol Environ* 4:364-390

Jordan VC and Gosden B (1982): Importance of the alkylaminoethoxy side-chain for the estrogenic and antiestrogen actions of tamoxifen and trioxifen in the immature rat uterus. *Mol Cell Endocrinol* 7:291-306

Jordan VC and Koerner S (1976): Tamoxifen as an antitumour agent: role of oestradiol and prolactin. *J Endocrinol* 68:305-310

Jordan VC and Murphy CS (1990): Endocrine pharmacology of antiestrogens as antitumor agents. *Endocr Rev* 11:578-610

Jordan VC, Phelps EL and Lindgren JU (1987): Effects of antiestrogens on bone in castrated and intact female rats. *Breast Cancer Res Treat* 10:31-35

Kamiya K, Sato T, Nishimura N, Goto Y, Kano K and Iguchi T (1995): Expression of estrogen receptor and proto-oncogene messenger ribonucleic acids in reproductive tracts of neonatally diethylstilbestrol-exposed female mice with or without postpubertal estrogen administration. *Exp Clin Endocrinol* (in press)

Kang YH, Anderson WA and DeSombre ER (1975): Modulation of uterine morphology and growth by estradiol-17ß and estrogen antagonist. *J Cell Biol* 64:682-691

Kincle FA (1990): *Hormones and Toxicity in the Neonate.* pp 334, Springer-Verlag, Berlin

Kirkland JL, Murphy L and Stancel GM (1993): Tamoxifen stimulates expression of the c-*fos* proto-oncogene in rodent uterus. *Mol Pharmacol* 43:709-714

Korach KS, Horigome T, Tomooka Y, Yamashita S, Newbold RR and McLachlan (1988): Immunodetection of estrogen receptor in epithelial and stromal tissues of neonatal mouse uterus. *Proc Natl Acad Sci USA* 85:3334-3337

Lecerf F, Nguyen B-L and Pasqualini JR (1988): Biological effects and ultrastructural alterations of cis-tamoxifen, N-desmethyltamoxifen and 4-hydroxytamoxifen in the uterus and vagina of newborn guinea pigs. *Acta Endocrinol* 119:85-90

Le Roy X, Escot C, Brouillet J-P, Theillet C, Maudelonde T, Simony-Lafontaine J, Pujol H and Rochefort H (1991): Decrease of c-*erb*B-2 and c-*myc* RNA levels in tamoxifen-treated breast cancer. *Oncogene* 6:431-437

Loose-Mitchell DS, Chiappetta C and Stancel GM (1988): Estrogen-regulation of c-*fos* messenger ribonucleic acid. *Mol Endocrinol* 2:946-951

Malfetano JH (1990): Tamoxifen-associated endometrial carcinoma in postmenopausal breast cancer patients. *Gynecol Oncol* 39:82-84

Mori T and Nagasawa H (eds) (1988): *Toxicity of Hormones in Perinatal Life.* p. 184, Boca Raton, Florida, CRC Press

Nephew KP, Polek TC, Akcali KC and Khan SA (1993): The antiestrogen tamoxifen induces c-*fos* and *jun*-B, but not c-*jun* or *jun*-D, protooncogenes in the rat uterus. *Br Med J* 309:1313-1314

Newbold RR and McLachlan JA (1982): Vaginal adenosis and adenocarcinoma in mice exposed prenatally or neonatally to diethylstilbestrol. *Cancer Res* 42:2003-2011

Newbold RR and McLachlan JA (1988): Neoplastic and non-neoplastic lesions in male reproductive organs following perinatal exposure to hormones and related substances. In: *Toxicity of Hormones in Perinatal Life*. Mori T and Nagasawa H (eds), CRC Press, Boca Raton, Florida, pp 89-109

Nguyen BL, Giambiagi N, Mayrand C, Lecerf F and Pasqualini JR (1986): Estrogen and progesterone receptors in the fetal and newborn vagina of guinea pig: Biological, morphological and ultrastructural responses to tamoxifen and estradiol. *Endocrinology* 119:978-988

Nishimura N, Goto Y and Iguchi T (1993): Tamoxifen induces expressions of oncogenes and estrogen receptor in genital tracts of female mice. *Zool Sci Suppl* 10:128

Noguchi S, Motomura K, Inaji H, Imaoka S and Koyama H (1993): Down-regulation of transforming growth factor-alpha by tamoxifen in human breast cancer. *Cancer* 72:131-136

Ohta Y (1982): Deciduoma formation in rats ovariectomized at different ages. *Biol Reprod* 27:303-311

Ohta Y (1985): Deciduomal response in prepubertal rats adrenalectomized-ovariectomized at different ages of early postnatal life. *Zool Sci* 2:89-93

Ohta Y (1995): Sterility in neonatally androgenized female rats and the decidual cell reaction. *Int Rev Cytol* 160:1-52

Ohta Y, Iguchi T and Takasugi N (1989): Deciduoma formation in rats treated neonatally with the anti-estrogens tamoxifen and MER-25. *Reprod Toxicol* 3:207-212

Ohta Y and Takasugi N (1974): Ultrastructural changes in the testis of mice given neonatal injections of estrogen. *Endocrinol Japan* 21:183-190

Ostrander PL, Mills KT and Bern HA (1985): Long-term responses of the mouse uterus to neontal diethylstilbestrol treatment and to later sex hormone exposure. *J Natl Cancer Inst* 74:121-135

Pasqualini JR and LEcerf F (1986): Ultrastructural modifications provokes by tamoxifen either along or combined with oestradiol in the uteri of fetal or newborn guinea-pigs. *J Endocrinol* 110:197-202

Pasqualini JR, Nguyen B-L, Mayrand C and Lecerf F (1986a): Oestrogen agonistic effects of tamoxifen in the uterus of newborn guinea pigs after short and long treatment. Biological and histological studies. *Acta Endocrinol* 111:378-386

Pasqualini JR, Nguyen B-L, Sumida C, Giambiagi N and Mayrand C (1986b): Tamoxifen and progesterone effects in target tissues during the perinatal period. *J Steroid Biochem* 25:853-857

Plapinger L (1982): Surface morphology of uterine and vaginal epithelia in mice during normal postnatal development. *Biol Reprod* 26:961-972

Plapinger L and Bern HA (1979): Adenosis-like lesions and other cervicovaginal abnormalities in mice treated perinatally with estrogen. *J Natl Cancer Inst* 63:507-518

Pollak M, Costantino J, Blauer S-A, Guyda H, Redmond C, Fisher B and Margolese R (1990): Effect of tamoxifen on serum insulin-like growth factor I levels in stage I breast cancer patients. *J Natl Cancer Inst* 82:1693-1697

Sakakibara K, Kan NC and Satyaswaroop PG (1992): Both 17ß-estradiol and tamoxifen induce c-*fos* messenger ribonucleic acid expression in human endometrial carcinoma grown in nude mice. *Am J Obstet Gynecol* 166:206-212

Sato T, Chiba A, Hayashi S, Okamura H, Ohta Y, Takasugi N and Iguchi T (1994a): Induction of estrogen receptor and cell division in genital tracts of male mice by neonatal exposure to diethylstilbestrol. *Reprod Toxicol* 8:145-153

Sato T, Ohta Y, Okamura H, Hayashi S and Iguchi T (1994b): Estrogen receptor mRNA expression in the genital tract of female mice by estrogen (DES) and antiestrogen (tamoxifen). *Zool Sci Suppl* 11:17

Sato T, Okamura H, Ohta Y, Hayashi S, Takamatsu Y, Takasugi N and Iguchi T (1992): Estrogen receptor expression in the genital tract of female mice treated neonatally with diethylstilbestrol. *In Vivo* 6:151-156

Satyaswaroop PG, Zaino RJ and Mortel R (1984): Estrogen-like effects of tamoxifen on human endometrial carcinoma transplanted into nude mice. *Cancer Res* 44:4006-4010

Selye H, Collip JB and Thomson DL (1933): On the effect of the anterior pituitary-like hormone on the ovary of the hypophysectomized rat. *Endocrinology* 17:494-500

Sutherland RL, Mester J and Baulien EE (1977): Tamoxifen is a potent 'pure' antiestrogen in chick oviduct. *Nature* 267:434-435

Taguchi O (1987): Reproductive tract lesions in male mice treated neonatally with tamoxifen. *Biol Reprod* 37:113-116

Taguchi O and Nishizuka Y (1985): Reproductive tract abnormalities in female mice treated neonatally with tamoxifen. *Am J Obstet Gynecol* 151:675-678

Takamatsu Y, Iguchi T and Takasugi N (1992): Effects of postpubertal treatment with diethylstilbestrol and tamoxifen on protein expression in the vagina and uterus of neonatally diethylstilbestrol-exposed mice. *In Vivo* 6:271-278

Takano-Yamamoto T and Rodan GA (1990): Direct effects of 17ß-estradiol on trabecular bone in ovariectomized rats. *Proc Natl Acad Sci USA* 87:2172-2176

Takasugi N (1963): Vaginal cornification in persistent-estrous mice. *Endocrinology* 72:607-619

Takasugi N (1976): Cytological basis for permanent vaginal changes in mice treated neonatally with steroid hormones. *Int Rev Cytol* 44:193-224

Takasugi N (1979): Development of permanently proliferated and cornified vaginal epithelium in mice treated neonatally with steroid hormones and the implication in tumorigenesis. *Natl Cancer Inst Monogr* 51:57-66

Takasugi N, Bern HA and DeOme KB (1962): Persistent vaginal cornification in mice. *Science* 138:438-439

Terenius L (1971): Structure-activity relationships of anti-oestrogens with regard to interaction with 17ß-oestradiol in the mouse uterus and vagina. *Acta Endocrinol Suppl* 66:431-447

Turner RT, Colvard DS and Spelsberg TC (1990): Estrogen inhibition of peiosteal bone formation in rat long bones: down-regulation of gene expression for bone matrix proteins. *Endocrinology* 127:1346-1351

Turner RT, Riggs BL and Spelsberg TC (1994): Skeletal effects of estrogen. *Endocr Rev* 15:275-300

Turner RT, Wakley GK, Hannon KS and Bell NH (1987): Tamoxifen prevents the skeletal effects of ovarian hormone deficiency in rats. *J Bone Min Res* 2:449-456

Turner RT, Wakley GK, Hannon KS and Bell NH (1988): Tamoxifen inhibits osteoclast-mediated resorption of trabecular bone in ovarian hormone deficient rats. *Endocrinology* 122:1146-1150

Uesugi Y, Ohta Y, Asashima M and Iguchi T (1992a): Comparative study of sexual dimorphism of the innominate bone in rodents and amphibians. *Anat Rec* 234:432-437

Uesugi Y, Taguchi O, Noumura T and Iguchi T (1992b): Effects of steroids on the development of sexual dimorphism in mouse innominate bone. *Anat Rec* 234:541-548

Uesugi Y, Sato T and Iguchi T (1993): Morphometric analysis of the pelvis in mice treated neonatally with tamoxifen. *Anat Rec* 235:126-130

Webb DK, Moulton BC and Kahn SA (1991): Estrogen induced expression of the c-*jun* protooncogene in the mature and immature rat uterus. *Biochem Biophys Res Commun* 175:480-485

Weisz A and Bresciani F (1988): Estrogen induces expression of c-*fos* and c-*myc* protooncogenes in rat uterus. *Mol Endocrinol* 2:816-824

Weisz A, Cicatiello L, Persico M and Bresciani F (1990): Estrogen stimulated transcription of c-*jun* proto-oncogene. *Mol Endocrinol* 4:1041-1050

Weisz A and Rosales R (1990): Identification of an estrogen response element upstream of the human c-*fos* gene that binds the estrogen receptor and the AP-1 transcription factor. *Nucleic Acids Res* 18:5097-5106

Yamashita S, Newbold RR, McLachlan JA and Korach KS (1989): Development pattern of estrogen receptor expression in female mouse genital tracts. *Endocrinology* 125:2888-2896

Yamashita S, Newbold RR, McLachlan JA and Korach KS (1990): The role of estrogen receptor in uterine epithelial proliferation and cytodifferentiation in neonatal mice. *Endocrinology* 127:2456-2463

9. THE COVALENT BINDING OF TAMOXIFEN TO PROTEINS AND DNA

David Kupfer

Tamoxifen is currently being used in adjuvant therapy for all stages of breast cancer (Jordan, 1995). Although initially Tamoxifen was earmarked for treatment of estrogen receptor (ER)-positive tumors, surprisingly and contrary to expectations a significant number of patients with ER-negative tumors also respond to Tamoxifen therapy. Of concern, however, are the findings that in the course of treatment a considerable number of breast tumors develop resistance to Tamoxifen therapy (see chapter 5) and that the mode of emergence of tumor resistance is not completely understood.

A noteworthy dilemma concerning Tamoxifen action arises from the observations that Tamoxifen exhibits different effects in different species; namely, Tamoxifen is a pure estrogen antagonist in the chicken, a partial agonist/antagonist in the rat and a pure agonist in the mouse (Harper and Walpole, 1967; Terenius, 1971; Sutherland et al., 1977; Furr and Jordan, 1984). Additionally, it is not understood why Tamoxifen is a partial agonist/antagonist in the uterus and an agonist in bone. Thus, the mechanism of action of Tamoxifen involving its reversible binding to the ER at the estradiol-binding site does not fully explain the complexity of its biological and pharmacological activity.

Recently, a large scale clinical trial was initiated to determine the potential for the prophylactic use of Tamoxifen against breast cancer in women considered at risk of contracting that disease (Fisher and Redmond, 1991; Jordan, 1992). However, of some concern are the observations that Tamoxifen treatment increases the incidence of endometrial cancer, and possibly of liver cancer in humans (Dauplat et al., 1990; Killackey et al., 1985; Fornander et al. 1989 - see chapter 4), and causes hepatocellular carcinoma in rats and p53 (tumor suppressor gene) mutations (Williams et al., 1993; Vancutsem, 1994). The mechanism of these carcinogenic manifestations associated with Tamoxifen treatment is not understood and consequently it is the subject of the current intensive investigation in several laboratories.

The above enigmas pertaining to the mechanism of action of Tamoxifen and of its side effects suggested the possibility that Tamoxifen metabolism, and particularly alteration of its metabolism, may play a role in the complexity of its activities. This chapter describes the observations that Tamoxifen metabolism results in the formation of reactive intermediate(s) that bind covalently to proteins and DNA. In turn, it is hypothesized that the mechanism of the Tamoxifen-associated carcinogenic effects involves the participation of Tamoxifen metabolites/ reactive intermediates and tamoxifen-macromolecular adducts.

Tamoxifen metabolism

Several studies demonstrated that Tamoxifen is metabolized by liver microsomes of animals and humans into a variety of compounds, most notably into the corresponding N-oxide (tam-N-oxide), N-desmethyl (N-desmethyl-tam), and 4-hydroxy (4-OH-tam) derivatives (Foster et al. 1980; Reunitz et al., 1984; McCague and Seago, 1986; Lyman and Jordan, 1986; Mani et al., 1993a; Kupfer and Dehal, 1996). Also, smaller amounts of 3,4-dihydroxy-tam, α-hydroxy-tam, α-hydroxy-tam-N-oxide, α-hydroxy-N-desmethyl-tam, 4-hydroxy-tam-N-oxide and Tamoxifen epoxide (Fig 1) have been detected (Reunitz et al., 1984; Lim et al., 1994; Phillips, 1994b; Poon et al., 1993; Poon et al., 1995). The hepatic enzymes, present in the endoplasmic reticulum, catalyzing the formation of the major Tamoxifen metabolites have been investigated. Our studies demonstrated that the N-demethylation and 4-hydroxylation of Tamoxifen are catalyzed by the hepatic cytochrome P450 (CYP) enzymes (Table 1) (Mani et al., 1993a).

Cytochrome P450 represents a superfamily of hemeproteins that catalyze the metabolism of xenobiotics (drugs, environmental pollutants and carcinogens) and the metabolism of a variety of endobiotics (steroid hormones, fatty acids and prostaglandins) (Kupfer, 1982; Waxman, 1988; Nelson et al., 1993). These reactions involve activation of molecular oxygen and its insertion into the substrates, rendering them more polar,

Table 1. Diminished Cytochrome P450 Catalyzed N-Demethylation and 4-Hydroxylation of Tamoxifen by Inhibitors of P450

% of Control[b]

Inhibitors	N-Desmethyl	4-hydroxy
SKF 525A, 0.5mM	17	8
Metyrapone, 0.5 mM	21	23
Benzylimidazole, 0.1 mM	28	18
Octylamine, 5.0 mM	25	0
CO/O_2 (1:1)[a]	85	50
CO/O_2 (4:1)[a]	49	32
CO/O_2 (10:1)[a]	42	28

[a] Control gaseous mixtures contained an atmosphere of N_2/O_2 , at the same ratio as CO/O_2.

[b] Control incubations were composed of liver microsomes from phenobarbital -treated rats (1 mg protein/ml) and 100 μM [^{14}C]-tamoxifen and NADPH. Results were compiled from Mani et al. (1993a).

and usually easier to excrete and less toxic. However, at times, the products are more toxic and even carcinogenic; examples of the latter are the carcinogenic metabolites of benzo[α]pyrene and aflatoxin B1 (Pitot, 1993; Aguilar, 1993; Bechtel, 1989)]. Among the various CYP enzymes examined, the CYP3A isoforms were found to catalyze N-demethylation (Jacolot et al., 1991; Mani et al., 1993a).

In rat liver, CYP3A includes at least two isoforms (3A1 and 3A2) that catalyze the 6ß-hydroxylation of androgens and glucocorticoids (Waxman, 1988). Human orthologs of the rat CYP 3A enzymes, having similar steroid hydroxylation activities, are CYP 3A3, 3A4 and 3A5. Catalysis of Tamoxifen 4-hydroxylation was found to be carried out by a P450 that was isolated from livers of TCDD or ß-naphthoflavone treated chick embryos and has been referred to as $P450_{TCDD}$ (Kupfer et al., 1994). However, the specific CYP isoform that catalyzes the 4-hydroxylation in mammals, has not been characterized. Nevertheless, there is weak evidence suggesting that in rats, CYP1A2 catalyzes the 4-hydroxylation of Tamoxifen (Kupfer and Dehal, unpublished) and there is indirect evidence, based on correlation studies, that human CYP 2C8, 2C9 and 2D6 catalyze the 4-hydroxylation (White et al., 1995). Also,

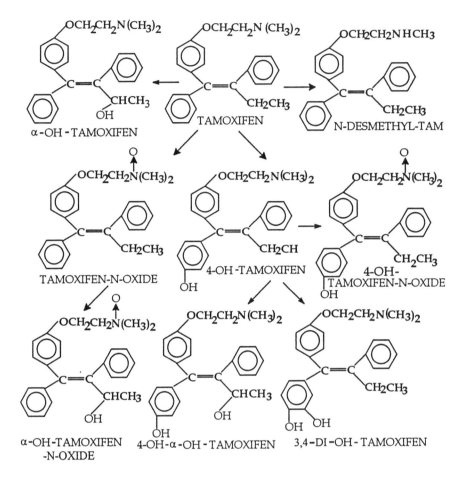

Figure 1. Pathways of Tamoxifen metabolism.

based on preliminary studies with classical P450 inhibitors, it appears that a CYP-like enzyme catalyzes the 3-hydroxylation of 4-OH-tam, yielding 3,4-di-OH-tam (Dehal and Kupfer, unpublished). The interest in identifying the enzyme(s) catalyzing the formation and metabolism of 4-OH-tam stems from the observations that 4-OH-tam exhibits a much higher affinity for the estrogen receptor than Tamoxifen, and that 4-OH-tam is a much more potent antiestrogen (Jordan et al., 1977; Borgna and Rochefort, 1981; Furr and Jordan, 1984). Also, 4-OH-tam is approximately 100-fold more potent than Tamoxifen in its anti-proliferation activity on normal breast cells and on MCF-7 breast cancer cells (Coezy et al., 1982; Vignon et al., 1987; Malet et al., 1988).

Thus, it has been speculated that Tamoxifen is indeed a prodrug and that 4-OH-tam may be the active antiestrogen and anti-breast cancer drug (Lyman and Jordan, 1986). However, direct evidence of whether the anti-tumorigenic activity is due to Tamoxifen per se or whether the active anti-cancer drug is indeed 4-OH-tam or its metabolite has not been obtained.

Whereas the major routes of metabolism are catalyzed by CYP enzymes, tamoxifen-N-oxidation is catalyzed by the hepatic flavin-containing monooxygenase (FMO), a non-P450 enzyme present in the endoplasmic reticulum (Mani et al., 1993b; Kupfer and Dehal, 1996). Since the metabolism of tam-N-oxide by hepatic enzymes occurs at an extremely slow rate and because tam-N-oxide can be enzymatically converted back to Tamoxifen with ease (Mani et al., 1993b), we speculate that the N-oxide may serve as a storage form of tamoxifen in body tissues.

Tamoxifen reactive intermediate and covalent binding

a. Covalent binding to proteins:
(i) Identification of the enzymes catalyzing covalent binding. In the course of investigating the metabolism of Tamoxifen by liver microsomal preparations of animals and man, we observed that Tamoxifen undergoes metabolic activation and yields a reactive intermediate (RI) that binds covalently to proteins (Table 2) (Mani and Kupfer, 1991). Cumulative evidence indicated that CYPs catalyze this covalent binding reaction. Namely, classical inhibitors of P450 (SKF 525A and carbon monoxide) strongly inhibited covalent binding to hepatic proteins (Table 3). Also, antibodies against the NADPH-P450 reductase markedly inhibited the N-demethylation and 4-hydroxylation of Tamoxifen, providing strong evidence for P450 catalysis of these reactions. NADPH-P450 reductase is a microsomal flavoprotein enzyme that transfers electrons from NADPH to the heme iron of P450s and the resultant reduction of the heme is necessary for P450-mediated activities. Thus, inhibition of the reductase activity by antibodies is expected to diminish the rate of a P450-mediated reaction.

Table 2. Covalent Binding of Tamoxifen Metabolite(s) to Hepatic Microsomal Proteins

	Species	Gender	Tamoxifen equivalents bound nmol/mg protein/60 min[b]
Exp. 1.	Rat	M	0.28±0.03
		F	0.49±0.06
Exp. 2.	Human	M,F[a]	0.07±0.01
	Mice	F	1.60±0.06
	Hamster	F	1.20
	Chicken	F	0.31±0.01

[a] Pooled sample from 4 donors. Results were compiled from Mani and Kupfer (1991) and Mani et al. (1994).
[b] Values represent mean ± S.D.

Most recently we demonstrated that CYP3A isoforms catalyze the covalent binding of Tamoxifen to liver proteins in rat and human (Tables 4,5) (Mani et al., 1994). This conclusion was based on several observations: (i) treatment of rats with phenobarbital, PCN or dexamethasone, inducers of hepatic CYP3A1 (Heuman et al., 1982; Ryan and Levin, 1990), dramatically enhanced covalent binding (Table 6) (Mani and Kupfer, 1991; Mani et al., 1994; Dehal and Kupfer, unpublished); (ii) antibodies against-CYP3A markedly inhibited covalent binding in rat and human liver microsomes; (iii) troleandomycin (TAO), a mechanism-based inhibitor of CYP3A, inhibited covalent binding in both rat and human liver microsomes, and (iv) in human liver, there appears to be a reasonable correlation between the levels of CYP3A-mediated enzymatic activity (i.e., testosterone 6ß-hydroxylation) and catalysis of Tamoxifen covalent binding (Mani et al., 1994). Most recently, White and coworkers suggested that, in addition to CYP3A4,

Table 3. Inhibition of Covalent Binding of Tamoxifen Metabolite(s) to Rat Liver microsomal Proteins by Inhibitors of Cytochrome P450 Catalyzed Reactions

Inhibitors , mM	Tamoxifen Equivalents Bound % Control [a]
SKF 525A, 0.5	7
Metyrapone, 0.5	8
Benzylimidazole, 0.1	14
Benzylimidazole, 1.00	2
Antibody to P450 Reductase [b]	25
$CO:O_2$ (4:1) vs $N_2:O_2$ (4:1)	10

[a] Incubations contained liver microsomes from phenobarbital treated male rats (1 mg protein/ml) and 100 μM of ^{14}C-tamoxifen. Results were compiled from Mani and Kupfer (1991).
[b] The ratio of antibodies to microsomal protein was 10:1.

Table 4. Evidence that CYP3A Isoforms Catalyze Covalent Binding of Tamoxifen Metabolite(s) to Liver Microsomal Proteins of Rat and Human

Species	Treatment	Addition	% of Control
Rat	PCN	Cortisol (0.25 mM) [a]	40
		Erythromycin (0.25 mM) [a]	35
		Antibodies to 3A1(5:1) [b]	25
Human	-	Cortisol (0.25 mM)	36
		Erythromycin (0.25 mM)	29
		Antibodies to 3A1(5:1) [b]	40

Results abstracted from Mani et al. (1994)
[a] Alternate substrates of CYP3A
[b] Ratio of antibodies to microsomal proteins

Table 5. **Time Dependent Inactivation by Troleandomycin (TAO) of Covalent Binding of Tamoxifen Metabolite(s) to Liver Microsomal Proteins in PCN treated rats**[a]

Preincubation[b]	% of Control
NADPH	100
TAO plus NADPH	28
TAO minus NADPH	100

[a] PCN = Pregnenolone-16α-carbonitrile induces cytochrome P450 3A1 (CYP3A1). TAO is a CYP3A1 inducer and a time dependent inactivator of CYP3A1 (Wrighton et al., 1985; Sonderfan et al.,1987).
[b] Preincubation of liver microsomes was conducted for 30 minutes, in the presence or absence of TAO (100 μM) at 37°C. Subsequently, the mixture was diluted 5 fold, supplemented with NADPH and tamoxifen (50 μM) and the incubation continued for an additional 30 minutes. Results abstracted from Mani et al. (1994).

Table 6. **Induction of Covalent Binding of Tamoxifen Metabolite(s) to Hepatic Microsomal Proteins by Treatment of Rats with Phenobarbital, Pregnenolone-16α-carbonitrile (PCN) and Dexamethasone**

Gender	Treatment[a]	Tamoxifen equivalents bound nmol/mg prot/60 min[b]	Ratio (t/c)[d]
M	-	0.28±0.03	
M	Phenobarbital	1.80±0.09[c]	6.4
F	-	0.49±0.06	
F	Phenobarbital	1.63±0.05[c]	3.3
M	-	0.64±0.04	
M	PCN	2.20±0.03[c]	3.4
F	-	0.21±0.10	
F	PCN	1.14±0.04[c]	5.4
F	-	0.41±0.02	
F	Dexamethasone	1.64±0.06[c]	4.0

[a] Phenobarbital was administered intraperitoneally (ip) to rats at 37.5mg/kg/dose, twice daily, for 4 days. PCN or Dexamethasone in corn oil were injected ip 50mg/kg daily for 3 days.
[b] Values represent a mean $\pm$ S.D. of 4-6 rats. [c] P $\leq$ 0.001
[d] t/c = treated/control
Results were abstracted from Mani and Kupfer (1991) and Mani et al. (1994) and from S. Dehal and D. Kupfer (unpublished results).

CYP2B6 also catalyzes the covalent binding of Tamoxifen to human liver microsomal proteins (White et al., 1995). However, the evidence for the catalysis by these P450 isoforms rested primarily on the observations that there is a significant correlation between the levels of human liver CYP3A4 and CYP2B6 and the covalent binding of Tamoxifen in these liver preparations. Hence, more direct studies are needed to substantiate these assertions. Interestingly, microsomes of human breast tumors were also able to activate Tamoxifen for covalent binding, albeit at an extremely low rate, being 7-fold lower than that of human liver microsomes (White et al., 1995). However, the significance of this minimal binding is not established. Of additional interest is our observation that the covalent binding may also involve catalysis by the hepatic FMO (Mani and Kupfer, 1991). This speculation is based on our observation that exposure of liver microsomes to 50^0C for 90 seconds, known to inactivate hepatic FMO but not P450, markedly diminished covalent binding of Tamoxifen and of 4-OH-tam (Mani and Kupfer, 1991; Dehal and Kupfer, unpublished). However, the possibility that a heat labile non-FMO enzyme, yet to be detected, is involved in catalysis of covalent binding or that the binding site of the acceptor protein is inactivated by heat, can not be ruled out.

Several studies indicated that Tamoxifen treatment of rats induces the levels of hepatic CYP3A (White et al., 1993; Nuwaysir et al., 1995). The finding that CYP3A catalyzes covalent binding (Mani et al., 1994) and the observation that an oral treatment of female rats with Tamoxifen (40 mg/kg/day for 4 days), increased the *in vitro* covalent binding of radiolabeled tamoxifen to hepatic microsomal proteins by 4-fold (White et al., 1995), if extrapolated to a human clinical setting, would suggest that Tamoxifen treatment could enhance its covalent binding to proteins and DNA and, consequently, may yield undesirable side effects.

(ii a) Identification of the Tamoxifen reactive intermediate binding to proteins. In attempts to identify the Tamoxifen metabolite that is most proximate to the reactive intermediate (RI), it was reasoned that the metabolite more proximate to the RI will bind covalently at a faster rate than metabolites that are more distant from the RI. Thus we determined the ability of several Tamoxifen derivatives/metabolites to undergo metabolic activation by liver microsomes and binding to proteins (Dehal and Kupfer, submitted for publication). To carry out those experiments, several radiolabeled tamoxifen derivatives were prepared. Results demonstrated that the rate of covalent binding of these Tamoxifen metabolites (tam-N-oxide, N-desmethyl-tam, 4-OH-tam and tam-N-oxide-epoxide) was approximately equal to or less than that of Tamoxifen. We were unable to synthesize radiolabeled tam-epoxide by $TiCl_3$ reduction of [3H]-tam-N-oxide-epoxide and thus were unable to determine the covalent binding of tam-epoxide. However, since the covalent binding of tam-N-oxide and tam-N-oxide-epoxide was not greater than that of Tamoxifen, it seems unlikely that tam-epoxide is the RI that binds to proteins. By contrast, we found that 4-OH-tam elicits a 3-5 fold more rapid covalent binding than the other compounds examined. Consequently, it was concluded that 4-hydroxylation represents a major route of Tamoxifen metabolism leading to its covalent binding to proteins (Dehal et al., 1994). It is conceivable that the reason for the low observable levels of 4-OH-tam in mammals (Poon et al., 1993; Jordan et al., 1977) is because of its subsequent hydroxylation into the 3,4-catechol, with resultant depletion of the latter due to its covalent binding. Indeed, certain laboratories detected only low levels of the 3,4-diOH-tam (catechol) *in vivo* and *in vitro* (Jordan et al., 1977; Borgna and Rochefort, 1981; Poon et al., 1993). Subsequently, the observation that 3,4-dihydroxy-tam catechol (3,4-di-OH-tam) is a metabolite of 4-OH-tam suggested that 3,4-di-OH-tam is more proximate to the RI than 4-OH-tam.

Previous studies, including our own, demonstrated that Tamoxifen metabolism yields a low or minimal accumulation of 3,4-di-OH-tam. However, by trapping the 3,4-di-OH-tam catechol as methyl ether, our studies demonstrated a significant formation of the catechol from Tamoxifen and 4-OH-tam in several species, including human. It is conceivable that the reason for the low levels of 3,4-di-OH-tam accumulation is that the catechol is continuously depleted by undergoing further metabolism, leading to its covalent binding to macromolecules and/or resulting in highly polar metabolites that are insoluble in the organic solvents employed and hence escape detection. Thus, to demonstrate the formation of the 3,4-di-OH-tam catechol from Tamoxifen or 4-OH-tam during incubation and to minimize its further metabolism, an indirect approach was developed that involves the *in situ* formation of a radiolabeled mono-methyl derivative from the radioinert catechol. That approach utilizes an enzymatic methylating system composed of endogenous (and occasionally added) catechol-α-methyl transferase (COMT) supplemented with [^{3}H]-S-adenosylmethionine ([^{3}H]-SAM) and the quantification of the [^{3}H]-monomethyl-3,4-di-OH-tam by scintillation spectrometry. Using that method, it was found that the formation of 3,4-di-OH-tam, represents a significant pathway of Tamoxifen metabolism in several species (Table 7). Of interest is our observation that the incubation of 4-OH-tam with liver microsomes from PCN-treated rats yielded three detectable metabolites (Dehal and Kupfer, manuscript submitted); one metabolite was identified as 4-OH-tam-N-oxide via its facile reduction back to 4-OH-tam by titanium(III) chloride. Another metabolite of 4-OH-tam was assumed to be the 3,4-dihydroxy-tam catechol (3,4-di-OH-tam), since the radiolabeled monomethylated catechol was observed when 4-OH-tam was incubated with liver microsomes in the presence of [^{3}H]-SAM and endogenous COMT. As expected, the rate of catechol formation from 4-OH-tam was higher (3-4 fold) than from Tamoxifen.

Table 7. Formation of 3,4-di-OH-tamoxifen catechol from 4-OH-tamoxifen by Liver Microsomes of Rats, Mice and Chicken

Species	Incubation time (min)	Methylated Catechol
Rat	30	1.2
Mice	20	2.0
Chicken	20	0.7

Incubations contained liver microsomes (1mg protein/ml), 4-OH-tamoxifen, [^{3}H]-SAM and NADPH (SS Dehal and D Kupfer, unpublished results)

(ii b) Evidence that 3,4-di-OH-tam is the metabolite proximate to the reactive intermediate (RI). It was reasoned that if the catechol were the most proximate metabolite to the reactive intermediate, then conditions that stimulate its depletion would reduce the formation of the reactive intermediate and consequently result in a lower rate of covalent binding and conditions that inhibit its covalent binding would enhance its accumulation. In fact, methylation of the 3,4-di-OH-tam by the addition of radioinert SAM to the incubations of [^{3}H]-tamoxifen, inhibited covalent binding by 17-23%. By contrast, inclusion of S-adenosyl-L-homocysteine (SAH), a potent inhibitor of COMT-mediated methylation of 3,4-di-OH-tam, essentially overcame the inhibition of the covalent binding by SAM. Additionally, ascorbic acid and glutathione, inhibitors of covalent binding of Tamoxifen, had little or no effect on Tamoxifen 4-hydroxylation, but produced an increase in accumulation of methylated catechol. These findings collectively indicate that 3,4-di-OH-tam is proximate to the ultimate RI that results in covalent binding to microsomal proteins. Our current findings indicate that the metabolic activation of Tamoxifen and its covalent binding to proteins involves the transformation of Tamoxifen into the 4-OH-tam and 3,4-di-OH-tam. Although the identity of the ultimate RI that binds to proteins is yet to be resolved, a likely possibility would be the oxidized products of 3,4-di-OH-tam, such as the semiquinone and quinone derivatives (Figure 2).

Our results of incubations of Tamoxifen with liver microsomes from PB-treated (Mani and Kupfer, 1991) and PCN- treated rats (Mani et al., 1994; Dehal and Kupfer, manuscript submitted) indicate that CYP3A is involved in the general catalysis of covalent binding to proteins. In addition, treatment of adult female rats with dexamethasone, a potent inducer of CYP3A, (Heuman et al., 1982) markedly elevated covalent binding of Tamoxifen (Dehal and Kupfer, unpublished). Similarly, others reported that dexamethasone treatment increases the covalent binding of Tamoxifen to proteins (White et al., 1995). We have demonstrated that the covalent binding of Tamoxifen to hepatic proteins in animals and humans involves catalysis by CYP3A (Mani et al., 1994). Inducers of CYP3A did not enhance the formation of 4-OH-tam in rats (Mani et al., 1993a; Dehal and Kupfer, unpublished results), hence we considered the possibility that CYP3A catalyzes the 3-hydroxylation of Tamoxifen, yielding the 3,4-di-OH-catechol. However, since catechol formation from 4-OH-tam was not elevated by treatment with phenobarbital or dexamethasone, it is highly unlikely that CYP3A catalyzes the

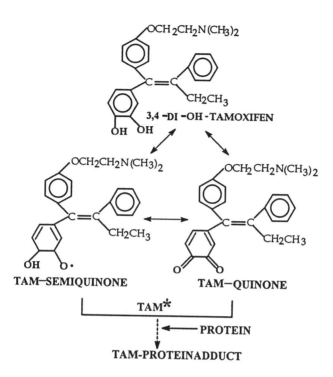

Figure 2. Putative reactive intermediate.

3-hydroxylation. Thus the mechanism of involvement of CYP3A in the covalent binding of Tamoxifen has not been resolved. Of interest and concern are the recent observations that Tamoxifen treatment of rats induces CYP2B1/2 and CYP3A1, indicating that Tamoxifen is a PB-like inducer (White et al., 1993; Nuwaysir et al., 1995). Thus, Tamoxifen treatment would be expected to enhance its own metabolism and its covalent binding to liver proteins. Human livers contain CYP2B6 (an ortholog of rat 2B), and CYP 3A3, 3A4, 3A5 (orthologs of rat 3A1/2) (Soucek and Gut, 1992; Mimura et al., 1993), which in turn may contribute to the covalent binding observed in the human microsomal preparations. Further studies are planned to identify the specific human P450s involved in covalent binding.

Estrogen-induced carcinogenesis has been postulated to occur by transformation of estrogens into catechol that may generate free radicals by metabolic redox reactions (Liehr, 1994; Liehr and Roy, 1990). The formation of hydroquinone and catechol from phenol by rat liver microsomes has been reported (Sawahata and Neal, 1983) and it was suggested that they are obligatory intermediates leading to reactive metabolites that bind covalently to microsomal proteins. Evidence suggests that certain semiquinones undergoing oxidation to quinones, reduce O_2 into superoxide [O_2^-] (Nelson, 1982). The observation that the metabolism of Tamoxifen by hepatocytes generates O_2^- (Turner et al., 1991), suggests that Tamoxifen semiquinone was formed and supports the above supposition that metabolism of Tamoxifen by hepatic enzymes generates oxidation products of the 3,4-di-OH-tam. Whether 3,4-di-OH-tam also undergoes metabolic redox transformation that may result in carcinogenicity has not been demonstrated.

The cumulative evidence supports our contention that 3,4-di-OH-tam is the penultimate metabolite that generates the RI that binds to proteins, possibly via the formation of semi-quinone and/or ortho-quinone. However, it appears that for DNA adduct formation other pathways for RI generation also exist, e.g., those involving the formation of the Ó-hydroxy-tam, tam-epoxide, 4-OH-tam, and metabolite E (a side chain dealkylated Tamoxifen); whether these RI's also bind to proteins is not known. Most importantly, the question of whether the 3,4-di-OH-tam is also a pro-RI that forms DNA adducts needs further exploration.

Tam-epoxide, although not fully characterized, was reported to be formed during the metabolism of Tamoxifen by liver microsomes (Reunitz et al., 1984), however, others could not demonstrate its presence (McCague and Seago, 1986). Nevertheless, Phillips et al. (1994a) demonstrated that synthetic tam-epoxide forms a DNA adduct that is indistinguishable from the DNA adduct formed in livers of Tamoxifen-treated rats and thus suggested the formation of tam-epoxide during Tamoxifen metabolism. Whether tam-epoxide is the reactive metabolite that also binds to proteins has not been investigated. Nevertheless, it appears unlikely that tam-epoxide is the RI that binds to proteins, since the covalent binding of tam-N-oxide and tam-N-oxide-epoxide to proteins was not greater than that of Tamoxifen. It is of prime interest that α-Hydroxy-tam, a minor metabolite of tamoxifen, produced a much greater levels of DNA adducts than Tamoxifen (Phillips et al., 1994b). Also, metabolite E is metabolically activated by rat liver microsomes to form DNA adducts (Pongracz et al., 1995). Furthermore, activation of metabolite E by horseradish peroxidase or by silver oxide resulted in the same DNA adducts; however, some of these adducts were different from those formed by incubation with

4-OH-tam (Pathak et al., 1995; Pongracz et al., 1995). The unavailability of radiolabeled α-hydroxy-tam and metabolite E precluded our investigation on the possible covalent binding of these compounds to proteins.

b. Covalent binding to DNA. In addition to the above observations on covalent binding to proteins, several groups have independently demonstrated the formation of Tamoxifen-derived DNA adducts *in vivo* and *in vitro*. Soon after Mani and Kupfer (1991) reported that Tamoxifen undergoes metabolic activation by liver P450 to form a reactive intermediate that binds to proteins, Han and Liehr (1992) published the key finding that treatment of female rats with a single injection of Tamoxifen elicits two hepatic DNA adducts. Moreover, multiple injections of Tamoxifen produced four additional liver adducts and there was an increase of up to 10-15 fold in the amount of DNA adducts formed as compared to a single injection. These findings indicated that a Tamoxifen reactive intermediate is formed *in vivo* and that it readily reacts with hepatic DNA. As a result of their findings, the authors introjected a word of caution that the accumulation of DNA adducts after Tamoxifen treatment "makes this drug a poor choice for the chronic preventive treatment of breast cancer". Subsequently, in the same year, White et al. (1992), demonstrated that the administration of Tamoxifen (45 mg/kg/day) for 7 days to rats or for 4 days to mice, produced hepatic DNA adducts. However, adducts could not be detected in kidney, lung, spleen, uterus or peripheral lymphocytes. The administration of pyrrolidinotamoxifen, a compound that cannot undergo N-demethylation, produced a similar level of DNA adduct formation as Tamoxifen. This indicated that N-demethylation is not necessary for adduct formation. The observation by Mani and Kupfer (1991) that N-demethylation was not involved in the generation of the reactive intermediate *in vitro* in its covalent binding to hepatic proteins, suggests similarity between the requirements for covalent binding to proteins and DNA. Of particular interest is the observation by White et al. (1992) that other Tamoxifen derivatives undergoing clinical trials (toremifene and droloxifene) do not form DNA adducts. However, whether these compounds could form reactive intermediates that bind to proteins, has hitherto not been investigated.

Several laboratories have been exploring the identity of the structure(s) of the Tamoxifen reactive intermediate that binds covalently to DNA. Tam-epoxide, although not fully characterized, was reported to be formed during the metabolism of Tamoxifen by liver microsomes

(Reunitz et al., 1984); however, others were unable to demonstrate its presence (McCague and Seago, 1986). Nevertheless, Phillips et al. (1994a) showed that the DNA adducts formed *in vivo* exhibit, after ^{32}P-postlabeling on PEI cellulose-chromatography, a similarity to adducts formed *in vitro* from a reaction of synthetic tamoxifen-1,2 epoxide with added DNA. By contrast, tam-N-oxide-epoxide formed only small amount of DNA adducts, evident from the faint radioactive spots. Consequently, Phillips et al., (1994a) suggested the formation of tam-epoxide during Tamoxifen metabolism. Whether tam-epoxide is the RI that also binds to proteins has not been studied so far.

Potter et al. (1994) hypothesized that the reactive intermediate that binds covalently to DNA and proteins, is α-hydroxy-tam (see Fig 1). They described a mechanistic scheme for generating the α-hydroxy-tam from Tamoxifen via a P450-mediated hydrogen abstraction. It is of interest that the α-hydroxy-tam has been detected as the N-oxide and not as the free amine. The authors suggest that the reason for the absence of the free amine derivative is because the diethylamine side-chain is better able to assist in the generation of the allylic carbocation by ipso-assisted electron release than the respective N-oxide. The authors also propose that the reason for Toremifene not readily forming DNA adducts is because the chlorine atom in the ethyl side chain prevents the α-hydroxylation. Additionally, they propose that 4-OH-tam is further metabolized by α-hydroxylation and that the 4-hydroxyl facilitates the α-hydroxylation. Indeed, the observation that 4-iodo-tam and iodoxifene do not form DNA adducts, suggests that α-hydroxylation alone is not responsible for the DNA adduct formation. Support for the involvement of α-hydroxylation in DNA adduct formation of Tamoxifen is provided by the findings of Phillips et al. (1994c), who observed a decrease in genotoxicity (DNA adduct formation) of Tamoxifen when the ethyl side chain contained 5 deuteriums. Namely, the administration of the [D_5 -ethyl]-tam to female Fisher rats yielded an approximately 2-fold decrease in hepatic DNA adducts as compared with the non-deuterated derivative. Similarly, treatment of human MCL-5 cell line with [D_5 -ethyl]-tam resulted in a 2-3 fold decrease in the number of micronuclei induction as compared with the non-deuterated Tamoxifen. The authors suggest that the reactive intermediate formed from Tamoxifen epoxide is the same allylic carbocation Tamoxifen that is formed from α-hydroxy-tam. Thus the putative reactive intermediate (Tam*) could be formed by direct oxidation of Tamoxifen, by dehydration of α-hydroxytam and by rearrangement of tamoxifen epoxide. A subsequent study by Phillips et al. (1994b) with female Fischer F344 rat hepatocytes compared the relative ability of α-hydroxy-tam and Tamoxifen to form DNA adducts. There was a 25 and 49 fold greater formation of DNA adducts with α-hydroxy-tam at 1 and 10 μM, respectively. In addition, α-hydroxy-tam was able to react with salmon sperm DNA *in vitro*, in the absence of metabolizing enzymes. This finding produces somewhat of an enigma, since other studies (see above) demonstrated that α-hydroxylation alone is not sufficient for DNA adduct formation and that 4-hydroxylation is required. Further evidence for involvement of α-hydroxylation in DNA adduct formation was obtained by Jarman et al. (1995), who observed a 3:1 higher ratio of the rate of α-hydroxylation in incubation of rat liver microsomes with unlabelled Tamoxifen versus [D_5-ethyl]-tam. This indicated a significant isotope effect in the α-hydroxylation that was similar to that previously observed when DNA adduct formation was assessed with these compounds. Indeed, these findings strongly suggest that the α-hydroxylation is an important pathway for the conversion of Tamoxifen into the reactive intermediate that binds to DNA. Of additional interest is the identification of both α-hydroxy-N-oxide-tam and α-hydroxy-N-desmethyl-tam as metabolites of Tamoxifen.

Pathak and Bodell (1994) demonstrated *in vitro* that hepatic microsomes from rat and human, in the presence of NADPH or cumene hydroperoxide (CuOOH), can activate Tamoxifen to form DNA adducts with added calf thymus DNA. Adduct formation was detected by ^{32}P-postlabeling. Pretreatment of rats with phenobarbital, increased several fold the microsomal catalyzed DNA adduct formation. With CuOOH as the cofactor, there were more adducts formed and they were different from the adducts generated when NADPH was the cofactor, indicating that the cofactor used dictates the nature of the reactive intermediates formed. The hepatic DNA adducts of Tamoxifen formed in rats and hamsters *in vivo* (White et al., 1992) appear similar to those generated *in vitro* when CuOOH is used and not when the native cofactor NADPH is employed (Pathak and Bodell, 1994). This interesting, albeit puzzling, finding needs further exploration. Also of interest is the observation that similar adducts were obtained *in vitro* from rat and human microsomal incubations of Tamoxifen, independent of whether NADPH or CuOOH was used. The observation that phenobarbital treatment increases DNA adduct formation (Pathak and Bodell, 1994) and the earlier findings that phenobarbital markedly induces adduct formation to liver microsomal proteins (Mani and Kupfer, 1991), suggest the possibility that similar Tamoxifen reactive intermediate(s) are involved in both DNA and protein adduct formation. Indeed, it was previously observed that Tamoxifen N-demethylation is not necessary for DNA adduct or protein adduct formation (Mani and Kupfer, 1991). Of additional interest is our observation that CYP3A enzyme catalyzes the Tamoxifen-protein adduct formation in rat and human liver microsomes (Mani et al., 1994). Since phenobarbital markedly induces CYP3A, we speculate that CYP3A is involved in both DNA and protein adduct formation.

Indirect evidence that phenolic and/or alcoholic Tamoxifen products are involved in DNA adduct formation was obtained by Randarath et al. (1994a). These authors reasoned that since such metabolites are potential substrates for sulfate conjugation, inhibition of sulfation by pentachlorophenol (a sulfotransferase inhibitor) would increase the formation of DNA adducts. Indeed, pentachlorophenol pretreatment of mice, followed by administration of Tamoxifen, yielded a 13-17 fold increase in the level of certain but not all DNA adducts, resulting in a 7-fold increase in overall DNA adduct formation. These findings suggest two pathways of adduct formation, one sensitive to pentachlorophenol and the other resistant. In a subsequent study, it was observed that the oral adminstration of Tamoxifen yielded more polar hepatic DNA adducts (group I) than the intraperitoneal administration which resulted in less polar products (group II) (Randarath et al., 1994b). These authors proposed that 4-OH-tam is a proximate metabolite *in vivo* in the formation of adducts that are intensified by pentachlorophenol. In addition, the results indicate that there are two routes of DNA adduct formation, one involving α-hydroxylation followed by sulfate conjugation and the other via 4-hydroxylation.

In a search for the identification of the reactive intermediate that binds covalently to DNA, Pongracz et al. (1995) demonstrated *in vitro* that Tamoxifen metabolite E, previously found in plasma of treated patients, can undergo activation by liver microsomes, in the presence of calf thymus DNA, to form two major (*a & b*) and up to six minor DNA adducts. Activation of metabolite E by horseradish peroxidase yielded the same *a & b* adducts. By contrast, microsomal activation of Tamoxifen yielded primarily a DNA adduct (referred to as adduct 6) and several minor DNA adducts; among the latter, two adducts were the same as *a & b*. The question of whether the DNA adducts formed *in vivo* from Tamoxifen are the same as adduct 6 or as *a & b* was addressed in another study by the same group (Pathak et al., 1995). The administration of Tamoxifen to rats for 7-days produced a complex pattern of DNA adducts that was similar to that produced *in vitro* by the hepatic microsomal activation of Tamoxifen with CuOOH as the cofactor, in the presence of calf thymus DNA. Interestingly, the principal DNA adduct 6 generated by microsomal incubation of Tamoxifen, in the presence of CuOOH, was the same as the principal adduct 6 formed in Tamoxifen-treated rats. In the same study, incubation of 4-hydroxy-tam with rat liver microsomes and NADPH or CuOOH, in the presence of calf thymus DNA, resulted in the formation of DNA adducts. It was observed that the same DNA adduct (*adduct a*) was formed, independent of whether NADPH or CuOOH was used. Interestingly, activation of 4-hydroxy-tam by horseradish peroxidase and lactoperoxidase, yielded a single DNA adduct that was identical to the adduct formed by liver microsomes. This finding demonstrated that peroxidases may be involved in catalysis of Tamoxifen adduct formation (Pathak et al., 1995). These investigators speculated that 4-OH-tam formed in the liver may accumulate at other tissue sites where it may be activated by peroxidase enzymes to form DNA adducts and that a similar process may be contributing to the induction of endometrial tumors in women on Tamoxifen therapy (Fischer et al., 1994; van Leeumne et al., 1994). Evidence to support such a possibility is provided by the findings of Davies et al. (1995). These investigators observed that incubation of Tamoxifen or Toremifene with horseradish peroxidase and H_2O_2 produced the corresponding N-desmethyl and N-oxide derivatives, but no 4-hydroxylated products were detected. Inclusion of calf thymus DNA during the incubation resulted in DNA damage. Both Tamoxifen and Toremifene caused comparable damage. The major DNA adducts derived from Tamoxifen exhibited similar R_f of two adducts formed by exposure of rats to Tamoxifen. They proposed that peroxidase metabolizes Tamoxifen and Toremifene into a putative reactive epoxide intermediate that is responsible for genotoxicity. Also, they suggested that Tamoxifen is metabolized by peroxidase into a carbon centered free radical which reacts with oxygen to form peroxy radicals. The authors speculated that the endometrial cancer associated with Tamoxifen treatment is due to activation by the peroxidase present in the respective extrahepatic tissue and not by the hepatic P450-mediated process. Interestingly, Davies et al. (1995) observed that peroxidases catalyze the covalent binding of Tamoxifen and Toremifene to albumin. However, we observed no effect on protein binding, when bovine serum albumin was present in the incubation of Tamoxifen with rat liver microsomes (Mani and Kupfer, unpublished). By contrast, there was a dramatic stimulation of covalent binding by albumin when the triphenylethylene, chlorotrianisene (TACE), was incubated with liver microsomes from methylcholanthrene-treated rats (Juedes et al., 1987; Juedes and Kupfer, 1990); binding was primarily to albumin.

Carthew et al. (1995) presented evidence for the persistence of tam-DNA adducts in rats, with a decrease of only 38% of adducts after 3 months after cessation of Tamoxifen treatment. Furthermore, phenobarbital treatment even after cessation of Tamoxifen treatment was found to promote high incidence of liver cancer. The authors suggested that the phenobarbital tumor promotion occurs because of the persistence of DNA adducts. However, since phenobarbital treatment can cause a marked increase in Tamoxifen-DNA adduct formation (Pathak and Bodell, 1994), the possibility that phenobarbital merely generated new Tamoxifen adducts (from residual Tamoxifen stored in tissues) and that these DNA adducts may be the cause for the phenobarbital-mediated tumor promotion, needs further exploration. These authors suggested that their findings may be of concern to women on Tamoxifen therapy because even when there is relatively small amount of Tamoxifen-induced liver DNA damage, other agents, like phenobarbital, could promote liver tumors.

Hemminki et al. (1995) compared the DNA-binding activity of Tamoxifen and Toremifene in rat *in vivo* and in human and rat liver microsomes *in vitro* and in cultured human lymphocytes by ^{32}P-postlabeling of the extracted DNA. Tamoxifen, but not Toremifene, caused DNA adducts in rat liver. Both compounds induced DNA adduct formation in rat and human liver microsomes and in cultured lymphocytes. However, Toremifene showed lower binding than Tamoxifen in all the systems studied. The authors cautioned that even though the results indicate large differences in the DNA-binding potencies between Tamoxifen and Toremifene, there is a possibility that the differences are misleading due to potentially large differences in ^{32}P-labeling efficiencies of the respective adducts. In a related study, Martin et al. (1995) compared livers of 7 women receiving Tamoxifen (20 mg once or twice daily) with livers of 7 women not receiving the drug. The hepatic DNA adducts were assayed by ^{32}P-postlabeling. The total level of DNA adducts in treated women was between 18-80 adducts/10^8 nucleotides. There was no difference in the DNA damage between Tamoxifen-treated and control groups. The pattern of DNA adducts in human subjects was different from those observed in rats exposed to Tamoxifen. Although only a limited number of patients have been examined, it appears that women are less susceptible to liver DNA damage by Tamoxifen than rats.

Discussion and conclusion

Recent findings demonstrated that subchronic and chronic treatment of rats with Tamoxifen induces their hepatic cytochrome P450s, CYP2B and CYP3A isoforms (White et al., 1993; Nuwaysir et al., 1995). The observations that CYP3A catalyzes the N-demethylation in rats and human livers (Jacolot et al., 1991; Mani et al., 1993a), suggests that patients undergoing Tamoxifen therapy may exhibit a faster rate of tamoxifen N-demethylation and possibly its further metabolism into a pharmacologically inactive form. Such an increase in Tamoxifen transformation could diminish Tamoxifen efficacy and hence may yield tumor resistance to this drug. We observed that CYP3A catalyzes Tamoxifen activation and covalent binding to proteins (Mani et al., 1994). More recently it was found that phenobarbital treatment, known to induce CYP3A and CYP2B (Ryan and Levin, 1990), increases Tamoxifen covalent binding to proteins and DNA (Mani et al, 1994; Pathak and Bodell, 1994). These observations suggest that Tamoxifen treatment could enhance the formation of its own reactive metabolites and of the subsequent covalent binding to macromolecules.

Adducts may be involved in the generation of a variety of side-effects associated with Tamoxifen treatment, such as endomerial tumor formation. Indeed, DNA adducts formed by a CYP-mediated generation of reactive intermediates of certain procarcinogens (e.g., benzo[α]pyrene and aflatoxin B_1), were found to be associated with tumor formation by such compounds (Pitot, 1993; Bechtel, 1989; Aguilar et al., 1993). Also, tissue necrosis after treatment with certain compounds, e.g., bromobenzene, is associated with a CYP-mediated formation of a reactive intermediate (bromobenzene epoxide) and its covalent binding to proteins (Brodie et al., 1971; Mitchell et al., 1971). Induction of CYP3A in patients on Tamoxifen therapy may occur due to the drug per se or by treatment with certain anti-inflammatory steroids, such as dexamethasone or antibiotics (rifampin). In fact, a subchronic dexamethasone treatment of rats markedly increases Tamoxifen covalent binding to proteins (see Table 6) (Dehal and Kupfer, unpublished; White et al., 1995). Thus, it appears that the induction of CYP3A in patients on Tamoxifen therapy could be an undesirable occurrence.

Although the formation of Tamoxifen-DNA adducts in rats and mice has been amply documented, the formation of such adducts in humans is still not satisfactorily verified. For instance, Martin et al. (1995) found no correlation between liver Tamoxifen levels and the total number of DNA adducts in humans. Also, there was no significant difference in the total number of DNA adducts between the Tamoxifen-treated and control groups. Additionally, they could not ascertain whether the DNA adducts were indeed associated with Tamoxifen, because there are no Tamoxifen-DNA standards available. Interestingly, they observed that the DNA adducts in human samples were different from those found in Tamoxifen treated rats.

The available information indicates that there is a considerable number of questions concerning Tamoxifen action, of basic and clinical relevance, that need resolution:

(i) The mechanism of the carcinogenic activity of Tamoxifen. Tumor generation in general is a multifactorial process and DNA damage is probably only the initial step in a multistep sequence. Most probably only certain DNA adducts participate in tumor generation and there are remarkable differences in species susceptibility to tumor formation. For instance, whereas Tamoxifen treatment of rats produced DNA adducts and hepatic tumors, the same treatment of mice also generated hepatic DNA adducts, but did not elicit liver tumor formation. Also, there is a dramatic difference in the levels of DNA adduct formation in rats and humans (humans appear to produce much fewer adducts), suggesting that humans should be markedly less at risk than rats of developing Tamoxifen-mediated liver tumors.

(ii) Identification of the reactive intermediate (RI). Despite the intensive investigation conducted on the Tamoxifen adduct formation and the multiplicity of evidence as to the nature of the reactive intermediates involved, the structure of the reactive intermediate (Tam*) that binds to proteins and DNA has not been characterized. Also, the question of whether the same reactive intermediate binds to proteins and DNA has not been answered. Because of the low level of the tam*-DNA adduct formed, it is unlikely that, with the current techniques available, the identification of the reactive intermediate bound to DNA can be achieved. By contrast, a considerable amount of Tamoxifen*-protein adduct is formed and hence it is much more likely that the identification of the RI will be obtained from determination of the molecular weight of the protein-adduct.

Among the various Tamoxifen derivatives tested, α-hydroxy-tam, tam-epoxide, 4-OH-tam, and metabolite E were found to bind covalently to DNA. However, the propensity of evidence points to the involvement of α-hydroxylation as being a major step in tam*-DNA adduct formation. Nevertheless, there exists a dilemma that still needs resolution; although α-hydroxy-tam was found to react directly with salmon sperm DNA *in vitro* (in the absence of metabolizing enzymes, Phillips et al., 1994b), certain studies demonstrated that α-hydroxylation alone is not sufficient for DNA adduct formation and that 4-hydroxylation may be required. By contrast, with respect to protein binding, tam-N-oxide, N-desmethyl-tam, tam-N-oxide-epoxide and 4-OH-tam were found to bind covalently. However, among these, 4-OH-tam was found to be by far the best substrate for covalent binding. Also, there is indirect evidence that points to the 3,4-di-OH-tam catechol, apparently derived from 4-OH-tam, as being proximate to the reactive intermediate that binds to proteins (Dehal and Kupfer, manuscript submitted). Most importantly, the question of whether the 3,4-di-OH-tam, could undergo metabolic activation and bind to DNA and whether that reaction represents a significant pathway for covalent binding to DNA, needs further exploration. Of additional interest would be the determination of whether α-hydroxy-tam could also bind effectively to proteins.

(iii) Does the same reactive intermediate participate in both protein and DNA adducts formation. The question of whether there exists a major common pathway of Tamoxifen metabolism that leading to a reactive intermediate that binds to both proteins and DNA has not been adequately addressed. Nevertheless, the observations that phenobarbital treatment increases Tamoxifen-DNA adduct formation (Pathak and Bodell, 1994), and the earlier findings (Mani and Kupfer, 1991; Mani et al., 1994) that phenobarbital markedly induces adduct formation of Tamoxifen to proteins, suggests that the same P450s and the same reactive intermediate(s) may be involved in both DNA and protein adduct formation. Additional support for such supposition is derived from the findings that 4-hydroxy-tam is a better substrate for both protein and DNA covalent binding. The findings that N-demethylation of Tamoxifen is not necessary for either DNA or protein adduct formation, provides further support for the view that the same reactive intermediates are involved in covalent binding of both DNA and proteins.

(iv) Characterization of the P450 isoform(s) that catalyzes the formation of protein and DNA adducts. The question of which cytochrome P450 isoform is the prime catalyst in covalent binding of

Tamoxifen, has been addressed. It appears that hepatic CYP3A in rats and humans catalyzes the overall covalent binding of Tamoxifen to liver proteins (Mani et al., 1994). However, the specific metabolic pathway of Tamoxifen catalyzed by CYP 3A that is involved in covalent binding, has not been identified. It has been suggested that α-hydroxylation of Tamoxifen is catalyzed by P450 and it appears that the 3-hydroxylation of 4-hydroxy-tam is mediated by P450; however, studies to determine whether P450 is indeed involved in these reactions and the characterization of the specific P450 isoforms catalyzing those reactions have not been carried out.

(v) Do toremifene, droloxifene and other triphenylethylenes form protein adducts. Although toremifene and droloxifene do not readily form DNA adducts and do not elicit tumorigenesis in rats, the question of whether they do form reactive intermediates that bind to proteins, needs further investigation. Another triphenylethylene, chlorotrianisene (TACE), is readily activated to form protein adducts (Juedes et al., 1987; Juedes and Kupfer, 1990), but the question of whether TACE forms DNA adducts has not been answered as yet.

(vi) Are the protein adducts of triphenylethylenes detrimental to the homeostasis of the human and the animal? We have demonstrated that the metabolic activation of TACE diminishes the level of the active form of the rat uterine estrogen receptor (ER), possibly due to covalent binding of the TACE reactive intermediate to the ER (Kupfer and Bulger, 1990). Also, we observed *in vitro*, that the proestrogenic pesticide methoxychlor undergoes a P450-mediated metabolic activation (Kupfer and Bulger, 1987) and binds covalently to hepatic iodothyronine 5'-deiodinase. *In vivo*, methoxychlor diminishes the activity of this enzyme, which is essential for generation of the active form of the thyroid hormone (Zhou et al., 1995). The question of whether Tamoxifen exhibits similar metabolic reactivity characteristics to TACE and methoxychlor, requires further studies.

ACKNOWLEDGMENTS

Financial support provided by United States Public Health Service grant (ES00834) from the National Institute for Environmental Health Sciences is gratefully acknowledged. The work performed in our laboratory has been carried out largely by Dr. Chitra Mani (my former associate) and by Dr. Shangara S. Dehal (my current associate), to both of whom I am highly indebted. Tamoxifen, Tamoxifen citrate, and 4-hydroxy-tam were obtained as a gift from

ICI Pharmaceuticals Group (Wilmington, DE). N-desmethyl-tam was kindly provided by Dr. John F. Stobaugh (University of Kansas, Lawerence, KS). The author is grateful to Mrs. Cathy Warren for the help with the word processing of this chapter.

REFERENCES

Aguilar F, Hussain SP, Cerutti P (1993): Aflatoxin B_1 induces the transversion of G→T in codon 249 of the p53 tumor suppressor gene in human hepatocytes. *Proc Natl Acad Sci USA* 90:8586-8590

Bechtel DH (1989): Molecular dosimetry of hepatic aflatoxin B_1-DNA adducts: Linear correlation with hepatic cancer risk. *Regul Toxicol Pharmacol* 10:74-81

Borgna J-L, Rochefort H (1981): Hydroxylated metabolites of tamoxifen are formed *in vivo* and bound to estrogen receptor in target tissues. *J Biol Chem* 256:859-868

Brodie BB, Reid W, Cho AK, Sipes IG, Gillette JR (1971): Possible mechanism of liver necrosis caused by aromatic organic compounds. *Proc Natl Acad Sci USA* 68:160-164

Carthew P, Martin EA, White INH, DeMatteis F, Edwards RE, Dorman BM, Heydon RT, Smith LL (1995): Tamoxifen induces short-term cumulative DNA damage and liver tumors in rats: Promotion by phenobarbital. *Cancer Res* 55:544-547

Coezy E, Borgna JL, Rochefort H (1982): Tamoxifen and metabolites in MCF-7 cells: correlation between binding to estrogen receptor and inhibition of cell growth. *Cancer Res* 42:317-323

Dauplat J, LeBouedec G, Achard JL (1990): Endometrial adenocarcinoma in 2 patients taking tamoxifen. *Press Med* 19:380-381

Davies AM, Martin EA, Jones RM, Lim CK, Smith LL, White INH (1995): Peroxidase activation of tamoxifen and toremifene resulting in DNA damage and covalently bound protein adducts. *Carcinogenesis* 16:539-545

Dehal SS, Mani C , Kupfer D (1994): Covalent binding of tamoxifen and its metabolites: 4-hydroxytamoxifen a proximate species to the reactive intermediate in rats and humans. *Proc of Intl Soc for the Study of Xenobiotics* 6:160

Fischer B, Costantino JP, Redmond CK, Fisher ER, Wickerham DL, Cronin WM (1994): Endometrial cancer in tamoxifen-treated breast cancer patients: Findings from the National Surgical Adjuvant Breast and Bowel Project (NSABP)B-14. *J Nat Cancer Inst* 86:527-537

Fisher B, Redmond C (1991): New perspective on cancer of the contralateral breast: a marker for assessing tamoxifen as a preventive agent. *J Natl Cancer Inst* 83:1278-1280

Fornander T, Cedermark B, Matteson A, Skoog L, Theve T, Askergren J, Rutqvist LE, Glas U, Silljverswaard C, Somell A, Wilking N, Hjolmar MJ (1989): Adjuvant tamoxifen in early breast cancer: occurrence of new primary cancers. *Lancet* I:117-119

Foster AB, Griggs LJ, Jarman M, vanMaanen MS, Schulten H-R (1980): Metabolism of tamoxifen by rat liver microsomes: formation of the oxide a new metabolite. *Biochem Pharmacol* 29:1977-1979

Furr BJA, Jordan VC (1984): The pharmacology and clinical uses of tamoxifen. *Pharmacol Ther* 25:127-205

Han X-L, Liehr JG (1992): Induction of covalent DNA adducts in rodents by tamoxifen. *Cancer Res* 52:1360-1363

Harper MJM, Walpole AL (1967): A new derivative of triphenylethylene: effect on implantation and mode of action in rats. *J Reprod Fertil* 13:101-119

Hemminki K, Widlak P, Hou S-M (1995): DNA adducts caused by tamoxifen and toremifene in human microsomal system and lymphocytes *in vitro*. *Carcinogenesis* 16:1661-1664

Heuman DM, Gallagher EJ, Barwick JL, Elshourbafy NA, Guzelian PS (1982): Immunochemical evidence for induction of a common form of hepatic cytochrome P450 in rats treated with pregnenolone-16Ó-carbonitrile or other steroidal or non-steroidal agents. *Mol Pharmacol* 21:753-760

Jacolot F, Simon I, Dreano Y, Beaune P, Riche C, Berthou F (1991): Identification of the cytochrome P-450 IIIA family as the enzymes involved in the N-demethylation of tamoxifen in human liver microsomes. *Biochem Pharmacol* 41:1911-1919

Jarman M, Poon GK, Rowlands MG, Grimshaw RM, Horton MN, Potter GA, McCague R (1995): The deuterium isotope effect for the α-hydroxylation of tamoxifen by rat liver microsomes accounts for the reduced genotoxicity of [D_5-ethy]tamoxifen. *Carcinogenesis* 16:683-688

Jordan VC, Collins MM, Rowsby L, Prestwich G (1977): A monohydroxylated metabolite of tamoxifen with potent antiestrogenic acitvity. *J Endocrinol* 75:305-316

Jordan VC (1992): The role of tamoxifen in the treatment and prevention of breast cancer. *Current Probl Cancer* 16:129-176

Jordan VC (1995): Tamoxifen: Toxicities and drug resistance during the treatment and prevention of breast cancer. *Ann Rev Pharmacol Toxicol* 35:195-211

Juedes MJ, Bulger WH, Kupfer D (1987): Monooxygenase-mediated activation of chlorotrianisene (TACE) in covalent binding to rat hepatic microsomal proteins. *Drug Metab Dispos* 15:786-793

Juedes MJ, Kupfer D (1990): Role of P-450c in the formation of a reactive intermediate of chlorotrianisene (TACE) by hepatic microsomes from methylcholanthrene-treated rats. *Drug Metab Dispos* 18:131-137

Killackey MA, Hakes TB, Price VK (1985): Endometrial adenocarcinoma in breast cancer patients receiving antiestrogens. *Cancer Treatment Rep* 69:237-238

Kupfer D (1982) In: Hepatic Cytochrome P-450 Monooxygenase System (Schenkman JB Kupfer D, eds.) pp 157-187, Pergamon Press Great Britain

Kupfer D, Bulger, WH (1987): Metabolic activation of pesticides with proestrogenic activity. *Federation Proc* 46:1864-1869

Kupfer D, Bulger WH (1990): Inactivation of the uterine estrogen receptor binding of estradiol during P-450 catalyzed metabolism of chlorotrianisene (TACE). Speculation that TACE antiestrogenic activity involves covalent binding to the estrogen receptor. *FEBS Letters* 261:59-62

Kupfer D, Mani C, Lee CA, Rifkind AB (1994): Induction of tamoxifen-4-hydroxylation by 2,3,7,8-tetrachlorodibenzo-p-dioxin(TCDD) ß-naphthoflavone (ßNF) and phenobarbital (PB) in avian liver: identification of P450 TCDD$_{AA}$ as catalyst of 4-hydroxylation induced by TCDD and ßNF. *Cancer Res* 54:3140-3144

Kupfer D, Dehal SS (1996): Tamoxifen metabolism by microsomal cytochrome P450 and flavin-containing monooxygenase. *Methods in Enzymology* (In press)

Liehr JG, Roy D (1990): Free radical generation by redox cycling of estrogens. *Free Radical Biol & Med* 8:415-423

Liehr JG (1994): Mechanisms of metabolic activation and inactivation of catecholestrogens: a basis of genotoxicity. *Polycyclic Aromatic Compounds* 6:229-239

Lim CK, Yuan Z-X, Lamb JH, White INH, De Matteis F, Smith LL (1994): A comparative study of tamoxifen metabolism in female rat, mouse and human liver microsomes. *Carcinogenesis* 15:589-593

Lyman SD, Jordan VC (1986): In: Metabolism of Non-steroidal Antiestrogens in Estrogen/Antiestrogen Action and Breast Cancer Therapy pp 191-219 Jordan VC ed Madison WI: The University of Wisconsin Press

Malet C, Compel A, Spritzer P, Bricout N, Yaneva H, Mowszowicz I, Kuttenn F, Mayvais-Jarvis P (1988): Tamoxifen and hydroxytamoxifen isomers versus estradiol effects on normal human breast cells in culture. *Cancer Res* 48:7193-7199

Mani C, Kupfer D (1991): Cytochrome P-450-mediated activation and irreversible binding of the antiestrogen tamoxifen to proteins in rat and human liver: possible involvement of flavin-containing monooxygenases in tamoxifen activation. *Cancer Res* 51:6052-6058

Mani C, Gelboin HV, Park SS, Pierce R, Parkinson A, Kupfer D (1993a): Metabolism of the antimammary cancer antiestrogenic agent tamoxifen. I. Cytochrome P-450-catalyzed N-demethylation and 4-hydroxylation. *Drug Metab Dispos* 21:645-656

Mani C, Hodgson E, Kupfer D (1993b): Metabolism of the antimammary cancer antiestrogenic agent tamoxifen. II. Flavin-containing monooxygenase-mediated N-oxidation. *Drug Metab Dispos* 21:657-661

Mani C, Pierce R, Parkinson A, Kupfer D (1994): Involvement of cytochrome P-4503A in catalysis of tamoxifen activation and covalent binding to rat and human liver microsomes. *Carcinogenesis* 15:2715-2720

Martin EA, Rich KJ, White INH, Woods KL, Powles TJ, Smith LL (1995): ^{32}P-postlabelled DNA adducts in liver obtained from women treated with tamoxifen. *Carcinogenesis* 16:1651-1654

McCague R, Seago A (1986): Aspects of metabolism of tamoxifen by rat liver microsomes. *Biochem Pharmacol* 35:827-834

Mimura M, Baba T, Yamazaki H, Ohmori S, Inui Y, Gonzalez FJ, Guengerich FP, Shimada T (1993): Characterization of cytochrome P-450 2B6 in human liver microsomes. *Drug Metab Dispos* 21:1048-1056

Mitchell JR, Reid WD, Christie B, Moskowitz J, Krishna G, Brodie BB (1971): Bromobenzene-induced hepatic necrosis: species differences and protection by SKF525A. *Res Comm Chem Pathol Pharmacol* 2:877-887

Nelson SD (1982): Metabolic activation and drug toxicity. *J Med Chem* 25:753-765

Nelson DR, Kamataki T, Waxman DJ, Guengerich FP, Estabrook RW, Feyereisen R, Gonzalez FJ, Coon MJ, Gunsalus IC, Gotoh O, Okuda K, Nebert DW (1993): The P450 superfamily: update on new sequences gene mapping accession numbers early trivial names of enzymes and nomenclature. *DNA Cell Biol* 12:1-51

Nuwaysir EF, Dragon YP, Jefcoate CR, Jordan VC, Pitot HC (1995): Effects of tamoxifen administration on the expression of xenobiotic metabolizing enzymes in rat liver. *Cancer Res* 55:1780-1786

Pathak DN, Bodell WJ (1994): DNA adduct formation by tamoxifen with rat and human liver microsomal activation system. *Carcinogenesis* 15:529-532

Pathak DN, Pongracz K, Bodell WJ (1995): Microsomal and peroxidase activation of 4-hydroxy-tam to form DNA adducts: Comparison with DNA adducts formed in Sprague-Dawley rats treated with tamoxifen. *Carcinogenesis* 16:11-15

Phillips DH, Hewer A, White INH, Farmer PB (1994a): Co-chromatography of a tamoxifen epoxide-deoxyguanylic acid adduct with a major DNA adduct formed in the livers of tamoxifen-treated rats. *Carcinogenesis* 15:793-795

Phillips DH, Carmichael PL, Hewer A, Cole KJ, Poon GK (1994b): α-Hydroxytamoxifen a metabolite of tamoxifen with exceptionally high DNA-binding activity in rat hepatocytes. *Cancer Res* 54:5518-5522

Phillips DH, Potter GA, Horton MN, Hewer A, Crofton-Sleigh C (1994c): Reduced genotoxicity of [D_5-ethyl]-tamoxifen implicates α-hydroxylation of the ethyl group as a major pathway of tamoxifen activation to a liver carcinogen. *Carcinogenesis* 15:1487-1492

Pitot HC (1993): Molecular Biology of Carcinogenesis. *Cancer Supplement* 72:962-969

Pongracz K, Pathak DN, Nakamura T, Burlingame AL, Bodell WJ (1995): Activation of the tamoxifen derivative metabolite E to form DNA adducts: Comparison with the adducts formed by microsomal activation of tamoxifen. *Cancer Res* 55:3012-3015

Poon GK, Chui YC, McCague R, Lonning PE, Feng R, Rowlands MG, Jarman M (1993): Analysis of phase I and phase II metabolites of tamoxifen in breast cancer patients. *Drug Metab Dispos* 21:1119-1124

Poon GK, Walter B, Lonning PE, Holton MN, McCague R (1995): Identification of tamoxifen metabolites in human hep G2 cell line human liver homogenate and patients on long-term therapy for breast cancer. *Drug Metab Dispos* 23:377-382

Potter GA, McCague R, Jarman M (1994): A mechanistic hypothesis for DNA adduct formation by tamoxifen following hepatic oxidative metabolism. *Carcinogenesis* 15:439-442

Randerath K, Bi J, Mabon N, Sriram P, Moorthy B (1994a): Strong intensification of mouse hepatic tamoxifen DNA adduct formation by pretreatment with the sulfotransferase inhibitor and ubiquitous environmental pollutant pentachlorophenol. *Carcinogenesis* 15:797-800

Randerath K, Moorthy K, Mabon N, Sriram P (1994b): Tamoxifen: evidence by ^{32}P-postlabeling and use of metabolic inhibitors for two distinct pathways leading to mouse hepatic DNA adduct formation and identification of 4-hydroxytamoxifen as a proximate metabolite. *Carcinogenesis* 15:2087-2093

Reunitz PC, Bagley JR, Pape CW (1984): Some chemical and biochemical aspects of liver microsomal metabolism of tamoxifen. *Drug Metab Dispos* 12:478-483

Ryan DE, Levin W (1990): Purification and characterization of hepatic microsomal cytochrome P-450. *Pharmacol Ther* 45:153-239

Sawahata T, Neal RA (1983): Biotransformation of phenol to hydroquinone and catechol by rat liver microsomes. *Mol Pharmacol* 23:453-460

Sonderfan AJ, Arlotto MP, Dutton DR, McMillen SK, Parkinson A (1987): Regulation of testosterone hydroxylation by rat liver microsomal cytochrome P450. *Arch Biochem Biophs* 255:27-41

Soucek P, Gut I (1992): Cytochromes P-450 in rats: structures functions properties and relevant human forms. *Xenobiotica* 22:83-103

Sutherland RL, Mester J, Baulieu EE (1977): Tamoxifen is a potent "pure" anti-oestrogen in chick oviduct. *Nature* (Lond) 267:434-435

Terenius L (1971): Structure-activity relationship of anti-oestrogens with regard to interaction with 17ß-oestradiol in the mouse uterus and vagina. *Acta Endocrinol* 66:431-447

Turner MJ, Fields CE, Everman DB (1991): Evidence for superoxide formation during hepatic metabolism of tamoxifen. *Biochem Pharmacol* 41:1701-1705

van Leeumne FE, Benraadt J, Coebergh JWW, Kiemeney LALM, Gimbrere CHF, Otter R, Schouten LJ, Damhuis RAM, Bontenbal M, Diepenhorst FW, van den Belt-Dusebout AW, van Tinteren H (1994): Risk of endometrial cancer after tamoxifen treatment of breast cancer. *Lancet* 343:448-452

Vancutsem PM, Lazarus P, Williams GM (1994): Frequent and specific mutations of the rat p53 gene in hepatocarcinomas induced by tamoxifen. *Cancer Res* 54:3864-3867

Vignon F, Bouton M-M, Rochefort H (1987): Antiestrogens inhibit the mitogenic effect of growth factors on breast cancer cells in the total absence of estrogens. *Biochem Biophys Res Commun* 146:1502-1508

Waxman D (1988): Interactions of hepatic Cytochromes P-450 with steroid hormones. *Biochem Pharmacol* 37:71-84

White INH, de Matteis F, Davies A, Smith LL, Crofton-Sleigh C, Venitt S, Hewer A, Phillips DH (1992): Genotoxic potential of tamoxifen and analogues in female Fischer F344/N rats DBA/2 and C57B1/G mice and in human MCL-5 cells. *Carcinogenesis* 13:2197-2203

White INH, Davis A, Smith LL, Dawson S, de Matteis F (1993): Induction of CYP2B1 and 3A1 and associated monooxygenase activities by tamoxifen and certain analogues in the livers of female rats and mice. *Biochem Pharmacol* 45:21-30

White INH, de Matteis F, Gibbs AH, Lim CK, Wolf CR, Henderson C, Smith LL (1995): Species differences in the covalent binding of [^{14}C]tamoxifen to liver microsomes and the forms of cytochrome P450 involved. *Biochem Pharmacol* 49:1035-1042

Williams GM, Iatropoulos MJ, Djordjevic MW, Kaltenberg OP (1993): The triphenylethylene drug tamoxifen is a strong carcinogen in the rat. *Carcinogenesis* 14:315-317

Wrighton SA, Maurel P, Schuetz EG, Watkins PB, Young B, Guzelian PS (1985): Identification of the cytochrome P-450 induced by macrolide antibiotics in rat liver as the glucocorticoid responsive cytochrome P-450p. *Biochemistry* 24:2171-2178

Zhou L-X, Dehal SS, Kupfer D, Morrell S, McKenzie BA, Eccleston ED, Holtzman JL (1995): Cytochrome P450 catalyzed covalent binding of methoxychlor to rat hepatic, microsomal Iodothyronine 5'-monodeiodinase, type I: Does exposure to methoxychlor disrupt thyroid hormone metabolism? *Arch Biochem Biophys* 322:390-394

10. TAMOXIFEN METABOLISM AND OESTROGEN RECEPTOR FUNCTION - IMPLICATIONS FOR MECHANISMS OF RESISTANCE IN BREAST CANCER

Stephen R.D. Johnston and Mitchell Dowsett

Introduction

As an endocrine agent for the treatment of breast cancer, Tamoxifen functions by competitively antagonising the mitogenic signal which results from the interaction of biologically active oestrogens with the oestrogen receptor (ER) in ER-positive cells. There are several pharmacological factors which may determine its ability to achieve this *in vivo*. These include the metabolism of Tamoxifen and the formation of various metabolites which may have different agonist/antagonist profiles, the bioavailability and pharmacokinetics of Tamoxifen, and the ability of these compounds to interact with ER and form inappropriate complexes which are no longer able to regulate the oestrogen-responsive genes involved in the growth pathway. It is as a consequence of the latter, namely Tamoxifen's interaction with ER, that the majority of pharmacological effects occur both *in vivo* and *in vitro*.

Tamoxifen is the most effective endocrine agent in the management of breast cancer which has been shown to prolong both disease free and overall survival in women following surgery for early breast cancer (EBCTCG 1992), and which is first line therapy in advanced breast cancer, particularly in women with ER-positive tumours (McGuire, 1978). However, many tumours are resistant *de novo* to Tamoxifen, and most tumours which initially respond eventually develop acquired resistance and progress on Tamoxifen. Until recently the biological basis for this resistance *in vivo* has been poorly understood.

An increased knowledge of how oestrogen regulate cell growth and the mechanism of action of oestrogens has provided targets for investigation within the ER-mediated growth pathway which may become defective in resistant cells. Two aspects which have been investigated extensively within the past few years have been Tamoxifen's metabolism and its interaction with ER, both of which may become altered in the context of resistance.

Pharmacology and metabolism of Tamoxifen

Pharmacological action. The pharmacological properties of Tamoxifen are complex. The drug can behave as an oestrogen (full agonist), a partial agonist or as an antagonist depending on the species or target organ studied and the biochemical end point which is measured (Furr and Jordan, 1984). The effects of Tamoxifen on the growth of human breast cancer have been studied intensely in cell lines, particularly the ER-positive MCF-7 breast cancer cell line. MCF-7 cells contain oestrogen receptors and are growth stimulated by oestradiol (Lippman et al., 1976). Tamoxifen inhibits MCF-7 cell growth as determined by cell numbers, DNA content and (^{3}H)thymidine incorporation (Lippman et al., 1976; Coezy et al., 1982). This can be reversed by addition of oestradiol suggesting that the growth inhibition is not cytotoxic. Subsequent studies of cell cycle kinetics have confirmed the cytostatic nature of Tamoxifen which reduces the proportion of cells in S phase and increases the number in G1 phase of the cell cycle (Osborne et al., 1983; Sutherland et al., 1983b), although at higher doses (10^{-5} M) the drug is cytotoxic and induces cell death. Hoever a biphasic growth response to Tamoxifen has also been noted, and at low doses (10^{-9} M) in oestrogen-depleted medium Tamoxifen stimulates cell growth in a manner similar to oestradiol (Reddel and Sutherland, 1984).

The mixed antagonist/agonist profile of Tamoxifen which is evident from study of the drug's pre-clinical pharmacology may have important therapeutic implications in clinical practice, particularly when considering long-term Tamoxifen therapy in either the adjuvant or chemo-preventive setting. There is evidence that the response to the drug *in vivo* varies depending on the target organ studied and that while in the breast the drug behaves as an antagonist, in other tissues including the bone and endometrium a predominantly agonist response may be seen.

The pharmacological response to Tamoxifen *in vivo*, therefore, may be species, dose or tissue dependent. In humans it is important to consider the metabolism of Tamoxifen and contribution of the respective metabolites to the overall action of the drug, as the metabolic profile may be relevant to the subsequent response of breast carcinomas to Tamoxifen *in vivo*.

Metabolism.

Metabolic pathways. The predominant metabolism of Tamoxifen occurs in the liver via cytochrome P-450 enzymes located in the microsomes (Jacolot et al., 1991). The two major metabolic pathways for Tamoxifen in humans are shown in Figure 1 and involve demethylation, deamination and hydroxylation of key positions on the phenyl groups of Tamoxifen. Demethylation of the tertiary amine results in the major metabolite found in human serum, N-desmethyltamoxifen (Adam et al., 1979). Further demethylation forms N,N-didesmethyltamoxifen (Kemp et al., 1983), and subsequent deamination results in the polar compound metabolite Y (Bain and Jordan, 1983). The alternative route of metabolism involves hydroxylation of Tamoxifen at the 4-position to form 4-hydroxytamoxifen, a potent antioestrogen (Fromson et al., 1973; Daniel et al., 1979).

Pharmacological activity of metabolites. All the major metabolites of Tamoxifen will bind oestrogen receptor *in vitro* and competitively inhibit oestradiol-stimulated growth on MCF-7 cells. However there is a considerable range in the relative binding affinity (RBA) for ER of the different metabolites. In particular metabolites which are hydroylated in the 4-position have a high RBA which is similar to oestradiol (Jordan et al., 1977), and are thus 100 times more potent than the parent compound Tamoxifen in inhibiting MCF-7 growth *in vitro* (Coezy et al., 1982). It is thought that all the major metabolites contribute to Tamoxifen's antioestrogenic activity *in vivo*. However some of the minor metabolites, namely metabolite E and bisphenol, appear to have significantly more agonist than antagonist properties in a variety of bioassay systems (Lyman and Jordan, 1985).

Isomers of 4-hydroxytamoxifen and metabolite E. Metabolites of Tamoxifen which are hydroxylated on the phenyl ring, namely 4-hydroxytamoxifen and metabolite E, are capable of undergoing time-temperature dependent isomerisation from the Z (trans) isomer to the E (cis) isomer (Jordan et al., 1981). The electron-withdrawing hydroxyl

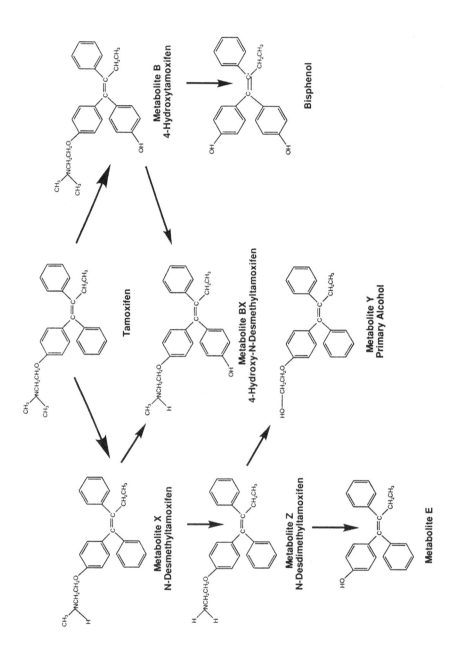

Figure 1. The metabolic pathway for Tamoxifen.

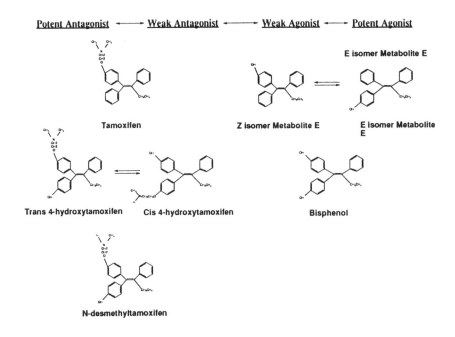

Potent Antagonist ◄─────► Weak Antagonist ◄─────► Weak Agonist ◄─────► Potent Agonist

Tamoxifen

Z isomer Metabolite E

E isomer Metabolite E

E isomer Metabolite E

Trans 4-hydroxytamoxifen   Cis 4-hydroxytamoxifen

Bisphenol

N-desmethyltamoxifen

Figure 2. The structural forms Tamoxifen's metabolites which may have either a predominantly agonist or antagonist effect upon interaction with ER.

group weakens the ethylene bond and permits the substituents attached to the carbon atoms to rotate around the double bond. These configurations are important when discussing the relative oestrogenic and antioestrogenic activities of these metabolites (Figure 2). The Z (trans)4-hydroxytamoxifen has a high RBA similar to that of oestradiol and is a potent antioestrogen, whereas E (cis) 4-hydroxytamoxifen has a low RBA and is a weaker antioestrogen (Katzenellenbogen et al., 1984).

The amine sidechain is thought to be essential for antioestrogenic activity of Tamoxifen (Jordan and Gosden, 1982). In metabolite E this sidechain is replaced by a hydroxyl group, and upon isomerisation to the E isomer the hydroxyl group occupies the same phenyl position as in Z-4-hydroxytamoxifen and consequently exhibits high binding affinity for the oestrogen receptor (Figure 2). However without the amine sidechain which determines antioestrogenic acitivity, the E isomer of metabolite E behaves as a potent oestrogen (Murphy et al., 1990). In contrast the Z isomer of metabolite, E has much lower binding affinity and is only a weak oestrogen.

Structure-activity relationships with oestrogen receptor. The transcriptional activity of the oestrogen receptor is mediated by at least two separate transactivation domains (TAFs) (Lees et al., 1989; Tora et al., 1989). TAF-1 is located near the N-terminal end of the receptor and appears to function constitutively when ER is bound to target DNA-binding sites, whereas TAF-2 which is located near the C-terminal end depends on oestradiol binding to initiate transcriptional activity (Figure 3). Thus different ER-regulated genes may be controlled through either TAF-1 or TAF-2 sites, and cooperation of activating or inhibiting transcription factors which may or may not be present within a cell may ultimately determine gene expression. Tamoxifen interaction with ER is thought to prevent gene expression via TAF-2, but not necessarily modulate TAF-1 activity. This in part may explain some of the mixed biochemical responses observed with the drug.

In addition to the effects of Tamoxifen on TAF function, a hypothetical model of ligand interaction with the oestrogen receptor has been developed in an attempt to explain the differential agonist and antagonist activities of Tamoxifen and its various metabolites (Jordan et al., 1984). Drug-receptor interaction comprises both binding of the drug, which is determined by the intrinsic activity of the drug-receptor complex. While an agonist ligand would bind to the receptor with the resulting complex having a high intrinsic activity, an ideal antagonist drug would retain a high affinity for the receptor, but result in a complex with low intrinsic activity (Belleau, 1964).

Marked differential effects can be envisaged using such a model if a comparison is made between the structural interaction of an agonist ligand (ie. oestradiol) and a antagonist drug (ie. 4-hydroxytamoxifen) with ER's ligand-binding site (Figure 4). Both compounds bind with a high affinity to ER, which for oestradiol may be primarily related to the C-3 phenolic group and for 4-hydroxytamoxifen to the phenol ring formed by hydroxylation of Tamoxifen at the 4 position. It is envisaged that oestrogen binding induces a conformational change in the tertiary structure which activates the receptor and allows the development of its intrinsic activity, namely binding to oestrogen response elements (EREs) within DNA, recruitment of accessory proteins and associated transcription factors, leading to transcription of oestrogen-regulated genes some of which include growth response genes (Figure 4a). In contrast 4-hydroxytamoxifen bound to the receptor prevents the formation of the necessary tertiary structure to allow receptor activation, such that the intrinsic activity of the complex is low. It is thought that the alkyl-

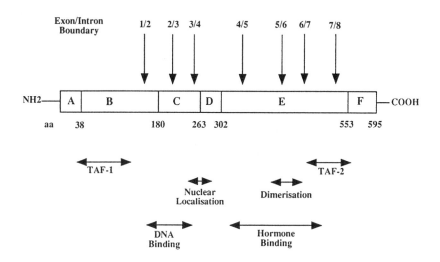

Figure 3. The six functional domains of the oestrogen receptor protein showing the location of the eight associated exon/intron boundaries of the ER gene, and the amino acid (aa) numbers of each domain. The relative position of each functional activity of the receptor is also shown.

aminoethoxy sidechain prevents the necesary changes in the receptor's tertiary structure by 'wedging' the ligand-binding site open such that the receptor, even though it can dimerise and bind to EREs, cannot recruit the accessory proteins and other transcription factors to the complex to result in transcription of growth response genes (Figure 4b). This interaction, therefore, is the basis of the drug's competitive antagonism.

This hypothetical model of structure-function relationships may also explain the relative oestrogenic and antioestrogenic activities of the various metabolites and isomeric forms of Tamoxifen (Figure 2). For example bisphenol, the metabolite formed after removal of the alkyl-aminoethoxy side chain of 4-hydroxytamoxifen, is a partial agonist *in vitro* (Jordan et al., 1984b). The loss of the side chain means that many receptor complexes may take the active form with high intrinsic activity. This would explain the observation that the side chain is important in governing the antioestrogenic action of the drug (Jordan and Gosden, 1982). In addition the relative position of the side chain, which differs between trans and cis isomers of 4-hydroxytamoxifen, may be important

Key to binding regions on ER

⬭ "Antioestrogen" binding site
◯ "Oestrogen" binding site
◯ Dimerisation site
⬤ DNA "zinc finger" binding site

A) Agonist Ligand

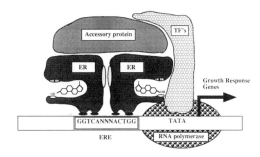

B) Antagonist Drug

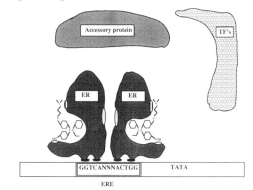

Figure 4. A hypothetical model of the structure-function relationships of the oestrogen receptor following binding of (a) agonist ligand (ie. oestrogen), or (b) antagonist drug (ie. 4-hydroxytamoxifen). Schematic diagram shows formation of ER homodimers after binding of oestradiol which bind to oestrogen response elements (ERE's) upstream of regulated genes. Recruitment of accessory proteins, transcription factors (TF's) and RNA polymerase results in gene transcription. While receptor occupancy by 4-hydroxytamoxifen allows dimerisation and DNA binding, an altered conformational structure prevents formation of the activated transcription complex and gene transcription is prevented. It is thought that the side chain of the drug is crucial in allowing binding to the antioestrogen site in the ligand-binding domain, which in turn keeps the ER tertiary structure 'wedged' open. (Adapted from Jordan et al., 1984a).

for this effect. In the cis-form the aminoethoxy side chain would lie adjacent from the so-called 'antioestrogen' region of the receptor site, thus preventing the 'wedging' of the receptor into an inactive form.

The overall metabolic profile and associated structure-activity relationships are aspects which may determine the oestrogenic/antioestrogenic activity of Tamoxifen *in vivo*. As discussed above, however, the differential response shown by separate tissues to the same compounds *in vivo* must also be considered. This suggests that the consequence of drug-receptor interaction differs between different tissues. This may be explained by altered transcription factors within these tissues which determine which genes are regulated by the activated receptor complex through either TAF-1 or TAF-2. An alternative explanation for such regulation is that the receptor structure itself differs between these tissues. To date these issues remain poorly understood.

Clinical pharmacology.

Serum pharmacokinetics. Following continuous treatment in humans, the serum level of Tamoxifen reaches steady state after approximately 4 weeks, although the concentration of the major metabolite N-desmethyltamoxifen rises more slowly and may take up to 8 weeks to achieve steady state (Patterson et al., 1980). N-desmethyltamoxifen is found at serum concentrations 1.5-2.0 times greater than the parent compound Tamoxifen, whereas the concentration of 4-hydroxytamoxifen is only about 2% of that of the parent drug. There are several reports in the literature which demonstrate the steady state levels of both Tamoxifen and its metabolites in breast cancer patients (Table 1). While individual patients vary greatly in their metabolic handling of the drug and wide ranges exist in the concentrations quoted in each study, in general these show excellent agreement and indicate linearity of drug concentrations over the dosage range of 20-40 mg daily. Once the steady state is achieved serum levels of Tamoxifen and its metabolites remain constant over many years of long-term therapy, and in particular the Tamoxifen/N-desmethyltamoxifen ratio remains remarkably constant (Langhan-Fahey et al., 1990). There is no evidence that the serum level of Tamoxifen achieved predicts for clinical response (Patterson et al., 1980; Bratherton et al., 1984).

Tissue Distribution. The majority of Tamoxifen and its metabolites are bound to serum proteins and only 2-5% is in the "free" unbound state

(Shah and Parsons, 1991). Because of this very little active drug gains access across the blood-brain barrier into the cerebrospinal fluid (Noguchi et al., 1988a). However, animal data suggest that levels of Tamoxifen and its metabolites in several tissues are much higher than those in the serum, with liver and uterine tissue accumulating much greater levels than skeletal muscle in studies performed in rats and mice (Robinson et al., 1991).

Tamoxifen resistance and metabolic tolerance

The biological effect of Tamoxifen *in vivo* is dependent of achieving adequate concentrations of drug within the target tissue to compete with oestradiol at the level of the oestrogen receptor. In considering breast cancer therapy in humans, situations in which insufficient intra-tumoural concentrations of Tamoxifen are achieved to antagonise the interaction of oestradiol with ER may be one method whereby cells escape growth inhibition by the drug. The phenomenon of metabolic tolerance has been used to describe such a potential mechanism where reduced cellular Tamoxifen levels develop, either through enhanced metabolism or impaired intra-cellular accumulation (Osborne et al., 1991; Osborne et al., 1994).

Intra-tumoural accumulation *in vivo*. There are only limited data in the literature on the normal tissue and intra-tumoural concentrations of Tamoxifen relative to serum in human breast cancer patients. In general this reflects the difficulty of getting adequate biopsy samples for these analyses. In a study from patients receiving 40 mg/day for at least 30 days (ie. steady state), Tamoxifen and its metabolites were found to accumulate in tissues 10-60 fold abover serum levels when expressed as ng/gm wet weight tissue to ng/ml serum (Lein et al., 1991). In a previous study of breast tumour homogenates, the relative intra-tumoural amounts of N-desmethyltamoxifen and 4-hydroxytamoxifen compared to Tamoxifen reflected the ratios found in the serum (Daniel et al., 1981). In other tumour types in which Tamoxifen therapy has been given, namely melanoma and squamous cell head and neck carcinoma, 4-fold (9100 ng/gm vs 2294 ng/ml) and 6-fold (9500 ng/gm vs 1646 ng/ml) uptake ratios, respectively, were observed relative to serum, albeit with much higher daily doses than used in breast cancer therapy (Trump et al., 1992). Taken together, all these previous studies suggest that human breast tumours accumulate Tamoxifen and its metabolites between 5 and 20 fold, relative to serum.

Although serum levels of Tamoxifen may remain constant during therapy *in vivo*, there is evidence that metabolic tolerance may occur as a consequence of reduced intra-tumoural accumulation. In MCF-7 xenografts in immune-deprived mice which had become resistant following 4-6 months prolonged therapy a near 10-fold reduction in intra-tumoural Tamoxifen compared with responding tumours was observed in the absence of any change in the serum concentrations (Osborne et al., 1991). In a small clinical study from the same investigators reduced intra-tumoural Tamoxifen concentrations were found in 8/11 "non-responsive tumours" treated with Tamoxifen for between 1 month and 6 years (Osborne et al., 1992), although serum Tamoxifen levels were not measured to exclude poor compliance.

We recently studied intra-tumoural Tamoxifen accumulation in a total of 51 Tamoxifen-resistant tumours (Johnston et al., 1993). In all cases a matched serum sample taken at the same time as the biopsy allowed an estimate to be made of tumour Tamoxifen accumulation relative to serum. There was no difference in the serum concentrations of Tamoxifen or N-desmethyltamoxifen in patients who developed either acquired Tamoxifen resistance after a median of 24 months, or were *de novo* resistant to the drug after a median of 4 months, or relapsed during adjuvant therapy after a median of 28 months. However, we found a significant reduction in intra-tumoural concentration of Tamoxifen in patients with acquired, but not *de novo*, resistance to the drug. This was represented in some patients by a ten-fold reduction in the ratio of tumour to serum Tamoxifen levels (Figure 5), a quantative difference similar to that observed by Osborne et al. (1991) in their xenograft model. This phenomenon was also observed in some tumours which relapsed during adjuvant therapy where the initial response to Tamoxifen was unknown, being observed particularly in tumours which were ER + ve and were associated with a longer disease-free interval.

Mechanism of reduced intra-tumoural accumulation. There are at least three potential mechanisms by which acquired Tamoxifen-resistant tumours may develop reduced intra-tumoural levels. Firstly, uptake of Tamoxifen into cells may become impaired by systemic factors which reduce either the drug's serum concentration or its bioavailability from the circulation. We have found no change in association with resistance in either the percentage of serum Tamoxifen in the protein-free form or in the concentration of alpha-1-acid glycoprotein (Johnston et al., 1994), a major serum protein whose concentration has been shown previously to affect Tamoxifen's bioavailability (Chatterjee and Harris, 1990).

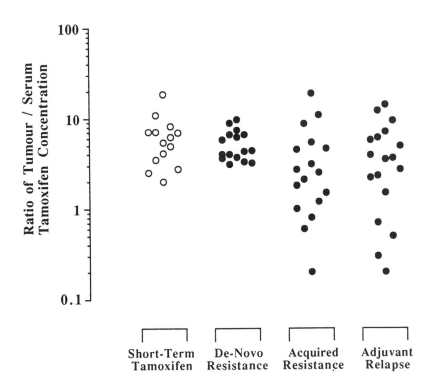

Figure 5. Ratio of intra-tumoural Tamoxifen (ng/gm) to serum Tamoxifen (ng/ml) in 51 patients with clinically defined Tamoxifen resistance and in 14 patients with primary breast cancer treated with short-term Tamoxifen for at least 2 weeks prior to surgery (reprinted with permission from Johnston et al., 1993).

Secondly, intra-tumoural levels could become lowered by increased intra-cellular metabolism of Tamoxifen, either to inactive compounds or to more oestrogenic metabolites. There is no reported evidence that breast carcinoma cell lines or tumours are able to metabolise Tamoxifen themselves (Borgna and Rochefort, 1981; Wiseman, 1994). However, an altered distribution of Tamoxifen metabolites has been reported in some Tamoxifen-resistant tumours (see below). In the 51 resistant patients we studied there appeared to be no significant change in the amounts of the major metabolites relative to Tamoxifen, and oestrogenic metabolites were not detected.

Finally, reduced intra-tumoural concentrations could be the result of transport pump mechanisms which actively exclude drugs from within the cell. Such a mechanism for acquired resistance to several cytotoxic drugs is well known, with overexpression of the membrane-associated 170 kD P-glycoprotein coded for by the MDR-1 gene being associated with reduction in intra-cellular drug concentrations below a therapeutic threshold (Juliano and Ling, 1976). Triphenylethylene antioestrogens have been implicated as P-glycoprotein substrates, and Tamoxifen is one of the agents known to reverse MDR-1 associated multi-drug resistance phenotype *in vitro* (Ramu et al., 1984). The possibility that Tamoxifen may induce over-expression of P-glycoprotein and thus reduce its own intra-cellular concentration has been the subject of one clinical study. A significant increase in expression of P-glycoprotein was observed in Tamoxifen-resistant tumours compared with tumours which responded to primary Tamoxifen (Keen et al., 1994). However, in the xenograft model of acquired resistance, enhanced expression of P-glycoprotein was not observed (Wiebe et al., 1995). Furthermore in a breast cancer cell line transfected with MDR-1 there was no evidence of reduced intra-tumoural Tamoxifen concentrations (Clarke et al., 1992). Thus the evidence is largely against an involvement of P-glycoprotein, but other pumps may exist which are capable of extruding Tamoxifen.

Metabolic tolerance and Tamoxifen-stimulated growth. Due to the mixed agonist/antagonist nature of Tamoxifen, it has been postulated that Tamoxifen failure may result from the development of Tamoxifen-stimulated growth (Howell et al., 1990). There is both clinical evidence to support this in terms of Tamoxifen-withdrawal responses observed in patients who relapse on Tamoxifen (Legault-Poisson et al., 1979; Canney et al., 1987; Howell et al., 1992), and experimental evidence from the xenograft model of dose-dependent stimulation of acquired resistant growth by Tamoxifen (Gottardis and Jordan, 1988) which may be antagonised by pure antioestrogens (Gottardis et al., 1989).

Oestrogenic metabolites. One mechanism for Tamoxifen stimulation may involve a relative increase in intra-tumoural concentration of more oestrogenic metabolites such as cis-4OHT, metabolite E or bisphenol. In the original xenograft model of acquired resistance (Osborne et al., 1991), a significant ($p < 0.005$) increase in the cis/trans-4-OHT ratio in resistant versus sensitive xenografts was noted (0.81Ý0.19 (SD) vs. 0.53Ý0.17, respectively). Subsequently the same group reported finding high cis/trans 4-OHT ratios in 6 Tamoxifen-resistant tumours (Osborne et al., 1992). In a further study of 5 patients with Tamoxifen non-responsive breast cancer the same investigators identified the oestrogenic metabolite

E (Wiebe et al., 1992), albeit at low concentrations (<50 ng/gm) compared with Tamoxifen and its antioestrogenic metabolites. However, the cis-isomer metabolite is unstable and high concentrations would be required *in vivo* to counter the inhibitory activity of Tamoxifen and its other antioestrogenic metabolites (Wolf et al., 1993).

The contribution of isomerisation, however, as a mechanism for Tamoxifen-stimulated growth *in vivo* has recently been questioned. Fixed-ring analogues of Tamoxifen have been synthesised in which the ethyl side-chain is replaced by a propyl group bonded from the pehnyl ring to the ethylene backbone, thus preventing isomerisation due to rotation around the double bond (McCague et al., 1986). Such fixed-ring derivatives of Tamoxifen have been demonstrated to equally stimulate growth of the Tamoxifen-resistant MCF-7 TAM xenografts compared with the parent compound, implying that isomerisation is not necessary for Tamoxifen-stimulated growth (Wolf et al., 1993). Furthermore analogues of Tamoxifen which are resistant to conversion to metabolite E (deoxytamoxifen) also stimulate growth (Osborne et al., 1994). These observations suggest that Tamoxifen-stimulated growth, in the xenograft model at least, is not due to isomerisation or metabolism of Tamoxifen to less antioestrogenic or more oestrogenic metabolites.

Biphasic dose-response.   Tamoxifen stimulation may occur as a consequence of known differential growth response to the drug which has been observed depending on its relative intra-cellular concentration. *In vitro* Tamoxifen has been shown to stimulate the proliferation of T-47D human breast cancer cells at low concentrations (10^{-9} M) in the presence of charcoal stripped fetal calf serum (Reddel and Sutherland, 1984). Likewise using the Courtenay-Mills clonogenic assay for MCF-7 cells in oestrogen-free conditions, Tamoxifen stimulated colony formation at low concentrations (10^{-6} M) (DeFriend et al., 1994). This biphasic response to Tamoxifen depending on dose, together with known pharmacokinetics of Tamoxifen and the prolonged time to reach steady-state, may explain the phenomenon of Tamoxifen flare following initiation of therapy. In support of this are the clinical observations that when menopausal status is specified, most reported cases of Tamoxifen flare are in postmenopausal women (McIntosh and Tynne, 1977; Plotkin et al., 1987) in which, as with the *in vitro* experiments, the relatively oestradiol-depleted conditions may allow Tamoxifen to exert is agonist effects. Furthermore there is biochemical evidence that in the first few days of Tamoxifen therapy when drug levels are rising, progesterone receptor levels rise, a response normally considered to be oestrogenic (Horwitz et al., 1978).

Cellular heterogeneity. Alterations in the ER-dependent growth pathway mean that some cells may inherently respond to Tamoxifen by being growth-stimulated rather than inhibited, perhaps due to specific alterations in the oestrogen receptor structure. Such cells may exist within a heterogenous ER+ tumour at low levels, but be selected for during Tamoxifen therapy to become the dominant type which results in Tamoxifen stimulated growth (Howell et al., 1992). There is experimental evidence that mutant forms of ER, particularly those with point mutations in the hormone binding domain, may have an altered response to Tamoxifen, perceiving the drug as an agonist (Mahfoudi et al., 1995). Evidence that these receptor mutants which have an altered response to Tamoxifen exist *in vivo* or play a significant role in the development of resistance is discussed below.

Clinical consequence of reduced intra-tumoural Tamoxifen. The above observations suggest that if following long-term therapy with Tamoxifen the intra-cellular concentrations of the drug become reduced, then the ligand's effect may be converted from that of an antagonist to an agonist. This could then account for the phenomenon of Tamoxifen-stimulated growth in tumours with acquired resistance. Alternatively, reduced intra-tumoural levels of Tamoxifen may be the cause of Tamoxifen failure clinically if these are insufficient to effectively antagonise the endogenous level of biologically active oestrogen. Whilst it has been previously estimated that the intra-tumoural levels of Tamoxifen are a 2-4 orders of magnitude greater than oestradiol (Nicholson et al., 1979), it is conceivable that in some patients intra-tumoural concentrations of Tamoxifen which are reduced by a factor of 10 may be insufficient to antagonise endogenous oestradiol. If such tumours remain hormone-sensitive, and the evidence from our data is that the majority are ER+ at relapse (Johnston et al., 1993), then one would expect them to re-grow in a hormone-dependent manner and to remain sensitive to further endocrine therapy with, for example, aromatase inhibitors. This would be consistent with the clinical observation that tumours with true acquired resistance following an initial response to Tamoxifen have response rates to second-line endocrine therapy of greater than 60%, whether it be pure antioestrogens, progestins or aromatase inhibitors that are used (Dowsett et al., 1995; Howell et al., 1995).

Tamoxifen's effect on ER function and expression

Markers of a functional ER pathway. It became clear from some of the original studies of endocrine therapy in breast cancer that the association between responsiveness and quantitative ER assessment is not absolute, and that many patients fail to respond to endocrine treatment despite high receptor levels in their tumour. An increased understanding of the molecular events following receptor activation came from the discovery of several cellular proteins in breast epithelia whose expression was clearly regulated through ER. The MCF-7 breast carcinoma cell line was found to contain receptors for a number of different steroid hormones, including the progesterone receptor (PgR) (Horwitz et al., 1975). It was subsequently shown that PgR expression was induced by oestrogen in ER+ve breast cancer cell lines (Horwitz et al., 1978). Several clinical studies have suggested that combined PgR expression in human breast cancers with ER status defines a better marker of hormone dependence (LeMaistre and McGuire, 1986; Ravdi et al., 1992). Oestrogen also induces the secretion of several other proteins in ER+ MCF-7 breast cancer cells including the lysosomal protease cathepsin D (Westley and May, 1987) and pS2 (Masiakowski et al., 1982). The pS2 gene encodes a 84-amino-acid precursor protein which is cleaved to yield a 7 kD protein which is cysteine-rich and has structural similarities to the Insulin Like Growth Factor II (Stack et al., 1988). Some clinical studies have suggested that pS2 expression is also a predictive factor for response to endocrine therapy (Henry et al., 1989; Skilton et al., 1989; Schwartz et al., 1991; Henry et al., 1991). However, in a recent larger Dutch study the data on pS2's ability to predict for endocrine responsiveness were less convincing (Foekens et al., 1994). This may be in part due to factors other than oestrogen regulating pS2 expression including peptide growth factors such as EGF and IGF (Cavailles et al., 1989).

Effect of Tamoxifen on ER expression and function *in vivo*. It was first reported that a significant fall in ER content followed endocrine therapy (Allegra et al., 1980; Taylor et al., 1982; Hull et al., 1983). In these early studies a ligand-binding assay was used to measure ER and it is probable that receptor occupancy by Tamoxifen resulted in a false negative ER assay for many tumours. The impact of such interference was recently demonstrated in a study were ER was detected more frequently by immuno-histochemical compared with ligand-binding assay in 34 patients on Tamoxifen (Encarnacion et al., 1993). Another confounding variable in many of these studies was the sequential comparison between different metastatic deposits of tumour, and it is possible that the ER phenotype of metastases may be different from the primary tumour. While in some *in vitro* studies Tamoxifen has been shown to upregulate ER expression (Kiang et al., 1989), the effect *in vivo* is less clear.

In vivo studies of paired biopsies have shown that short-term Tamoxifen may increase PgR expression in ER+ve, but not ER-ve tumours (Namer et al., 1980). In one study of 52 patients with locally advanced or recurrent breast cancer the initial rise in PgR following Tamoxifen predicted for a response to endocrine therapy (Howell et al., 1987). Studies have indicated that this effect of Tamoxifen on PgR induction is maximal within the first week of therapy, and that following 14 days no induction is seen and levels subsequently fall over time in responding tumours (Noguchi et al., 1988b). It is unclear whether this initial induction of PgR during the first few days of therapy is a consequence of the agonist activity of Tamoxifen at low doses prior to sufficient intra-tumoural levels being reached to antagonise ER.

The effects of Tamoxifen therapy on pS2 expression *in vivo* have not been studied extensively. Available *in vitro* data suggest that while Tamoxifen alone may have a partial oestrogenic effect on pS2 expression, it can effectively antagonise oestrogen-induced synthesis of pS2 suggesting a classical ER-dependent regulation of pS2 (Johnson et al., 1989). On this basis if pS2 expression in primary tumours is indicative of a hormone-sensitive tumour, levels should fall following Tamoxifen. However, data exist which show that in the absence of oestradiol, Tamoxifen can still inhibit EGF- or IGF-induced pS2 gene expression (Chalbos et al., 1993). These data further support the observation that pS2 may also be regulated by alternative pathways which are separate from the direct transcriptional effects of oestradiol.

ER expression and function in Tamoxifen-resistant breast cancer. The current literature suggests that *in vivo* Tamoxifen may have a complex effect on ER expression and function within the primary tumour. Tamoxifen acts mainly as an anti-proliferative agent on ER+cells, and as ER expression is heterogenous within a tumour, the possibility that continued therapy may lead to the selective outgrowth of ER-negative cell clones has been an attractive hypothesis. This clonal selection could become manifest as an ER-negative recurrent tumour, such that changes in ER expression and function could explain the development of Tamoxifen resistance. However, the clinical observation that many patients which develop acquired resistance to Tamoxifen remain sensitive to further endocrine therapies (Smith et al., 1981), including pure antioestrogens, aromatase inhibitors and progestins, suggests that the ER-mediated growth pathway remains functional in many of these tumours.

Change in ER phenotype. We recently analysed the expression of ER, PgR and pS2 by immuno-histochemical assay in 72 paired tumour biopsies taken before treatment and at relapse or progression on Tamoxifen. Overall the frequency of ER expression was reduced in Tamoxifen-resistant tumours from 51% pretamoxifen to 29% at progression or relapse, with a significant reduction in the quantitative level of ER (Johnston et al., 1995). The majority of resistant ER+ tumours still appeared functional as determined by PgR and pS2 expression. In these tumours even if Tamoxifen initially down-regulated PgR and pS2, at relapse these proteins continued to be expressed in tumours which were progressing on Tamoxifen. Analysis showed that the persistence of ER+PgR/pS2+phenotype was predominantly confined to tumours which acquired resistance following an initial objective response to Tamoxifen (median of 24 months), whereas tumours which progressed during primary Tamoxifen (median 4 months) were predominantly ER-ve. These data in themselves suggest a fundamental difference in the mechanism of Tamoxifen resistance between these two groups, one of which is associated with a functional ER pathway and the other which is related to non-ER pathways.

    All of the 20 non-responders in our study which progressed on Tamoxifen were Er-ve, yet six tumours were found to express PgR and/or pS2 despite the absence of ER at progression (Figure 6). Comparison with the pre-Tamoxifen biopsy showed that four of these tumours had been completely negative for ER, PgR and pS2. While previous studies have attributed this ER-Pgr+phenotype in Tamoxifen treated tumours to a false negative ER assay (Holdaway and Bowditch, 1983), a similar observation was recently noted by Osborne's group using an immuno-histochemical assay with 3 different monoclonal antibodies (Encarnacion et al., 1993). They noted 6/30 patients with documented Tamoxifen resistance in whom the tumour was clearly ER-ve by both ligand-binding and immuno-histochemical assays, but strongly positive for PgR. This phenotype has been found to be associated with increased levels of a variant form of ER mRNA in which exon 5 of the ER gene, which codes for the hormone binding domain, is spliced out during transcription (Fuqua et al., 1991). The potential significance of this variant and its possible association with Tamoxifen resistance are discussed below.

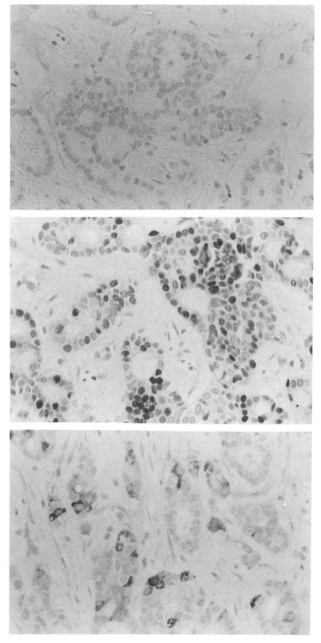

Figure 6. Immunohistochemical staining of adjacent sections of a Tamoxifen-resistant breast carcinoma which was negative for ER, but positive for PgR and pS2 (x400). (Reprinted with permission from Johnston et al., 1995).

In tumours which relapses during adjuvant therapy, resistant tumours were more like to be ER-/PgR-/pS2- (Johnston et al., 1995). Many of these tumours represented either regional or metastatic recurrences, and previous studies have found a drift towards this phenotype in secondary sites of disease compared with primary tumours (Holdaway and Bowditch, 1983). It could be argued that this phenotype, known to be *de novo* resistant to Tamoxifen, correlates with a more metastatic tumour cell which could be disseminated already at the time of primary surgery and which survives and grows through adjuvant Tamoxifen.

pS2 discordance. In light of the evidence that pS2 expression may be regulated by factors other than oestradiol, together with inconclusive clinical studies of pS2's predictive value for endocrine response (Foekens et al., 1994), we recently examined the concordance of pS2 with ER in a cohort of 110 primary untreated tumours and 160 Tamoxifen-resistant tumours. Only 34/56 (60%) resistant compared with 29/34 (85%) untreated pS2+tumours were ER+(p=0.01). This loss was particularly seen in tumours which progressed on primary therapy with *de novo* resistance where in all 8 cases pS2 was expressed in the absence of ER. In contrast 23/29 (80%) pS2+tumours with acquired resistance were also ER-positive. Our findings are in agreement with the only previous study of pS2 expression in 21 Tamoxifen-resistant tumours; of 11 tumours which were treated with Tamoxifen and responded for 9-30 months before subsequently relapsing, 8 (73%) were pS2+ at relapse compared with only 1/10 tumours which progressed with *de novo* resistance after 3-8 months (Henry et al., 1989).

The continued expression of pS2 in many acquired resistant tumours could be due to its continued hormone regulation together with ligand-induced stimulation by endogenous oestradiol, agonist activity of Tamoxifen, or other unidentified components of the ER-dependent pathway. It is of interest to note that *in vitro* Tamoxifen may stimulate pS2 expression at low concentrations in MCF-7 cells (Johnson et al., 1989). Furthermore in Tamoxifen-resistant MCF-7 varient cells, antioestrogens may induce expression of oestrogen-regulated genes at doses where no such effect is seen in parent cells (Vignon et al., 1984). Thus, it is possible that in tumours with acquired resistance Tamoxifen itself stimulates pS2 expression via an ER-dependent pathway, which in turn may be associated with an agonist growth response to the drug possibly at lower concentrations.

In tumours with *de novo* resistance the emergence of pS2 discordance with ER may indicate an alternative pS2-associated mechanism for resistance. In variant MCF-7 cells which develop hormone-independence *in vitro* during prolonged passage (ie. LCC1), elevated baseline levels of ER expression (Brunner et al., 1993). These LCC1 cell lines exhibit a more malignant phenotype *in vivo* than parental MCF-7 cells, and comparison between them showed an altered pattern of gene expression with constitutive expression of oestrogen-regulated proteins were not associated with gene amplification in the resistant cell lines, but rather suggested transcriptional (pS2) or translational (PgR) alterations in association with resistance. It is unclear whether pS2 expression in these circumstances is associated with up-regulation or constitutive activation of growth factor pathways.

Oestrogen receptor variants

Although several mechanisms to explain Tamoxifen resistance in breast cancer have been proposed, there is increasing evidence that activation of the molecular events involved in the oestrogen/ER regulated pathway may facilitate hormone escape. Constitutive activity of ER independent of oestrogen is one such potential mechanism for hormone-independent growth. Recent evidence suggests that some variant forms of ER may stimulate expression of oestrogen-regulated genes independent of ligand, and that these could function as types of 'oncogene' in some forms of breast cancer with over-expression rendering a tumour hormone-resistant (Sluyser and Mester, 1985).

As a ligand controlled-transcription factor, any structural alteration in ER may cause an uncoupling of either the protein's hormonal regulation or its DNA-binding function. In some breast cancer cells this may result in a non-functional ER which is transcriptionally inactive. These cells will be unresponsive to hormonal therapy with Tamoxifen as growth would not be dependent on the ER mediated pathway. Alternatively, an unconstrained ER may exist which is transcriptionally active independent of ligand and which functions to drive cell proliferation, and is unresponsive to Tamoxifen. Several molecular changes in the transcription of the ER gene may account for the development of variant ERs with so-called 'oncogenic' potential, some of which could represent a mechanism for Tamoxifen resistance.

ER DNA mutations. Unlike many other oncogenes there is no evidence for ER gene amplification or re-arrangement in breast cancer to account for aberrant ER function (Koh et al., 1989). Specific point mutations in the ER gene resulting in an amino acid mismatch have been detected in the B domain of some ER+ve tumours, although the functional significance of these remains unclear (Garcia et al., 1989). It has been possible to show that point mutations in specific regions of ER generated by site-directed mutaganesis *in vitro* can significantly alter the function of the receptor. In particular a point mutation in the hormone-dependent transactivation region of the receptor (TAF-2) not only reduces oestrogen-dependent transactivation, but alters the pharmacological response of ER to Tamoxifen from that of an antagonist to a full agonist (Mahfoudi et al., 1995). It is presumed that the conformational change induced by such mutations alters the interaction of the receptor/drug complex with associated transcription factors, accessory proteins and RNA polymerase II such that gene transcription via TAF-2 is activated rather than suppressed. These data imply a possible role for receptor mutants in rendering a tumour 'resistant' to Tamoxifen.

The majority of changes in the ER gene which have been detected in tumours, however, are found in introns and do not directly encode the mRNA or protein. Furthermore two recent studies have suggested that mutations of the ER gene as detected by single-stranded chain polymorphism (SSCP) occur at a very low frequency and do not account for hormone-independent, Tamoxifen-resistant breast cancers (Karnick et al., 1994; Roodi et al., 1995). However SSCP only detects 80-90% of genomic mutations, and other more sensitive screening approaches may be required to detect ER gene mutations.

ER mRNA splice variants. During transcription of the ER gene and synthesis of its mRNA, alternative splicing with delections of whole exons can occur which generates shorter mRNA transcripts. A variety of different ER mRNA splice variants involving precise deletions of whole exons (2, 3, 4, 5, 6 or 7) have been identified in human breast tumours (Fuqua et al., 1991; Wang and Miksicek, 1991; Fuqua et al., 1992; Zhang et al., 1993; Pfeffer et al., 1995). The location of the splicing junctions flanking each exon determines whether the resulting spliced transcript in either in frame, or instead results in a frameshift whereby a new codon reading sequence is introduced. The latter occurs after splicing out of exon 5, and results in a novel peptide sequence (7 amino acids) followed by the early introduction of a stop codon with premature termination of translation yielding a truncated ER protein (Figure 7).

The variant receptors formed by alternative splicing may have a range of different properties within the cell depending on the consequence of each deletion on the functional activity of the receptor (McGuire et al., 1991). The ER varient may be completely inactive, as occurs with the exon 2 deletion variant (ER▲E2) where a frameshift results in premature termination of translation within examon 3 and a truncated protein which is transcriptionally inactive (Wang and Miksicek, 1991). However, the ER variant may behave as a "dominant negative" receptor which is capable of inhibiting the transcriptional activity of the wild-type receptor. This occurs with the ER▲E3 variant in which a precise in-frame deletion of examon, which encodes the second 'zinc finger' within the DNA binding domain, generates a variant protein which is unable to bind DNA or activate transcription. However as the receptor is otherwise intact (exons 1-2 and 4-8), it can slo heterodimerise with wild-type receptor and interfere with its transcriptional activity (Miksicek et al., 1993).

Alternatively variant mRNA transcripts may code for a "dominant-positive" receptor which is constitutively active, as exemplified by the ER▲E5 variant which has been shown *in vitro* to be transcriptionally active independent of oestradiol (Fuqua et al., 1991). The ability to activate oestrogen-regulated genes independent of oestradiol is a potential explanation for the high levels of PgR found in a small subset of ER-negative tumours. Horwitz (1981) first suggested that a permanently activated ER might explain the high persistent levels of PgR in T47D tissue culture cells, and the discovery of the ER▲E5 variant in an ER- PgR+tumour provided the first evidence to support this is as a molecular explanation for this rare phenotype.

Potential function of variant ERs. Variant ERs with dissociated hormone binding and DNA binding functions may offer an explanation for some of the known anomalies between ER status and hormone responsiveness in breast cancer. It is possible that one or several of these varient transcripts may occur alongside wild-type mRNA within a given tumour, and that the relative balance of variant and wild-type receptor may dicate the interaction with Tamoxifen and determine the degree of hormone responsiveness which is observed.

DNA binding. Two studies of primary breast cancer have examined the ER protein's ability to bind a labelled synthetic ERE oligonucleotide probe in a gel-retardation assay as an indicator of its functional DNA binding capacity. Foster et al. (1991) showed that 40% of tumours which were apparently ER- by ligand-binding assay still had protein which could bind ERE and which could be recognised by anti-ER antibodies.

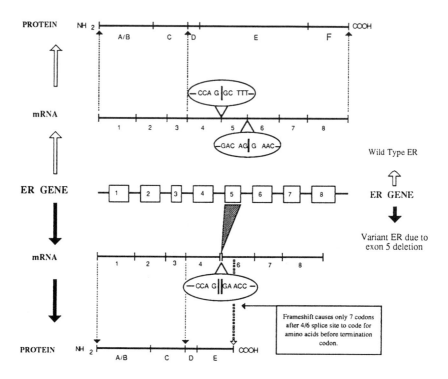

Figure 7. Transcription of oestrogen receptor gene with splicing of introns to form mRNA, followed by translation of mRNA into ER protein. Transcription of both wild-type ER and variant ER in which exon 5 is spliced out is shown. Numbers 1-8 refer to the eight known exons of the ER gene, which in turn code for the six functional domains of the ER protein (A-F). Loss of exon 5 during splicing results in a frameshift in translation of the nucleotide sequence of exon 4 into exon 6, with a truncated ER protein of approximately 40 kDa which lacks a major part of the ligand-binding domain, but which can still bind DNA through domain C.

These tumours, some of which expressed PgR in apparent absence of ER, may contain truncated but constitutively active variant ER protein. In addition, 19% of apparent ER+tumours were unable to bind ERE and failed to express PgR. Such tumours may contain defective ER with intact hormone binding but impaired DNA binding or transcriptional activity. Scott et al. (1991) used a panel of ER monoclonal truncated forms of DNA binding and non-DNA binding ER. While on theoretical grounds Tamoxifen would fail to interact with these receptors, to date no clinical study has correlated such DNA binding activity with Tamoxifen resistance *in vivo*.

Constitutive activity. The potential function of the constitutively active ER▲E5 varient has been investigated following stable transfection into ER+ MCF-7 cells (Fuqua and Wolf, 1995). These transfected cells produced a truncated ER protein of approximately 40 kDa size which was able to induce oestrogen-responsive gene expression (PgR) in the absence of an oestrogenic stimulus, in contrast to control cells which required the addition of oestradiol. In a study of 27 tumours of varying phenotypes analysed by ribonuclease protection assay, ER▲E5 was confirmed to be the predominant RNA in ER-/PgR+ tumours, but was also detected to a varying extent in ER+/PgR+ and ER+/PgR- tumours (Zhang et al., 1993). We recently examined the expression of ER▲E5 variant in relation to PgR-pS2 in a series of 120 tumours, and demonstrated that both ER- PgR+ pS2+ tumours expressed significantly greater levels of % ▲5/WT ER compared with other phenotypes (Daffada et al., 1995).

Role in Tamoxifen resistance. An oestrogen receptor which lacks a regulatory ligand domain but which can constitutively activate ER-dependent proteins could, in theory, activate ER-dependent growth signal pathways independent of oestradiol and be resistant to Tamoxifen. This has been confirmed *in vitro* where ▲5 ER transfected into hormone-dependent MCF-7 cells resulted in an increase in oestradiol-independent growth together with resistance to Tamoxifen, but interestingly not to the pure antioestrogen ICI 164,384 (Fuqua et al., 1994; Fuqua and Wolf, 1995). These data imply that while overexpression of ▲5 ER may alter the response of previously hormone-sensitive cells to Tamoxifen, there may be a diferent interaction of other antioestrogens with this variant protein which may allow its constitutive activity to be modulated.

In vivo we have demonstrated no overall increase in ▲5 ER expression in Tamoxifen resistant compared with untreated primary breast cancers, although in some resistant ER+ tumours in which PgR or pS2 was expressed ▲5 levels were increased (Daffada et al., 1995). In support of our observations, a recent report has investigated the expression of ER▲E5 in a MCF-7 cell line which acquired resistance to Tamoxifen following long-term culture (Madsen et al., 1995). Resistant cells (MCF-7/TAM^R-1) remained ER + for both protein and RNA, but RT/PCR confirmed a number of mRNA splice variants including deletions of exons 2, 4, 5, 7 in addition to splicing of exons 4 and 7 together. Semi-quantiative RT-PCR showed that while one particular splice variant was increased in resistant compared with parental MCF-7 cells (exon 2 deletion), the ER▲E5 variant was actually decreased in resistant cells. Taken together these data imply that acquired Tamoxifen resistance is unlikely to be explained by an overexpression of the exon 5-deletion mRNA splice variant.

Conclusions

In summary, Tamoxifen is an effective yet complex antioestrogen whose pharmacological action and molecular interaction with oestrogen receptor is now being understood in consideration detail. The numerous metabolites of Tamoxifen contribute to the overall activity of the drug *in vivo*, and these compounds in themselves may have effects which differ from the parent drug. Ultimately the interaction of Tamoxifen and its metabolites with the receptor determines the intrinsic activity of the receptor complex and dictates to what extent the transcription of oestrogen-regulated genes, including the genes involved in the growth pathway, is modulated.

Resistance to Tamoxifen *in vivo* has been shown to be associated with reduced intratumoural concentrations of Tamoxifen which may either induce a stimulatory growth response, or alternatively may fail to antagonise the effect of endogenous oestradiol. Tumours which acquire resistance to Tamoxifen often appear to retain a functional ER, despite the fact that the drug can no longer inhibit growth. Targets within the ER-mediated growth pathway which may become active independent of ligand/Tamoxifen control include the expression of pS2. Constitutively active ER receptor variants may also bypass the control of Tamoxifen, although evidence suggests that they do not play a major role in Tamoxifen-resistance *in vivo*. Other factors which are outside the scope of this chapter such as autonomous growth factor activity may also contribute.

An increased understanding of Tamoxifen's action together with the mechanisms involved in resistance to the drug may provide new targets for the design of therapeutic agents which can both effectively antagonise the ER-dependent growth pathway, as well as circumvent or prevent the emergence of inevitable resistance to the drug *in vivo*.

Table 1.   Mean serum concentrations of Tamoxifen and its metabolites (ng/ml) in breast cancer patients receiving chronic administration of either 20 mg, 30 mg or 40 mg per day for at least 2 months. (Adapted from Furr and Jordan, 1984 and Langhan-Fahey et al., 1994).

Dose TAM (mg/day)	N-dMT	4-OH	Z	4-OH N-dMT	Y	Reference
20						
167	-	3.4	-	-	-	Daniel et al., 1979
125	160	-	-	-	-	Wilkinson et al., 1980
159	-	-	-	-	-	Bratherton et al., 1984
113	214	-	-	-	18	Jordan et al., 1983
148	290	-	-	-	-	Langhan-Fahey et al., 1990
163	314	-	75	-	-	Johnston et al., 1993
30						
144	-	-	-	-	-	Fabian et al., 1980
145	343	6.5	55	-	35	Milano et al., 1987
113	242	<5	33	-	26	Stevenson et al., 1988
141	220	3.5	51	9.3	34	Lien et al., 1989
40						
285	477	-	-	-	-	Patterson et al., 1980
300	462	6.7	-	-	-	Daniel et al., 1981
310	481	-	-	-	49	Kemp et al., 1983
273	-	-	-	-	-	Bratherton et al., 1984
214	246	-	-	-	-	McVie et al., 1986

(TAM = tamoxifen; N-dMT = N-desmethyltamoxifen; 4-OH = 4-hydroxytamoxifen; Z = N,N-didesmethyltamoxifen; 4-OH-N-dMT = 4-hydroxy-N-desmethyltamoxifen; Y = metabolite Y)

REFERENCES

Adam HK, Douglas EJ, Kemp JV (1979): The metabolism of tamoxifen in humans. *Biochem Pharmacol* 27:145-147

Allegra JC, Barlock A, Huff KK, Lippman ME (1980): Changes in multiple or sequential estrogen receptor determinations in breast cancer. *Cancer* 45:792-794

Bain RR, Jordan VC (1983): Identification of a new metabolite of tamoxifen in patient serum during breast cancer therapy. *Biochem Pharmacol* 32:373-375

Belleau B (1964): A molecular basis for drug action. *J Med Chem* 7:776-784

Borgna JL, Rochefort H (1981): Hydroxylated metabolites of tamoxifen are formed *in vivo* and bound to estrogen receptor in target tissues. *J Biol Chem* 256:859-868

Bratherton DG, Brown CH, Buchanan B, Hall V, Pillers EMK, Wheeler TK et al. (1984): A comparison of two doses of tamoxifen (Nolvadex) in post-menopausal women with advanced breast cancer. *Br J Cancer* 50:199-205

Brunner N, Boulay V, Fojo A, Freter CE, Lippman ME, Clarke R (1993): Acquisition of hormone-independent growth in MCF-7 cells is accompanied by increased expression of estrogen-regulated genes but without detectable DNA amplifications. *Cancer Res* 53:283-290

Canney PA, Griffiths T, Latief TN (1987): Clinical significant of tamoxifen withdrawal response. *The Lancet* i:36

Cavailles V, Garcia M, Rochefort H (1989): Regulation of cathespin-D and pS2 gene expression by growth factors in MCF-7 human breast cancer cells. *Mol Endocrinol* 3:552-553

Chalbos D, Philips A, Galtier F, Rochefort H (1993): Synthetic antioestrogens modulate induction of pS2 and cathespin-D messenger ribonucleic acid by growth factors and adenosine 3'5'-monophosphate in MCF-7 cells. *Endocrinology* 133(2):571-576

Chatterjee M, Harris AL (1990): Reveral of acquired resistance to adriamycin in CHO cells by tamoxifen and 4-hydroxytamoxifen; role of drug interaction with alpha 1 acid glycoprotein. *Br J Cancer* 62:712-717

Clarke RB, Currier S, Kaplan O, Lovelace E, Boulay V, Gottesman MM et al. (1992): Effect of P-glycoprotein expression on sensitivity to hormones in MCF-7 human breast cancer cells. *J Natl Cancer Inst* 84:1506-1512

Coezy E, Borgna J-L, Rochefort H (1982): Tamoxifen and Metabolites in MCF-7 Cells: Correlation between Binding to Estrogen Receptor and Inhibition of Cell Growth. *Cancer Res* 42:317-323

Daffada AAI, Johnston SRD, Smith IE, Detre S, King N, Dowsett M (1995): Exon 5 deletion variant estrogen receptor messenger RNA expression in relation to tamoxifen resistance and progestrone receptorpS2 status in human breast cancer. *Cancer Res* 55:288-293

Daniel P, Gaskel SJ, Bishop H, Campbell C, Nicholson RI (1979): Determination of tamoxifen and an hydroxylated metabolite in plasma from patients with advanced breast cancer using gas chrmatography-mass spectrometry. *J Endocrinol* 83:401-408

Daniel P, Gaskell SJ, Bishop H, Campbell C, Robertson RI (1981): Determination of tamoxifen and biologically active metabolites in human breast tumours and plasma. *Eur J Cancer Clin Oncol* 17(11):1183-1189

DeFriend DJ, Anderson E, Bell J, Wilks DP, West CML, Mansell RE et al. (1994): Effects of 4-hydroxytamoxifen and a novel pure antioestrogen (ICI 182780) on the clonogenic growth of human breast cancer cells *in vitro*. *Br J Cancer* 70:204-211

Dowsett M, Johnston SRD, Iveson TJ, Smith IE (1995): Response to pure antioestrogen (ICI 182,780) in tamoxifen-resistant breast cancer. *Lancet* 345:525

EBCTCG (1992): Systemic treatment of early breast cancer by hormonal, cytotoxic or immune therapy. *The Lancet* 339:1-15,71-85

Encarnacion CA, Ciocca DR, McGuire WL, Clark GM, Fuqua SAW, Osborne CK (1993): Measurement of steroid hormone receptors in breast cancer patients on tamoxifen. *Breast Cancer Res Treat* 26:237-246

Fabian C, Sternson L, Barnett M (1980): Clinical pharmacology of tamoxifen in patients with breast cancer: comparison of traditional and loading dose schedules. *Cancer Treat Rep* 64:765-773

Foekens JA, Portengen H, Look MP, Van Putten WLJ, Thirion B, Botenbal M, et al. (1994): Relationship of PS2 with response to tamoxifen therapy in patients with recurrent breast cancer. *Br J Cancer* 70:1217-1223

Foster BD, Cavener DR, Parl FF (1991): Binding analysis of the oestrogen receptor to its specific DNA target site in human breast cancer tissue. *Cancer Res* 51:3405-3410

Fromson JM, Pearson S, Bramah S (1973): The metabolism of tamoxifen (ICI 46,474). Part 1. In laboratory animals. *Xenobiotica* 3:693-709

Fuqua SAW, Fitzgerald SD, Allred DC, Elledge RM, Nawaz Z, McDonnell DP, et al. (1992): Inhibition of estrogen receptor action by a naturally occurring variant in human breast tumors. *Cancer Res* 52:483-486

Fuqua SAW, Fitzgerald SD, Chamness GC, Tandon AK, McDonnell DP, Nawaz Z, et al. (1991): Variant human breast tumour estrogen receptor with constitutive transcriptional activity. *Cancer Res* 51:105-109

Fuqua SAW, Wilschke C, Castles C, Wolf D, Allred DC (1994): A role for estrogen-receptor variants in endocrine resistance. *Endocrine-Related Cancer* 2:19-25

Fuqua SAW, Wolf DM (1995): Molecular aspects of estrogen receptor variants in breast cancer. *Breast Cancer Res Treat* 35:233-241

Furr BJA, Jordan VC (1984): The pharmacology and clinical uses of tamoxifen. *Pharmac Ther* 25:127-205

Garcia T, Sanchez M, Cox JL, Shaw PA, Ross JBA, Lehrer S, et al. (1989): Identification of a variant form of the oestrogen receptor with an amino acid replacement. *Nucleic Acids Res* 17:8364-8365

Gottardis M, Jordan VC (1988): Development of tamoxifen-stimulated growth of MCF-7 tumors in athymic mice after long-term antioestrogen administation. *Cancer Res* 48:5183-5187

Gottardis MM, Jiang SY, Jeng MH, Jordan VC (1989): Inhibition of tamoxifen-stimulated growth of an MCF-7 tumor variant in athymic mice by novel steroidal antiestrogens. *Cancer Res* 49(15):4090-4093

Henry JA, Nicholson S, Hennesey C, Lennard TWJ, May FEB, Westley BR (1989): Expression of the oestrogen regulated pNR-2 mRNA in human breast cancer: relation to oestrogen receptor mRNA levels and response to tamoxifen therapy. *Br J Cancer* 61:32-38

Henry JA, Piggott NH, Mallick UK, Nicholson S, Farndon JR, Westley BR, et al. (1991): pNR-2/pS2 immunohistochemical staining in breast cancer: correlation with prognostic factors and endocrine response. *Br J Cancer* 63:615-622

Holdaway IM, Bowditch JV (1983): Variation in receptor status between primary and metastatic breast cancer. *Cancer* 52:479-485

Horwitz KB (1981): Is a functional estrogen receptor always required for progesterone receptor induction in breast cancer? *J Steroid Biochem* 15:209-217

Horwitz KB, Costlow ME, McGuire WL (1975): A human breast cancer cell line with estrogen, androgen, progesterone and glucocortiocoid receptors. *Steroids* 26:785-795

Horwitz KB, Koseki Y, McGuire WL (1978): Estrogen control of progesterone receptor in human breast cancer: role of estradiol and antiestrogen. *Endocrinology* 103:1742-1751

Howell A, De Friend D, Robertson J, Blamey R, Walton P (1995): Response to the pure antioestrogen ICI 182,780 in tamoxifen resistant breast cancer. *The Lancet* 345:29-30

Howell A, Dodwell DJ, Anderson H, Radford J (1992): Response after withdrawal of tamoxifen and progestins in advanced breast cancer. *Ann Oncol* 3(8):611-617

Howell A, Dodwell DJ, Laidlaw I, Anderson H, Anderson E (1990): Tamoxifen as an agonist for metastatic breast cancer. In: Endocrine Therapy of Breast Cancer. Ed. A Goldhirsch. New York, Springer-Verlad pp 49-58

Howell A, Harland RNL, Barnes DM, Baildam AD, Wilkinson MJS, Hayward E, et al. (1987): Endocrine therapy for advanced carcinoma of the breast: relationship between the effect of tamoxifen upon concentrations of progesterone receptor and subsequent response to treatment. *Cancer Res* 47:300-304

Hull DF, Clark GM, Osborne CK, Chamness GC, Knight WA, McGuire WL (1983): Multiple estrogen receptor assays in human breast cancer. *Cancer Res* 43:413-416

Jacolot F, Simon I, Dreano Y, Beaune P, Riche, Berthou F (1991): Identification of the cytochrome p450 IIIa family as enzymes involved in the N-demethylation of tamoxifen in human liver microscomes. *Biochem Pharmacol* 41:1911-1919

Johnson MD, Westley BR, May FEB (1989): Oestrogenic activity of tamoxifen and its metabolites on gene regulation and cell proliferation in MCF-7 breast cancer cells. *Br J Cancer* 59:727-738

Johnston SRD, Haynes BP, Smith IE, Jarman M, Sacks NPM, Ebbs SR, et al. (1993): Acquired tamoxifen resistance in human breast cancer and reduced intra-tumoural drug concentration. *The Lancet* 342:1521-1522

Johnston SRD, Saccani-Jotti G, Smith IE, Salter J, Newby J, Coppen M, et al. (1995): Changes in estrogen receptor, progesterone receptor and pS2 expression in tamoxifen-resistant human breast cancer. *Cancer Res* 55:3331-3338

Johnston SRD, Tillyer C, Smith IE, Dowsett M (1994): Serum alpha-1-acid glycoprotein concentrations in tamoxifen-resistant breast cancer. *Br J Cancer* 69(Suppl XXI):29

Jordan VC, Bain RR, Brown RR, Gosden B, Santos MA (1983): Determination and pharmacology of a new hydroxylated metabolite of tamoxifen observed in patient sera during therapy for advanced breast cancer. *Cancer Res* 43:1446-1450

Jordan VC, Collins MM, Rowsby L, Prestwich G (1977): A monohydroxylated metabolite of tamoxifen with potent antioestrogen activity. *J Endocrinology* 75:305-316

Jordan VC, Gosden B (1982): Importance of the alkylaminoethoxy side chain for the estrogenic and antiestrogenic actions of tamoxifen and trioxifene in the immature rat uterus. *Molec Cell Endocrinol* 27:291-306

Jordan VC, Haldemann B, Allen KE (1981): Geometric isomers of substituted triphenylethylenes and antiestrogen action. *Endocrinology* 108:1353-1361

Jordan VC, Koch R, Lieberman ME (1984a): Structure-activity relationships of nonsteroidal estrogens and antiestrogens. In: Estrogen/Antiestrogen Action and Breast Cancer Therapy. Ed. VC Jordan. Madison, University of Wisconsin Press:19-41

Jordan VC, Lieberman ME, Cormier E, Koch R, Baley JR, Reunitz PC (1984b): Structural requirements for the pharmacological activity of non-steroidal antiestrogens *in vivo*. *Mol Pharmacol* 26:272-278

Juliano RL, Ling V (1976): A surface glycoprotein modulating drug permeability in Chinese hamster ovary cells mutants. *Biochem Biophys* 455:152-162

Karnick PS, Kulkarni S, Liu X-P, Budd GT, Bukowski RM (1994): Estrogen receptor mutations in tamoxifen-resistant breast cancer. *Cancer Res* 54:349-353

Katzenellenbogen BS, Norman MJ, Eckert RL, Peltz SW, Mangel WF (1984): Bioactivities, estrogen receptor interactions, and plasminogen activator-inducing activities of tamoxifen and hydroxytamoxifen isomers in MCF-7 human breast cancer cells. *Cancer Res* 44:112-119

Keen JC, Miller EP, Bellamy C, Dixon JM, Miller WR (1994): P-glycoprotein resistance to tamoxifen. *The Lancet* 343:1047-1048

Kemp JV, Adam HK, Wakeling AE, Slater R (1983): Identification and biological activity of tamoxifen metabolites in human serum. *Biochem Pharmacol* 32:2045-2052

Kiang DT, Kollander RE, Thomas T, Kennedy BJ (1989): Up-regulation of estrogen receptors by non-steroidal antioestrogens in human breast cancer. *Cancer Res* 49:5312-5316

Koh EH, Wildrick DM, Hortobagyi GN, Blick M (1989): Analysis of the oestrogen receptor gene structure in human breast cancer. *Anticancer Res* 9:1841-1846

Langhan-Fahey SM, Tormey DC, Jordan VC (1990): Tamoxifen metabolites in patients on long-term adjuvant therapy for breast cancer. *Eur J Cancer* 26(8):883-888

Lees JA, Fawell SE, Parker MG (1989): Identification of two transactivation domains in the mouse oestrogen receptor. *Nucleic Acids Res* 17:5477-5488

Legault-Poisson S, Jolivet J, Poisson R, Beretta-Piccoli M, Band PR (1979): Tamoxifen-induced tumor stimulation and withdrawal response. *Cancer Treat Rep* 63:1839-1841

LeMaistre CF, McGuire WL (1986): Progestrone receptor determinations: a refinement of predictive tests for hormone dependency of breast cancer. In: Estrogen/Antiestrogen Action and Brest Cancer Therapy. Ed. VC Jordan. Madison, University of Wisconsin Press:341-354

Lien EA, Solheim E, Lea OA, Lundgren S, Kvinnsland S, Ueland PM (1989): Distribution of 4-hydroxy-N-desmethyltamoxifen and other tamoxifen metabolites in human biological fluids during tamoxifen treatment. *Cancer Res* 49:2175-2183

Lein EA, Solheim E, Ueland PM (1991): Distribution of tamoxifen and its metabolites in rat and human tissue during steady state treatment. *Cancer Res* 51:4837-4844

Lippman ME, Bolan G, Huff K (1976): The effects of estrogens and antiestrogens on hormone responsive human breast cancer in long-term tissue culture. *Cancer Res* 36:4595-4601

Lyman SD, Jordan VC (1985): Metabolism of tamoxifen and its uterotrophic activity. *Biochem Pharmacol* 34:2787-2794

Madsen MW, Reiter BE, Lykkesfeldt AE (1995): Differential expression of estrogen receptor mRNA splice variants in the tamoxifen resistant human breast cancer cell line, MCF-7/TAM[R]-1 compared to the parental MCF-7 cell line. *Mol Cell Endocrinol* 109:197-207

Mahfoudi A, Roulet E, Dauvois S, Parker MG, Wahli W (1995): Specific mutations in the estrogen receptor change the properties of antiestrogens to full agonists. *Proc Natl Acad Sci USA* 92:4206-4210

Masiakowski P, Breathnack R, Bloch J, Gannon F, Chambon P (1982): Cloning of cDNA sequences of hormone-regulated genes from MCF-7 human breast cancer cell line. *Nucleic Acid Res* 10:7895-7903

McCague R, Kuroda R, LeClerq G, Stoessel S (1986): Synthesis and estrogen receptor binding of 6,7-dihydro-8-phenyl-9[4-[2-(dimethylamino)ethoxy[phenyl]5H-benzocycloheptene,anon-isomerisable analogue of tamoxifen. X-ray crystallographic studies. *J Medic Chem* 29:2053-2058

McGuire WL (1978): Hormone receptors; their role in predicting prognosis and response to endocrine therapy. *Semin Oncol* 5:428-433

McGuire WL, Chamness GC, Fuqua SAW (1991): Estrogen receptor variants in clinical breast cancer. *Mol Endocrinol* 5:1571-1577

McIntosh IH, Thynne (1977): Tumour stimulation by antioestrogens. *Br J Surg* 64:900-901

McVie JG, Simonetti GPC, Stevenson D, Briggs RJ, Guelen PJM, de Vos D (1986): The bioavailability of tamoplex (tamoxifen). Part 1. A pilot study. *Methods and Findings in Exp Clin Pharmacol* 8:505-512

Miksicek RJ, Lei Y, Wang Y (1993): Exon skipping gives rise to alternatively spliced forms of the estrogen receptor in breast tumor cells. *Breast Cancer Res Treat* 26:163-174

Milano G, Etienne MC, Frenay M, Khater R, Formento JL, Renee N, et al. (1987): Optimised analysis of tamoxifen and its main metabolites in the plasma and cytosol of mammary tumours. *Br J Cancer* 55:509-512

Murphy CS, Langan FS, McCague R, Jordan VC (1990): Structure-function relationships of hydroxylated metabolites of tamoxifen that control the proliferation of estrogen-responsive T47D breast cancer cells *in vitro*. *Mol Pharmacol* 38(5):737-743

Namer M, Laianne C, Baulieu E-E (1980): Increase of progesterone receptor by tamoxifen as a hormonal challenge test in breast cancer. *Cancer Res* 40:1750-1752

Nicholson RI, Syne JS, Daniel CP, Griffiths K (1979): The binding of tamoxifen to oestrogen receptors under equilibrium and non-equilibrium conditions. *Eur J Cancer* 15:317-329

Noguchi S, Miyauchi K, Imaoka S, Koyama H (1988a): Inability of tamoxifen to penetrate into cerebrospinal fluid. *Breast Cancer Res Treat* 12:317-318

Noguchi S, Miyauchi K, Nishizawa, Koyama H (1988b): Induction of progesterone receptor with tamoxifen in human breast cancer with special reference to its behaviour over time. *Cancer* 61:1345-1349

Osborne CK, Boldt DH, Clark GM, Trent JM (1983): Effects of tamoxifen on human breast cancer cell kinetics: accumulation of cells in early G1 phase. *Cancer Res* 43:3583-3585

Osborne CK, Coronado E, Allred DC, Wiebe V, DeGregorio M (1991): Acquired tamoxifen resistance: correlation with reduced breast tumor levels of tamoxifen and isomerisation of trans-4-hydroytamoxifen. *J Natl Cancer Inst* 83:1477-1482

Osborne CK, Jarman M, McCague R, Coronado EB, Hilsenbeck SG, Wakeling AE (1994): The importance of tamoxifen metabolism in tamoxifen-stimulated breast tumor growth. *Cancer Chemother Pharmacol* 34:89-95

Osborne CK, Wiebe VJ, McGuire WL, Ciocca DR, De Gregoria MW (1992): Tamoxifen and the isomers of 4-hydroxytamoxifen-resistant tumors from breast cancer patients. *J Clin Oncol* 10:304-310

Patterson JS, Settatree RS, Adam HK, Kemp JV (1980): Serum concentrations of tamoxifen and major metabolites during long-term Nolvadex therapy, correlated with clinical response. Breast Cancer - Experimental and Clinical Aspects. HT Mouridsen, Palshof T. Oxford, Pergamon Press:89-92

Pfeffer U, Fecarotta E, Vidali G (1995): Coexpression of multiple estrogen receptor variant messenger RNAs in normal and neoplastic breast tissues and in MCF-7 cells. *Cancer Res* 55:2158-2165

Plotkin D, Lechner JJ, Jung WE, Rosen PJ (1978): Tamoxifen flare in advanced breast cancer. *JAMA* 240:2644-2646

Ramu A, Glaubiger D, Fuks Z (1984): Reversal of acquired resistance to daunorubicin in P388 murine leukaemia cells by tamoxifen and other triparanol analoques. *Cancer Res* 44:4392-4395

Ravdin PM, Green S, Melink Dorr T, McGuire WL, Fabian C, Pugh RP, et al. (1992): Prognostic significant of progesterone receptor levels in oestrogen-receptor positive patients with metastatic breast cancer treated with tamoxifen: results of a prospective Southwest Oncology Group study. *J Clin Oncol* 10:1284-1291

Reddel RR, Sutherland RL (1984): Tamoxifen stimulation of human breast cancer cell proliferation *in vitro*: a possible model for tamoxifen tumour flare. *Eur J Cancer Clin Oncol* 20:(11)1419-1424

Robinson SP, Langhan-Fahey SM, Johnson DA, Jordan VC (1991): Metabolites, pharmacodynamics and pharmacokinetics of tamoxifen in rats and mice compared to the breast cancer patient. *Drug Metab Dispos* 19:(1)36-43

Roodi N, Bailey LR, Kao W-Y, Verrier CS, Yee CJ, Dupont WD, et al. (1995): Estrogen receptor gene analysis in estrogen receptor-positive and receptor-negative primary breast cancer. *J Natl Cancer Inst* 87:446-451

Schwartz LH, Koerner FC, Edgerton SM, Sawicka JM, Rio MC, Bellocq J-P, et al. (1991): pS2 expression and response to hormonal therapy in patients with advanced breast cancer. *Cancer Res* 51:624-628

Scott GK, Kushner P, Vigne J-L, Benz CC (1991): Truncated forms of DNA-binding estrogen receptors. *J Clin Invest* 88:700-706

Shah IG, Parsons DL (1991): Human albumin binding of tamoxifen in the presence of a perfluorochemical erythrocyte substitute. *J Parhm Pharmacol* 43:790-793

Skilton RA, Luqmani YA, McClelland RA, Coombes RC (1989): Characterisation of a messenger RNA selectively expressed in human breast cancer. *Br J Cancer* 60:168-175

Sluyser M, Mester J (1985): Oncogenes homologous to steroid receptors? *Nature* 315:546

Smith IE, Harris AL, Morgan M (1981): Tamoxifen versus aminoglutethimide in advanced breast carcinoma: a randomised cross-over trial. *Br Med J* 283:1432-1434

Stack G, Kumar V, Green S, Ponglikimongkol M, Berry M, Rio MC, et al. (1988): Structure and function of the pS2 gene and estrogen receptor in human breast cancer cells. In: Breast Cancer: Cellular and Molecular Biology. Ed. ME Lippman and RB Dickson. Boston, Kluwer Academic Publishers:185-206

Stevenson D, Briggs RJ. Chapman DJ, de Vos D (1988): Determination of tamoxifen and five metabolites in plasma. *J Pharmaceut Biomed Analysis* 6:1065-1068

Sutherland RL, Green MD, Hall RD, Reddell RR, Taylor IW (1983): Tamoxifen induced accumulation of MCF-7 human mammary carcinoma cells in the G0/G1 phase of the cell cycle. *Eur J Cancer Clin Oncol* 19:615-621

Taylor RE, Powles TJ, Humphreys J, Bettelheim R, Dowsett M, Casey AJ, et al. (1982): Effects of endocrine therapy on steroid receptor content of breast cancer. *Br J Cancer* 45:80-85

Tora L, White J, Brou C, Tasset D, Webster N, Scheer E, et al. (1989): The human estrogen receptor has two independent non-acidic transcriptional activation functions. *Cell* 59:477-487

Trump DL, Smith DC, Ellis PG, Rogers MP, Schold SC, Winer EP, et al. (1992): Vinblastine and high dose tamoxifen, a potential multidrug resistance reversal agent: a phase I trial in combination with vinblastine. *J Natl Cancer Inst* 84:1811-1816

Vignon F, Lippman ME, Nawata H, Derocq D, Rochefort H (1984): Induction of two estrogen-responsive proteins by antiestrogens in R27, a tamoxifen-resistant clone of MCF-7 cells. *Cancer Res* 44:2084-2088

Wang Y, Miksicek RJ (1991): Identification of a dominant negative form of the human estrogen receptor. *Mol Endocrinol* 5:1707-1715

Westley BR, May FEB (1987): Oestrogen regulates cathespin D mRNA levels in oestrogen responsive human breast cancer cells. *Nucleic Acid Res* 15:3773

Wiebe VJ, De Gregorio MW, Osborne CK (1995): Tamoxifen metabolism and resistance. In: Drug and Hormonal Resistance in Breast Cancer. Ed. RB Dickson and ME Lippman. London, Ellis Horwood:115-131

Wiebe VJ, Osborne CK, McGuire WL, DeGregorio MW (1992): Identification
    of estrogenic tamoxifen metabolite(s) in tamoxifen-resistant human breast
    tumors. *J Clin Oncol* 10:990-994
Wilkinson P, Ribiero G, Adam H, Patterson J (1980): Clinical pharmacology of
    tamoxifen and N-desmethyltamoxifen in patients with advanced breast
    cancer. *Cancer Chemother Pharmacol* 5:109-111
Wiseman H (1994): Metabolism and toxicology of tamoxifen: an overview. In:
    Tamoxifen, Molecular Basis of Use in Cancer Treatment and Prevention.
    Ed. H Wiseman. Chichester, John Wiley and Sons:19-30
Wolf DM, Langhan-Fahey SM, Parker CJ, McCaque R, Jordan VC (1993):
    Investigation of the mechanism of tamoxifen-stimulated breast tumor
    growth with nonisomerisable analogues of tamoxifen and metabolites. *J
    Natl Cancer Inst* 85:806-812
Zhang Q-X, Borg A, Fuqua SAW (1993): An exon 5 deletion variant of the
    estrogen receptor frequently coexpressed with wild-type estrogen receptor
    in human breast cancer. *Cancer Res* 53:5882-5884

11. TAMOXIFEN AND THE E-CADHERIN/CATENIN COMPLEX

Marc E. Bracke, Frans M. Van Roy, Vincent Castronovo and Marc M. Mareel

The prognosis of breast cancers is determined by the invasive and metastatic capabilities of the neoplastic cells. In malignant tumor invasion promoters, such as cell-substrate adhesion molecules, matrix proteases and motility factors appear to outbalance -at least temporarily- the function of invasion suppressor molecules, such as protease inhibitors and cell-cell adhesion molecules (Mareel et al., 1993a). One of the most powerful invasion suppressors in epithelial cell populations is the cell-cell adhesion molecule E-cadherin (Takeichi, 1993; Birchmeier and Behrens, 1994). During recent years, our and other laboratories have studied the downregulation of this molecule in invasive cancer cells, both to understand the mechanisms of downregulation and to find upregulating agents that may be useful therapeutically. In this chapter, we will first describe the complex between E-cadherin and the catenins, which are the connecting molecules with the cytoskeleton, and we will provide evidence for the invasion-suppressor function of this complex in mammary epithelium. Next, the possibility to modulate the function of the complex will be envisaged, and finally the effects of antiestrogens (i.e. Tamoxifen) on the E-cadherin/complex will be described.

The E-cadherin/catenin complex in mammary tumors

Human E-cadherin (identical to cell-CAM 120/80, and homologous to L-CAM and to mouse E-cadherin or uvomorulin) is a 120-kDa transmembrane glycoprotein encompassing three major parts (Fig. 1).

The extracellular part has five well conserved repeat domains ("CAD repeats") with four calcium-binding sites, presumably involved in stabilization of the conformation (Overduin et al., 1995). Recent data indicate that the homophilic interactions between cadherins in opposing plasma membranes occur as dimer-dimer associations with a major role for the HAV-sequence in the first CAD repeat (Shapiro et al., 1995). The membrane-spanning part connects the extracellular part of E-cadherin to the cytoplasmic part, which contains the recognition sites for the catenins.

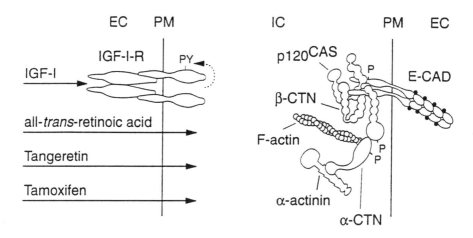

Figure 1. Correction of the defective function of the E-caherin/catenin complex in human mammary carcinoma cells (MCF-7/6) by external agents. At the right side, the E-cadherin/catenin complex is drawn schematically with the plasma membrane (PM) as a vertical line. E-cadherin (E-CAD) is a transmembrane glycoprotein possessing five repeated domains and four binding sites for calcium (black dots) in it extracellular (EC) part. Its cytoplasmic part binds to beta-catenin or gamma-catenin (CTN), and to p120^{cas}. alpha-Catenin forms the link with alpha-actinin and F-actin. At the left side, four molecules that can activate the function of the complex, are indicated. Note that insulin-like growth factor I (IGF-I) interacts with its transmembrane receptor (IFG-I-R) to induce tyrosine (PY) phosphorylation of the receptor. The signal transduction from the activating molecules, including Tamoxifen, towards the E-cadherin/catenin complex has not been elucidated.

Three types of catenins form a complex with E-cadherin by means of non-covalent interactions (Kemler, 1993). Both beta-catenin (homologous with plakoglobin and with the product of the segment polarity gene *armadillo* in *Drosophila*) and gamma-catenin (presumably identical to plakoglobin) can bind to the cytoplasmic part of E-cadherin. alpha-Catenin (homologous with vinculin) connects beta-catenin to alpha-actinin and to the actin cytoskeleton. A fourth catenin-like molecule, coined p120^{cas}, was recently found to be part of the complex, and four isoforms have been detected up to now (Reynolds et al., 1992; Reynolds et al., 1994; Daniel and Reynolds, 1995). The link between E-cadherin and the cytoskeleton via the cantenins does not exclude, however, that the catenins associated with the plasma membrane complex can be exchanged for free molecules from the cytoplasm, and that the latter can form complexes with other molecules than E-cadherin (e.g. with the adenomatous polyposis coli [APC] proteins).

The concept of E-cadherin as an invasion suppressor stems from correlation studies that showed downregulation in invasive tumors, and from experimental up- or downregulation leading to, respectively, inhibition and induction of invasion (Bracke et al., 1995). Homogeneous or heterogeneous downregulation of E-cadherin was studied in histological sections of a variety of human carcinomas, and this phenomenon correlated with malignancy parameters, such as tumor progression, loss of differentiation, invasion, metastatic potential and bad prognosis. Data obtained from mammary carcinomas have confirmed this correlation (Shiozaki et al., 1993; Rasbridge et al., 1993; Moll et al., 1993; Oka et al., 1993; Lipponen et al., 1994). The factors responsible for this downregulation are still a matter of speculation. An autocrine-motility-factor-like molecule (Ishisaki et al., 1994), transforming growth factor-beta (Miettinen et al., 1994), *erb*B-2 (D'Souza and Taylor-Papadimitriou, 1994) and the *Slug* gene production (Nieto et al., 1994) have been proposed as possible candidates.

Strong evidence supporting the concept that E-cadherin is an invasion suppressor are derived from invasion experiments with cell lines (including mammary cell lines) differing in their expression of E-cadherin. The invasion assays used include: (a) the formation of invasive and metastatic tumors in syngeneic or immunodeficient laboratory animals, (b) confronting cultures with living embryonic chick heart fragments, and (c) penetration into non-living substrates such as Matrigel and type I collagen gels (Mareel et al., 1993b). Although the presence of potentially up- and downregulating factors of E-cadherin may differ substantially among these assays, the overall results appear to confirm an inverse correlation between E-cadherin expression and invasion. With mammary epithelioid cells, invasion was inhibited by transfection of the E-cadherin cDNA into constitutively E-cadherin-negative variants (Frixen et al., 1991; Vleminckx et al., 1991). Induction of invasion in constitutively E-cadherin positive variants was achieved by antagonizing the expression of the molecule via transfection with a plasmid encoding E-cadherin-specific antisense mRNA (Vleminckx et al., 1991), or via the application of antibodies that neutralize the adhesion function of E-cadherin (Doki et al., 1993; Chen and Öbrink, 1991; Behrens et al., 1989). In mammary carcinoma cells, downregulation of E-cadherin seems to be necessarily associated to expression of the intermediate filament component vimentin (typical for epithelial to mesenchymal transitions) for invasion to occur (Sommers et al., 1991). E-cadherin may, however, "override"the vimentin-associated invasiveness (Thompson et al., 1994).

Exceptions to the rule of inverse correlation between E-cadherin expression and invasion have been reported. For instance, human MCF-7/6 mammary carcinoma cells can give rise to invading and metastasizing tumors in nude mice (Correc et al., 1990). Both the primary tumors and the metastases, however, show homogeneous expression of E-cadherin, as evident from immunohistochemistry. Invasion *in vitro* with homogeneous E-cadherin expression was also found with this mammary cell line (Bracke et al., 1991). Together with data from non-mammary tumor cells, these findings suggest that invasion can also be the result of functional inactivity or inactivation of E-cadherin at the tumor cell surface.

Modulation of the function of the E-cadherin/catenin complex in mammary cells by extracellular agents

The function of E-cadherin in mammary cells can be defective for several reasons: (a) genomic mutations in any of the components of the complex with functional implications, (b) downregulation of the expression of one of the catenins, or (c) tyrosine phosphorylation of the complex. A point mutation in exon 7 of E-cadherin with possible functional impact (Asn - > Ser) was recently detected in two cases of invasive mammary carcinoma (Kania et al., 1994). Protein truncation mutations were found at high frequency (4 out of 7) in the E-cadherin gene of infiltrative lobular breast carcinomas (Berx et al., 1995). Downregulation of alpha-

or gamma-catenin have both been found in mammary carcinomas (Ochiai et al., 1994b; Sommers et al., 1994), while a deletion in the N-terminal region of beta-catenin was only detected in stomach cancer cells so far (Oyama et al., 1994; Kawanishi et al., 1995). Those inactivating events can be considered as virtually irreversible.

Tyrosine phosphorylation of the E-cadherin/catenin complex, however, appears to be a rapid and reversible mechanism to downregulate its function. Transformation experiments with the v-*src* oncogene have shown that the tyrosine kinase activity of its gene product preferentially increases beta-catenin tyrosine phosphorylation, and this lead to impaired cell compaction (Matsuyoshi et al., 1992) and induced invasiveness *in vitro* (Behrens et al., 1993). In addition, a number of tyrosine kinase receptors have been implicated in the regulation of the E-cadherin/catenin complex, such as the receptors for hepatocyte growth factor/scatter factor, for epidermal growth factor (Shibamoto et al., 1994; Hoschuetzky et al., 1994) and for heregulin (Ochiai et al., 1994a).

From both a scientific and a therapeutical point of view correction of the defective function of the E-cadherin/catenin complex appears to be an interesting goal. Therefore, we examined a number of variants of the human MCF-7 cell line, which was originally derived from the pleural effusion of a metastasizing mammary adenocarcinoma (Soule et al., 1973). Variants were obtained from different laboratories and their MCF-7 origin was confirmed by specific immunoreactive markers (Coopman et al., 1991). All variants were confronted *in vitro* with embryonic chick heart fragments, cultured in suspension for 8 days, and their interaction was evaluated by histologic analysis (Mareel et al., 1979). Some variants (e.g. MCF-7/6) invaded the heart tissue, while others (e.g. MCF-7/AZ) failed to do so (Bracke et al., 1991). The presence of an apparently intact E-cadherin/catenin complex at the plasma membrane of both MCF-7/6 and MCF-7/AZ cells was demonstrated with multiple techniques (immunocytochemistry, immunohistochemistry, co-immunoprecipitation, flow cytometry and Western blotting). From these data we concluded that the E-cadherin/catenin complex was unable to exert its invasion suppressor function in MCF-7/6 cells (Bracke et al., 1993).

The comparison between invasive MCF-7/6 and non-invasive MCF-7/AZ cells revealed differences in cell-cell adhesion *in vitro* (Bracke et al., 1993). A fast aggregation assay, modified after the techniques of Takeichi (1977) and Kadmon et al. (1990), starts by detaching cells from their plastic tissue culture substrate under conditions that should leave the E-cadherin/catenin complex functionally intact. By Coulter counter measurements, the initial number of particles in suspension is compared with the number after 30 min of aggregation. In this assay, MCF-7/7 cells showed poor aggregation in contrast with their non-invasive MCF-7/AZ counterparts. MCF-7/AZ aggregation was specifically inhibited in the presence of monoclonal antibodies directed against a functional domain of E-cadherin (HECD-1, MB2), but not by other monoclonals binding to other glycoproteins of the plasma membrane (e.g. 5D10). These results indicate that E-cadherin at the surface of MCF-7/6 cells is unable to mediate cell-cell adhesion and prevent invasion *in vitro*.

We have shown that insulin-like growth factor I (IGF-I), at near-physiological serum concentrations, can correct the defective cell-cell adhesion function of the E-cadherin/catenin complex in the invasive MCF-7/6 cell variant (Bracke et al., 1993). Fast aggregation is stimulated by IGF-I within 30 minutes, and the effect is independent from *de novo* protein synthesis. This increased aggregation is mediated by E-cadherin, since it can be blocked by the monoclonal anti-E-cadherin antibodies HECD-1 and MB2. IGF-I interacts with the IGF-I receptor on the MCF-7 cell surface, and the anti-IGF-I receptor monoclonal antibody alpha-IR3 completely inhibits the effect of IGF-I on MCF-7/6 aggregation. MCF-7 cells express in addition insulin receptors that show homology to the IGF-I receptor, and insulin is indeed able to mimick the IGF-I effect on cell aggregation, but at supraphysiological concentrations only. The insulin effect is not blocked by the monoclonal antibody alpha-IR3, indicating that insulin does not act via the IGF-I receptor, but presumably via its own receptor. It is not excluded that our MCF-7/6 cells possess a hybrid of the IGF-I and the insulin receptor, which is less sensitive to the IGF-I and insulin that the proper IGF-I or insulin receptors, respectively. Insulin-like growth factor II (IGF-II), having its own type of receptor, is not able to induce fast cell aggregation of MCF-7/7 cells.

Signal transduction from the triggered IGF-I receptor starts with switching on its intracellular tyrosine kinase activity, which leads to autophosphorylation of the receptor in our MCF-7/6 cells and to phosphorylation of (a) cytoplasmic substrate(s) (Jacobs et al., 1983; Kadowaki et al., 1987). For the insulin receptor, these phosphorylations have been shown to result in *ras* activation through a cascade of rapid molecular interactions (Skolnik et al., 1993; Baltensperger et al., 1993). We have shown that activation of E-cadherin-mediated aggregation of MCF-7/6 cells can be blocked by a number of tyrosine kinase inhibitors: genistein (25 micromoles), me-2, 5-diOH cinnamate (50 micromoles) and 2-OH-5-(2,5 diOH benzyl) aminobenzoic acid (10 micromoles). We have tried to reveal possible alterations of the phosphorylation of the E-cadherin/complex by IGF-I treatment in well controlled experiments, but failed to find any effect.

When added to the culture medium of confronting cultures between MCF-7/6 cells and chick heart fragments, IGF-I exerted an anti-invasive effect, which was reversible upon removal of the factor. Again this effect appeared to be mediated by the IGF-I receptor, because it could be blocked by a monoclonal antibody against the IGF-I receptor. Our finding that IGF-I receptor triggering prevents invasion *in vitro*, should be related to studies on human mammary tissue samples showing production of IGF-I by stromal cells of non-maligant specimens, and production of IGF-II by stromal cells of invasive carcinomas (Cullen et al., 1991; Paik, 1992). Furthermore, expression of high levels of IGF-I receptor in mammary tumors has been claimed to be an indicator of better prognosis (Peyrat and Bonneterre, 1992; Papa et al., 1993). However, since IGF-I is a growth factor for breast cancer cells, it is difficult to advocate this molecule as a therapeutic agent.

Some flavonoids are interesting tools to study the mechanisms of mammary tumor invasion. Examples are genistein (Martin et al., 1978; Akiyama et al., 1987), quercetin (Graziani, 1986), (+)-catechin(Bracke et al., 1987), 3,7-dimethoxy flavone (Parmar et al., 1994), and flavone acetic acid (Ching and Baguley, 1987). Tangeretin, a flavonoid extractable from citrus plants, was retained in a screening program for potential anti-invasive molecules in the assay with embryonic chick heart. This molecule inhibited the invasion of virus-transformed MO4 mouse cells and of MCF-7/6 cells (Bracke et al., 1994a). Tangeretin corrects the defective function of the E-cadherin/catenin complex in MCF-7/6 cells in a way that resembles the effect of IGF-I and induces MCF-7/6 fast cell aggregation. This phenomenon is mediated by E-cadherin, since it can be blocked by the anti-E-cadherin monoclonal antibodies HECD-1 and MB2, and it is not dependent on *de novo* protein synthesis, since cycloheximide does not inhibit the tangeretin effect. The flavonoid effect, however, differs from the IGF-I effect in that it does not seem to require triggering of the IGF-I receptor, as evidenced by the lack of effect of alpha-IR3, the monoclonal antibody that inhibits the function of this receptor. Furthermore, tangeretin does not induce tyrosine autophosphorylation of the IGF-I receptor.

All-*trans*-retinoic acid (RA) exerts opposite effects on invasion depending on the type of MCF-7 cells under study. When added to the medium of confronting embryonic chick heart cultures, RA inhibits invasion of MCF-7/6 cells, but induces invasion in the non-invasive cell variant MCF-7/AZ (Bracke et al., 1993). RA affects multiple functions of MCF-7/6 cells: it decreased fast plasma membrane motility and increased the enzymatic activity of tissue-type transglutaminases (Bracke et al., 1992) and cell-cell adhesion. So, the anti-invasive effect of RA on MCF-7/6 can be explained as induction of a less motile, more rigid and more strongly adherent phenotype.

Fast aggregation of MCF-7/6 cells was increased by addition of RA to the medium. This effect was about maximal after pretreatment of the cells for 4h, and was concentration-dependent. Using the anti-E-cadherin monoclonal antibiodies HECD-1 and MB2, we were able to demonstrate that RA specifically corrects the defective function of the E-cadherin/catenin complex in these cells. Like with IGF-I and tangeretin the RA effect was not sensitive to cycloheximide, which shows that *de novo* protein synthesis is not required.

The action mechanism of RA on MCF-7/6 cells is not well understood. RA is transported in the cytoplasm towards the nucleus via the cytoplasmic RA-binding protein (CRABP). Interaction with the nuclear RA receptors modulates gene transcription, and other molecules can interact with this zinc-finger mediated phenomenon (Mader et al., 1993). Cycloheximide insensitivity makes classical promotion of DNA transcription/translation of relevant genes by RA rather improbable. Up to now we have also gathered arguments to believe that RA does not act via triggering of the IGF-I receptor, because neither blocking of this receptor by the monoclonal antibody alpha-IR3, nor inhibition of its tyrosine kinase activity diminish the effect of RA on fast aggregation.

Effects of antiestrogens on invasion and cell-cell adhesion of mammary carcinoma cells in vitro

We have observed an anti-invasive effect with three antiestrogens: Tamoxifen, ICI 164,384 and ICI 182,760 (the latter two pure anti-estrogens were gifts from Dr. Alan Wakeling, ZENECA Pharmaceuticals, Macclesfield, Cheshire, U.K.). Since these effects have been published extensively for Tamoxifen (Bracke et al., 1994b) and ICI 164,384 (Bracke et al., 1993), we will illustrate here our data with ICI 182,760 as an example. When MCF-7/6 cells were confronted with embryonic chick heart fragments in organ culture for 10 days, invasion was inhibited by ICI 182,760 at concentrations of 10^{-9}M or higher in the culture medium (Table I). This inhibition was obvious from serial hitological sections of the confronting cultures, stained with Hematoxylin-eosin or with an immunohistochemical technique to reveal chick heart antigens (Fig. 2). The anti-invasive effect of ICI 182,760 could be competed out by a higher than equimolar concentration of estradiol, which indicates that both compounds possess a common target, presumably the estrogen receptor. Omission of the drug from the culture medium after 10 days of treatment and culturing for another 7 days in drug-free medium showed that the anti-invasive effect was fully reversible: invasion resumed during the second culture period, and this indicated that the anti-invasive effect of ICI 812,760 cannot be ascribed to cytotoxicity on the MCF-7/6 cells.

Table I. Anti-invasive effect of the antiestrogen ICI 182,780

Treatment		Result
E2	ICI 182,780 (M)	Grade (n^0 of cultures)
0	0	III (1), IV (4)
0	10^{-10}	III (3), IV (1)
0	10^{-9}	II (4)
0	10^{-8}	II (3)
0	10^{-7}	II (3)
0	10^{-6}	II (4)
10^{-10}	0	IV (3)
10^{-9}	0	IV (3)
10^{-8}	0	IV (3)
10^{-10}	10^{-9}	II (2)
10^{-9}	10^{-9}	II (3)
10^{-8}	10^{-9}	IV (3)

Confronting cultures of MCF-7/6 with chick heart fragments were incubated for 10 days in DMEM/HamF12(50:50) supplements with 10% steroid-stripped fetal bovine serum. Grade II indicates absence of invasion, while grades III and IV correspond to invasion (Bracke et al., 1984).

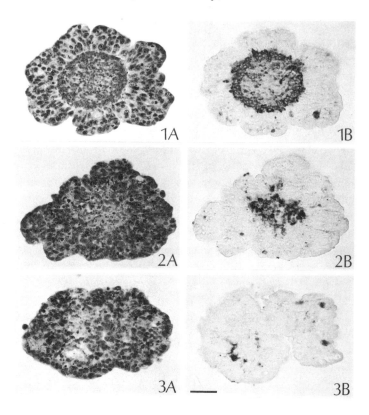

Figure 2. Histological sections from 10-day old confronting cultures between human MCF-7/6 mammary carcinoma cells and embryonic chick heart fragments. Panels on the left (A) were stained with hematoxylin-eosin, and those on the right (B) with an immunohistochemical technique to reveal chick heart antigens (darkly stained tissue). The cultures were treated with 10^{-9}M ICI 182,760 (1A and 1B), with the solvent only (2A and 2B) or with a combination of 10^{-9}M ICI 182,760 and 10^{-8} estradiol (3A and 3B). The pure antiestrogen has an anti-invasive activity, which can be competed out by an excess of estradiol. Scale bar $=50$ micromoles.

The anti-invasive effect of Tamoxifen *in vitro* seems to contrast with the results of another paper, in which this molecule was found to stimulate MCF-7 cell invasion (Thompson et al., 1988). Apart from possible differences in the MCF-7 variants and in the assays for invasion used in both studies, the control (drug-free) cultures were not similar as far as the presence of estrogens was concerned. In our study with

Tamoxifen the control cultures were kept in culture medium supplemented with fetal bovine serum, and showed invasion. In the other study, the controls were kept in serum-free medium and showed no invasion. So, depending on the presence of serum estrogens in the control cultures, one can observe an anti-invasive or an invasion-promoting effect of Tamoxifen. The latter effect may be ascribed to the slight estrogenic activity of Tamoxifen.

Not all effects of antiestrogens on invasion of MCF-7/6 cells can be attributed to an activation of the E-cadherin/catenin complex. Here Tamoxifen rather stands as an exception (Bracke et al., 1994b). Fast aggregation of these cells was increased by Tamoxifen at anti-invasive concentrations (10^{-6}M), and the effect was rapidly observable (within 30 min). Tamoxifen-induced aggregation was sensitive to inhibition by HECD-1 and MB2 monoclonal antibodies against the extracellular part of E-cadherin. This observation showing that E-cadherin was implicated in the activation of MCF-7/6 cell aggregation, was confirmed by the calcium-dependency in the extracellular medium of the effect. *De novo* protein synthesis was not required, since cycloheximide did not affect the Tamoxifen action on fast aggregation. Blocking of the IGF-I receptor with the monoclonal antibody alpha-IR3 did not inhibit the Tamoxifen-induced fast cell aggregation, which indicated that triggering of the extracellular part of this receptor is not part of the signalling pathway of Tamoxifen. Moreover, we found that Tamoxifen, unlike IGF-I, was not able to increase tyrosine phosphorylation of the IGF-I receptor in MCF-7/6 cells. This issue may be somewhat controversial, since another group has published recently that Tamoxifen sensitizes some MCF-7 variants to the proliferative effects of IGF-I possibly by induction of the IGF-I receptor (Wiseman et al., 1993). The latter effects on proliferation, however, differ from those on cell aggregation by their kinetics: activation of the E-cadherin/catenin complex by Tamoxifen is completed within minutes, and makes an indirect pathway via receptor induction rather unlikely.

In contrast with the IGF-I receptor the estrogen receptor appears to be implicated in the effect of Tamoxifen on fast cell aggregation. One argument could be found in the insensitivity of estrogen-receptor negative mammary cell lines, such as HBL-100 and SK-BR-3, to the Tamoxifen effect on cell aggregation.

One could argue that very high concentrations of Tamoxifen (10^{-6}M or higher) are required for the effects described above. Studies on intratumoral Tamoxifen concentrations, however, have shown that 10^{-6}M is usually exceeded in human mammary carcinomas after daily oral intake of 20 mg of Tamoxifen (Johnston et al., 1993). We therefore believe that the restoration of the E-cadherin function in human mammary carcinoma cells may contribute to the established therapeutic benefit of Tamoxifen in breast cancer patients.

The major metabolites of Tamoxifen, 4-OH-Tamoxifen and N-desmethyl-Tamoxifen, were inactive in both the assay for invasion *in vitro* and in the fast aggregation assay. Remarkably, the pure antiestrogens ICI 164,384 and ICI 182,760 showed a clear anti-invasive effect, but were unable to increase the fast aggregation on MCF-7/6 cells. This finding suggests that the pure antiestrogens owe their effect on invasion to another mechanism than activation of the E-cadherin/catenin complex. Video-microscope measurements of the fast plasma membrane motility of MCF-7/6 cells have demonstrated an inhibitory effect of ICI 164,384, which opens the possibility that at least this anti-estrogen blocks invasion through slowing down cell motility (Bracke et al., 1993).

Conclusion

The E-cadherin/catenin complex is a powerful invasion suppressor in epithelial cells. Although downregulation of the elements of the complex at the transcriptional level is a frequent phenomenon in mammary carcinomas, posttranslational modifications of the complex also occur, and they can result in functional inactivation and lead to the invasive phenotype of the mammary cells. Loss of function is an interesting target for upregulation by external agents, that may become useful as drugs in both therapeutic and preventive regimens for breast cancer. Insulin-like growth factor-I, retinoic acid and the citrus flavonoid tangeretin are examples of molecules that can activate the E-cadherin/catenin complex and inhibit invasion of human MCF-7 mammary carcinoma cells *in vitro*. Antiestrogens possess an anti-invasive activity, but their action mechanisms may be different. Tamoxifen is a rapid activator of the E-cadherin/catenin complex, and this may contribute to its therapeutic benefit in breast cancer patients. The mechanism of the anti-invasive activity of the pure antiestrogens ICI 164,384 and ICI 182,760 awaits further investigation.

ACKNOWLEDGEMENTS

Parts of our study were supported by the Department of Citrus of the State of Florida, the FGWO, Brussels, Belgium, the Sportvereniging tegen Kanker, Brussels, Belgium and the G.O.A. van de Vlaamse Gemeenschap, Brussels, Belgium. Frans M. Van Roy is Research Director with the Belgian N.F.W.P. Vincent Castronovo is Research Associated with the Belgian F.N.R.S.,and is partly supported by l'Association contre le Cancer. The authors thank Stefan Vermeulen, Krist'l Vennekens, Erik Bruyneel, Georges De Bruyne, Caroline Labit, Veerle Van Marck, Geert Berx, Annick Keirsebilck, Friedel Nollet, Jolanda van Hengel and Ann Van Landschoot for helpful discussions.

REFERENCES

Akiyama T, Ishida J, Nakagawa S, Ogawara H, Watanabe S, Itoh N, Shibuya M, Fukami Y (1987): Genistein, a specific inhibitor of tyrosine-specific protein kinases. *J Biol Chem* 262:5592-5595

Baltensperger K, Kozma LM, Cherniack AD, Klarlund JK, Chawla A, Banerjee U, Czech MP (1993): Binding of the *ras* activator son of sevenless to insulin receptor substrate-1 signaling complexes. *Science* 260:1950-1952

Behrens J, Mareel MM, Van Roy FM, Birchmeier W (1989): Dissecting tumor cell invasion: epithelial cells acquire invasive properties following the loss of uvomorulin-mediated cell-cell adhesion. *J Cell Biol* 108:2435-2447

Behrens J, Vakaet L, Friis R, Winterhager E, Van Roy F, Mareel MM, Birchmeier W (1993): Loss of epithelial morphotype and gain of invasiveness correlates with tyrosine phosphorylation of the E-cadherin/beta-catenin complex in cells transformed with a temperature-sensitive v-*src* gene. *J Cell Biol* 120:757-766

Berx G, Cleton-Jansen A-M, Nollet F, de Leeuw WJF, can de Vijver MJ, Cornelisse C, Van Roy F (1995): E-cadherin is a tumor/invasion suppressor gene mutated in human lobular breast cancer. *EMBO J* (In Press)

Birchmeier W, Behrens J (1994): Cadherin expression in carcinomas: role in the formation of cell junctions and the prevention of invasiveness. *Biochim Biophys Acta* 1198:11-26

Bracke M, Romijn H, Vakaet L Jr, Vyncke B, De Mets M, Mareel M (1992): The use of spheroids in the study of invasion. In: Spheroid Culture in Cancer Research, R. Bjerkvig R, ed. CRC Press Inc., pp. 73-105

Bracke ME, Bruynell EA, Vermeulen SJ, Vennekens K, Van Marck V, Mareel MM (1994a): Citrus flavonoid effect on tumor invasion and metastases. *Food Technology* 48:121-124

Bracke ME, Castronovo V, Van Cauwenberge RM-L, Vakaet L Jr, Strojny P, Foidart J-M, Mareel MM (1987): The anti-invasive flavonoid (+)-catechin binds to laminin and abrogates the effect of laminin on cell morphology and adhesion. *Exp Cell Res* 173:193-205

Bracke ME, Charlier C, Bruyneel EA, Labit C, Mareel MM, Castronovo V (1994b): Tamoxifen restores the E-cadherin function in human breast cancer MCF-7/6 cells and suppresses their invasive phenotype. *Cancer Res* 54:4607-4609

Bracke ME, Van Cauwenberge RM-L, Mareel MM (1984): (+)-Catechin inhibits the invasion of malignant fibrosarcoma cells into chick heart *in vitro*. *Clin Exp Metastasis* 2:161-170

Bracke ME, Van Larebeke NA, Vyncke BM, Mareel MM (1991): Retinoic acid modulates both invasion and plasma membrane ruffling of MCF-7 human mammary carcinoma cells *in vitro*. *Br J Cancer* 63:867-872

Bracke ME, Van Roy FM, Mareel M (1995): The E-cadherin/catenin complex in invasion and metastasis. *Curr Top Microbiol Immunol* (In Press)

Bracke ME, Vyncke BM, Bruyneel EA, Vermeulen SJ, De Bruyne GK, Van Larebeke NA, Vleminckx K, Van Roy FM, Mareel MM (1993): Insulin-like growth factor I activates the invasion suppressor function of E-cadherin in MCF-7 mammary carcinoma cells *in vitro*. *Br J Cancer* 68:282-289

Chen W, Öbrink B (1991): Cell-cell contacts mediated by E-cadherin (Uvomorulin) restrict invasive behaviour of L-cells. *J Cell Biol* 114:319-327

Ching LM, Baguley BC (1987): Induction of natural killer cell activity by the antitumor compound flavone acetic acid (NSC 34512). *Eur J Cancer Clin Oncol* 23:1047-1050

Coopman PJ, Bracke ME, Lissitzky JC, De Bruyne GK, Van Roy FM, Foidart J-M, Mareel MM (1991): Influence of basement membrane molecules on directional migration of human breast cell lines *in vitro*. *J Cell Sci* 98:395-401

Correc P, Fondanèche M-C, Bracke M, Burtin P (1990): The presence of plasmin receptors on three mammary carcinoma MCF-7 sublines. *Int J Cancer* 46:745-750

Cullen KJ, Smith HS, Hill S, Rosen N, Lippman ME (1991): Growth factor messenger RNA expression by human breast fibroblasts from benign and malignant lesions. *Cancer Res* 51:4978-4985

D'Souza B, Taylor-Papadimitriou J (1994): Overexpression of *erb*B2 in human mammary epithelial cells signals inhibition of transcription of the E-cadherin gene. *Proc Natl Acad Sci USA* 91:7202-7206

Daniel JM, Reynolds AB (1995): The tyrosine kinase substrate p120^{cas} binds directly to E-cadherin but not to the adenomatous polyposis coli protein or alpha-catenin. *Mol Cell Biol* 15:4819-4824

Doki Y, Shiozaki H, Tahara H, Inoue M, Oka H, Iihara K, Kadowaki T, Takeichi M, Mori T (1993): Correlation between E-cadherin expression and invasiveness *in vitro* in a human esophageal cancer cell line. *Cancer Res* 53:3421-3426

Frixen UH, Behrens J, Sachs M, Eberle G, Voss B, Wards A, Löchner D, Birchmeier W (1991): E-cadherin-mediated cell-cell adhesion prevents invasiveness of human carcinoma cells. *J Cell Biol* 113:173-185

Graziani Y (1986): In: Plant Flavonoids in Biology and Medicine: Biochemical, Pharmacological and Structure-Activity Relationships, Cody V, Middleton E Jr, Harborne JB, eds. New York: Alan R. Liss Inc., pp. 301-313

Hoschuetzky H, Aberle H, Kemler R (1994): ß-catenin mediates the interaction of the cadherin-catenin complex with epidermal growth factor receptor. *J Cell Biol* 127:1375-1380

Ishisaki A, Oida S, Momose F, Amagasa T, Rikimaru K, Ichijo H, Sasaki S (1994): Identification and characterization of autocrine-motility-factor-like activity in oral squamous-cell-carcinoma cells. *Int J Cancer* 59:783-788

Jacobs J, Kull FC Jr, Earp HS, Svoboda ME, Van Wyck JJ, Cuatrecasas P (9183): Somatomedine-C stimulates the phosphorylation of the ß subunit of its own receptor. *J Biol Chem* 258:9581-9584

Johnston SRC, Haynes BP, Smith IE, Jarman M, Sacks NPM, Ebbs SR, Dowsett M (1993): Acquired tamoxifen resistance in human breast cancer and reduced intra-tumoral drug concentration. *Lancet* 342:1521-1522

Kadmon G, Korvitz A, Altevogt P, Schachner M (1990): The neural cell adhesion molecule N-CAM enhances L1-dependent cell-cell interactions. *J Cell Biol* 110:193-208

Kadowaki T, Koyasu S, Nishida E, Tobe K, Izumi T, Takaku F, Sakai H, Yahara I, Kasuga M (1987): Tyrosine phosphorylation of common and specific sets of cellular proteins rapidly induced by insulin, insulin-like growth factor I, and epidermal growth factor in an intact cell. *J Biol Chem* 262:7342-7350

Kanai Y, Oda T, Tsuda H, Ochiai A, Hirohashi S (1994): Point mutation of the E-cadherin gene in invasive lobular carcinoma of the breast. *Jpn J Cancer Res* 85:1035-1039

Kawanishi J, Kato J, Sasaki K, Fujii S, Watanabe N, Nittsu Y (1995): Loss of E-cadherin-dependent cell-cell adhesion due to mutation of the ß-catenin gene in a human cancer cell line, HSC-39. *Mol Cell Biol* 15:1175-1181

Kemler R (1993): From cadherins to catenins: cytoplasmic protein interactions and regulation of cell adhesion. *TIG* 9:317-321

Lipponen P, Saarelainen E, Ji H, Aaltomaa S, Syrjanen K (1994): Expression of E-cadherin (E-CD) as related to other prognostic factors and survival in breast cancer. *J Pathol* 174:101-109

Mader S, Leroy P, Chen JY, Chambon P (1993): Multiple parameters control the selectivity of nuclear receptors for their response elements. Selectivity and promiscuity in response element recognition by retinoic acid receptors and retinoic X receptors. *J Biol Chem* 268:591-600

Mareel M, Kint J, Meyvisch C (1979): Methods of study of the invasion of malignant C3H mouse fibroblasts into embryonic chick heart *in vitro*. *Virchows Arch B Cell Pathol* 30:95-111

Mareel MM, Van Roy FM, Bracke ME, (1993a): How and when do tumor cells metastasize? *Crit Rev Oncogenesis* 4:559-594

Mareel MM, Van Roy FM, Bracke ME, De Baetselier P (1993b): Molecular mechanisms of cancer invasion. *Encyclopedia* (In Press)

Martin PM, Hamaguchi M, Tanigushi S, Nagafuchi A, Tsukita S, Takeichi M (1992): Cadherin-mediated cell-cell adhesion is perturbed by v-*src* tyrosine phosphorylation in metastatic fibroblasts. *J Cell Biol* 118:703-714

Miettinen PJ, Ebner R, Lopez AR, Derynck R (1994): TGF-ß induced transdifferentiation of mammary epithelial cells to mesenchymal cells: involvement of type I receptors. *J Cell Biol* 127:2021-2036

Moll R, Mitze M, Frixen UH, Birchmeier W (1993): Differential loss of E-cadherin expression in infiltrating ductal and lobular breast carcinomas. *Am J Pathol* 143:1731-1742

Nieto MA, Sargent MG, Wilkinson DG, Cooke J (1994): Control of cell behavior during vertebrate development by *Slug*, a zinc finger gene. *Science* 264:835-839

Ochiai A, Akimoto S, Kanani Y, Shibata T, Oyama T, Hirohashi S (1994a): c-*erb*B-2 gene production associates with catenins in human cancer cells. *Biochem Biophys Res Commun* 205:73-78

Ochiai A, Akimoto S, Shimoyama Y, Nagafuchi A, Shoichiro T, Hirohashi S (1994b): Frequent loss of alpha catenin expression in scirrhous carcinomas with scattered cell growth. *Jpn J Cancer Res* 85:266-273

Oka H, Shiozaki H, Kobayashi K, Inoue M, Tahara H, Kobayashi T, Takatsuka Y, Matsuyoshi N, Hirano S, Takeichi M, Mori T (1993): Expression of E-cadherin cell adhesion molecules in human breast cancer tissues and its relationship to metastasis. *Cancer Res* 53:1696-1701

Overduin M, Harvey TS, Bagby S, Tong KI, Yau P, Takeichi M, Ikura M (1995): Solution structure of the epithelial cadherin domain responsible for selective cell adhesion. *Science* 267:386-389

Oyama T, Kanai Y, Ochiai A, Akimoto S, Oda T, Yanagihara K, Nagafuchi A, Tsukita S, Shibamoto S, Ito F, Takeichi M, Matsuda H, Hirohashi S (1994): A truncated ß-catenin disrupts the interaction between E-cadherin and alpha-catenin: a cause of loss of intercellular adhesiveness in human cancer cell lines. *Cancer Res* 54:6282-6287

Paik S (1992): Expression of IGF-I and IGF-II mRNA in breast tissue. *Breast Cancer Res Treat* 22:31-38

Papa V, Gliozzo B, Clark GM, McGuire WL, Moore D, Fujita-Yamaguchi Y, Vigner R, Goldfine ID, Pezzino V (1993): Insulin-like growth factor-I factors are overexpressed and predict a low risk in human breast cancer. *Cancer Res* 53:3736-3740

Parmar VS, Jain R, Sharma SK, Vardhan A, Jha A, Taneja P, Singh S, Vyncke BM, Bracke ME, Mareel MM (1994): Anti-invasive activity of 3,7-dimethoxyflavone *in vitro*. *J Pharm Sci* 83:1217-122

Peyrat JP, Bonneterre J (1992): Type I IGF receptor in human breast diseases. *Breast Cancer Res Treat* 22:59-67

Rasbridge SA, Gillett CE, Sampson SA, Walsh FS, Millis RR (1993): Epithelial (E-) and placental (P-) cadherin cell adhesion molecule expression in breast carcinoma. *J Pathol* 169:245-250

Reynolds AB, Daniel J, McCrea PD, Wheelock MJ, Wu J, Zhang Z (1994): Identification of a new catenin: the tyrosine kinase substrate p120^{cas} associates with E-cadherin complexes. *Mol Cell Biol* 14:8333-8342

Reynolds AB, Herbert L, Cleveland JL, Berg ST, Gaut JR (1992): p120, a novel substrate of protein tyrosine kinase receptors and of p60v-*src*, is related to cadherin-binding factors ß-catenin, plakoglobin and armadillo. *Oncogene* 7:2439-2445

Shapiro L, Fannon AM, Kwong PD, Thompson A, Lehmann MS, Grübel G, Legrand JF, Als-Nielsen J, Colman DR, Hendrickson WA (1995): Structural basis of cell-cell adhesion by cadherins. *Nature* 374:327-337

Shibamoto S, Nayakawa M, Takeuchi K, Hori T, Oku N, Myoazawa K, Kitamura N, Takeichi M, Ito F (1994): Tyrosine phosphorylation of ß-catenin and plakoglobin enchanced by hepatocyte growth factor and epidermal growth factor in human carcinoma cells. *Cell Adhesion and Communication* 1:295-305

Shiozaki H, Doki Y, Oka H, Iihara K, Miyata M, Kadowaki T, Matsui S, Tamura S, Inoue M, Mori T (1993): The function of GRB2 in linking the insulin receptor to *ras* signaling pathways. *Science* 260:1953-1055

Sommers CL, Gelmann EP, Kemler R, Cowin P, Byers SW (1994): Alterations in ß-catenin phosphorylation and plakoglobin expression in human breast cancer cells. *Cancer Res* 54:3544-3552

Sommers CL, Thompson EW, Torri JA, Kemler R, Gelmann EP, Beyers SW (1991): Cell adhesion molecule uvomorulin expression in human breast cancer cell lines: relationship to morphology and invasive capacities. *Cell Growth Differ* 2:365-372

Soule HD, Vazquez J, Long A, Albert S, Brennan M (1973): A human cell line from pleural effusion derived from a breast carcinoma. *J Natl Cancer Inst* 51:1409-1416

Takeichi M (1977): Functional correlation between cell adhesive properties and some cell surface proteins. *J Cell Biol* 75:464-474

Takeichi M (1993): Cadherins in cancer: implications for invasion and metastasis. *Current Opin Cell Biol* 5:806-811

Thompson EW, Reich R, Shima TB, Albini A, Graf J, Martin GR, Dickson RB, Lippman ME (1988): Differential regulation of growth and invasiveness of MCF-7 breast cancer cells by anti-estrogens. *Cancer Res* 48:6764-6768

Thompson EW, Torri J, Sabol M, Sommers CL, Dickson RB (1994): Oncogene-induced basement membrane invasiveness in human mammary epithelial cells. *Clin Exp Metastasis* 12:181-194

Vleminckx K, Vakaet L Jr, Mareel M, Fiers W, Van Roy F (1991): Genetic manipulation of E-cadherin expression by epithelial tumors cells reveals an invasion suppressor role. *Cell* 66:107-119

Wiseman LR, Johnson MD, Wakeling AE, Lykkesfeldt AE, May FE, Westley BR (1993): Type I IGF receptor and acquired tamoxifen resistance in oestrogen-responsive human breast cancer cells. *Eur J Cancer* 29A:2256-2264

12. REGULATION OF GROWTH FACTOR GENE EXPRESSION BY TAMOXIFEN

Liam J. Murphy and Leigh C. Murphy

Introduction

Estrogens exert multiple different actions in a wide variety of tissues. The recent availability of specific immunological and molecular probes have demonstrated that estrogen receptors (ER) are expressed in a variety of cell types and tissues not usually considered to be classical estrogen targets. The functions of estrogen in these tissues remain elusive in many cases. Amongst the best studied estrogen action is estrogen-induced cellular proliferation. However, the mechanisms by which estrogens promote the growth of various target tissues remain unclear. Both *in vitro* and *in vivo* data suggest that a major component of this effect of estrogen is mediated via the regulation of expression of locally acting stimulatory and inhibitory autocrine/paracrine growth factors and their receptors (Lippman and Dickson, 1989). The antiestrogens, of which Tamoxifen is the best known, antagonize the estrogen induced growth of estrogen target tissues and inhibit the effect of estrogen.

It has been generally thought that the basis of the antiproliferative effect of Tamoxifen results from its ability to competitively inhibit the binding of estrogen to estrogen receptors, therefore inhibiting estrogen signal transduction and specific expression of particular growth factor genes. In support of this notion are the many reports that exogenous growth factors can reverse the antiproliferative effects of antiestrogens on various cell lines in culture. However, as will be discussed below, some recent intriguing reports would suggest that this may be an oversimplificiation. For example, Tamoxifen is able to inhibit cellular proliferation induced by a variety of growth factors in addition to those induced by estrogen.

Tamoxifen can have modest agonist or estrogenic activity in addition to its antiestrogenic activity. The relative ratio of estrogenic activity versus antiestrogenic activity demonstrates considerable species variability. However, even within a single species there is also tissue specificity with Tamoxifen having modest estrogenic activity in, for example, the human uterus but antagonist effects at the levels of pituitary and breast (Malet et al., 1988; Holinka et al., 1986). Furthermore, there appear to be differences between *in vitro* activities of Tamoxifen on cellular proliferation and those observed *in vivo*, indicating that the contribution from adjacent stromal tissue and/or hormonal factors may be very important in determining the overall effect of Tamoxifen in a given setting and its clinical efficacy. These tissue specific differences may be explained in terms of differences in tissue uptake and/or metabolism of Tamoxifen and thus the relative ratios of estrogens and Tamoxifen in different tissues (Osborne et al., 1991) or tissue differences in the interaction of antiestrogen-ER and estrogen-ER with the transcriptional machinery (Webb et al., 1995) or possibly the existence of multiple forms of ER (Wiltschke and Fuqua, 1995).

In this review we will discuss the effects of Tamoxifen and other antiestrogens on growth factor pathways in a variety of tissues and cell lines and the underlying mechanisms responsible for the differences and similarities of estrogen and Tamoxifen action. Current data support an interaction of growth factors and estrogen/antiestrogen action at two main levels: 1. The regulation of expression of the growth factor and/or its receptor by estrogen/antiestrogen, and 2. Cross-talk between polypeptide growth factor signal transduction pathways and steroid hormone receptor signal transduction pathways.

Growth factors as mediators of estrogen and antiestrogen action

Experiments using antireceptor antibodies and antisense oligonucleotide technology have provided convincing evidence that local growth factor expression is important in estrogen-induced proliferation. Indeed, in many cases either a single growth factor or a combination of growth factors can result in a response comparable to that seen with estrogen. The most dramatic *in vivo* example of this is the demonstration that epidermal growth factor (EGF) administered to ovariectomized mice can induce all the morphological and biochemical changes in the uterus which occur in the estrogenized uterus (Nelson et al., 1990). This effect is thought to be mediated via the ER and is inhibited by pure antiestrogens (Ignar-Trowbridge et al., 1992). These types of experiments do not however exclude direct effects of estrogen on expression of genes which coordinate the transition into and through the cell cycle nor do they demonstrate unequivocally the role of a particular growth factor in estrogen action. Rather, they demonstrate that a growth factor, or combination of growth factors (often at supraphysiological concentrations) can induce a response comparable to estrogen. The example cited above is particularly apt in this regard. Clearly the increase in uterine expression and accumulation of EGF in the ovariectomized or immature mouse after estrogen administration is far too delayed to be directly responsible for estrogen induced uterine proliferation (DiAugustine et al., 1988).

In addition to any direct role growth factors have in mediating estrogen action, estrogen-induced modulation of autocrine/paracrine growth factor pathways may amplify the estrogen effects. Interactions of these growth factor pathways themselves may serve to amplify the initial mitogenic signal. For example, estrogen is able to induce expression of insulin-like growth factor-I (IGF-I), c-*fos* and c-*jun* in uterine tissue (Murphy et al., 1988a; Weisz and Bresciani, 1988). IGF-I itself can induce c-*fos* and c-*jun* in a variety of cell types including smooth muscle cells and fibroblasts. Thus activation of expression of IGF-I may amplify estrogen induced expression of genes with appropriate response elements, in this case AP1 response elements, by increasing the nuclear concentration of c-*fos*/c-*jun* heterodimers. Indeed an AP1 sequence present in the IGF-I has been implicated in the transcriptional regulation of IGF-I and may be involved in the estrogen induction of transcription of the IGF-I gene. In estrogen responsive MCF-7 cells, it is possible to demonstrate this type of synergism between insulin acting through the IGF-IGF-I receptor and estradiol. Using MCF-7 cells in steroid hormone depleted culture conditions, van der Burg and colleagues have shown that insulin enhances the effects of estrogen on MCF-7 DNA synthesis (van der Burg et al., 1989). Under their culture conditions estradiol, in the absence of insulin or IGF-I is able to stimulate c-*fos* and m-*myc* expression but results in only a modest stimulation of DNA synthesis. While estrogen has no effect on c-*jun* expression in this tissue, insulin or IGF-I alone stimulates both c-*jun* and c-*fos* expression and markedly enhances the mitogenic effect of estrogen. Although the activated, liganded ER complex is the initial trigger to the estrogen-induced proliferative response in the uterus, a rapid increase in expression of a variety of proto-oncogenes and other trans-acting factors can be demonstrated following estrogen administration.

In addition to this interaction at the nuclear level, estrogen-induced growth factor expression may indirectly activate other growth factor or cytokine systems. For example both EGF and IGF-I have been shown to induce reciprocal expression of each other. That is, in the ovariectomized mouse uterus local administration of IGF-I induces EGF expression and vice versa (Hana and Murphy, 1994a). Activated steroid hormone receptors can interact synergistically with several other trans-acting factors including CP1, Sp1, OTF and NF1 (Schule et al., 1988; Meyer et al., 1989). Thus, some of the demonstrable effects of estrogen on growth factor transcription may not necessarily be due to a direct interaction of the liganded ER to a classical estrogen response element. It has been suggested that estrogen-induced IGF-I expression involves activation of transcription with direct ER binding to IGF-I genomic DNA.

Since it is becoming increasingly apparently that classical estrogen response elements are not present in many genes which appear to be transcriptionally regulated by estrogen, the transcriptional millieu in different tissues may be very important in determining the effects of estrogen and antiestrogens such as Tamoxifen. For example, Berry et al., (1989) have recently proposed that Tamoxifen acts an an estrogen agonist when it promotes estrogen receptor binding to a target gene from which transcription is activated by TAF-1 whereas it acts as an antagonist when the activation of a given promoter is dependent on TAF-2.

Effects of Tamoxifen on the insulin-like growth factor system

Over the last half decade we have come to realize that the steroid hormones are inimately involved in the regulation of both IGF-I and IGF-II expression in normal and malignant uterine and mammary tissue and in the liver (Huff et al., 1986; Murphy and Friesen, 1986; Murphy and Ghahary, 1990). Furthermore, other components of the IGF system such as the IGF-I receptor and some of the IGF binding proteins can also be regulated by steroid hormones in a variety of tissues (Murphy and Ghahary, 1990). Studies in rodents demonstrated that both IGF-I and IGF-II mRNA levels are increased in the uteri of ovariectomized rats following estrogen administration and this effect is mimicked by Tamoxifen which has predominantly estrogen agonist effects in the rodent uterus. This response is pituitary-independent, transcriptional and does not require continuing protein synthesis (Murphy and Ghahary, 1990).

The IGF system appears to be important in a variety of malignant disease including both breast and uterine cancer. Both breast and uterine cancer cells in culture are responsive to the IGFs and both IGF-I-like and IGF-II-like proteins have been detected in conditioned media of these cell lines (Huff et al., 1986). Blockage of the IGF-I receptor inhibits the effect of IGF-I and IGF-II and at least partially inhibits estrogen induced proliferation of human breast cancer cells (Osborne et al., 1989). In breast cancer cells estrogen increases and Tamoxifen inhibits secretion of an IGF-I-like protein (Huff et al., 1986). Although the presence of authentic IGF-I in conditioned medium from breast cancer cells remains controversial, the fact that exogenous IGF-I is a potent growth stimulator of breast cancer cell growth *in vitro* suggests that estrogen-antiestrogen regulation of breast stromal cell production of this growth factor (Yee et al., 1989) and of the circulating levels of IGF-I (Colletti et al., 1989), may contribute to modulation of breast tumour growth *in vivo*. In situ hybridization and immunohistochemical techniques have demonstrated that IGF-I is predominantly expressed in stromal tissue (Yee et al., 1989). In contrast to IGF-I, IGF-II expression by human breast cancer tissue has been consistently demonstrated by several groups and expression is upregulated by estrogen (Osborne et al., 1989; Yee et al., 1988). Furthermore, overexpression of IGF-II in MCF-7 human breast cancer cells was associated with loss of estrogen dependent growth (Cullen et al., 1992). In T61 human breast cancer xenografts, Tamoxifen inhibited both IGF-II expression and growth (Brunner et al., 1993).

In Ishikawa human endometrial cancer cells both estradiol and Tamoxifen enhanced IGF-I mRNA levels and increased IGF-I secretion but had no significant effect on IGF-II expression (Hana and Murphy, 1994b). This induction of IGF-I expression was partially reversed by the pure antiestrogen ICI 182,780, indicating that the Tamoxifen effect in this cell line was likely to be due to its intrinsic estrogenic effects on endometrial tissue.

An additional complexity to the IGF system is the presence of high affinity binding proteins which can complete with the receptor for binding of IGFs. They can both enhance and inhibit the action of IGF-I in various *in vitro* assay systems. So far six binding proteins have been identified and characterized. Of these, IGFBP-1 and IGFBP-3 appear to be regulated by estrogen (Molnar and Murphy, 1994; Hana and Murphy, 1994b). IGFBP-2 and -5 may also be regulated by estrogens under some circumstances (Yee et al., 1991; Sheikh et al., 1993). Furthermore there is now some convincing evidence that regulation of IGFBPs by Tamoxifen may be important in the therapeutic effect of this agent in the treatment of breast cancer. Expression of IGFBP-1 and IGFBP-3 are downregulated by estradiol in ovariectomized rats and in cycling rats, expression is highest in diestrus (Molnar and Murphy, 1994). Tamoxifen has a similar effect on this tissue. In human breast cancer cells, ER negative cell lines tend to secrete IGFBP-1, -3, and -4 white ER positive cell lines secrete IGFBP-2 and -4 but not IGFBP-3 or -1 (Clemmons et al., 1990). IGFBP-3 expression has also been shown to be higher in ER negative breast cancer biopsies than in ER positive biopsies (Shao et al., 1992). Interestingly, recombinant IGFBP-3 has been shown to inhibit proliferation of human breast cancer cells in culture (Oh et al., 1993). Although this may simply involve competition with the IGF-I receptor for IGF-I binding, an IGF-I independent inhibition of cell proliferation has been demonstrated in some cell lines (Cohen et al., 1993).

Serum levels of IGF-I are increased in women with breast cancer compared to age-matched controls (Peyrat et al., 1993). Patients treated with Tamoxifen show a reduction in plasma IGF-I levels (Yee et al., 1989; Pollack et al., 1990; Lien et al., 1992). This effect may be due to the known inhibitory effect of estrogen on hepatic IGF-I expression [21]. If this is the case, it would suggest that the estrogenic effects of Tamoxifen predominate in the human liver, as is the case in the uterus. However the majority of the IGF-I present in plasma is bound to IGFBP-3 and reductions of the plasma IGF-I levels of the magnitude observed following Tamoxifen treatment would necessitate reduction in IGFBP-3 levels.

The effects of Tamoxifen on the transforming growth factor-alpha system

The transforming growth factor-alpha (TGF-alpha) is a 50 amino acid, single chain polypeptide which is structurally very similar to epidermal growth factor and interacts with the EGF receptor. It is synthesized as a large precursor and conversion to the mature 5.6 kDa TGF-alpha involves proteolytic cleavage by an elastase-like protease. Since prepro-TGF-alpha is present on the cell surface it can function in a juxtacrine manner by interacting with the EGF receptors on adjacent cells. TGF-alpha stimulates cellular proliferation of a variety of cells including human breast and endometrial adenocarcinoma cells and in human and rodent endometrium (Derynck, 1988). In the Ishikawa human endometrial cancer cells, TGF-alpha expression is upregulated by estrogen and downregulated by antiestrogens and progestins (Gong et al., 1992). A functional estrogen responsive element has been identified in the 5'-flanking sequences of the human TGF-alpha gene. A 58 bp sequence lying between positions -194 and -241 of the human TGF-alpha gene contains two imperfect palindromes separated by 20 bp and this sequence can confer estrogen inducibility on a CAT reporter gene in transient expresison assays (El-Ashry et al., 1991).

In the Ishikawa cell line, antiserum to the EGF-receptor is able to block cellular proliferation suggesting that TGF-alpha, or some other ligand produced by these cells functions in an autocrine manner in this cell line (Gong et al., 1994). In estrogen replete medium, Tamoxifen causes a dramatic reduction in both TGF-alpha expression by Ishikawa cells and inhibits cellular proliferation (Gong et al., 1992). In estrogen-depleted medium both Tamoxifen and estradiol stimulate cell proliferation but have quite different effects on TGF-alpha expression. Estradiol enhances expression whereas, even under these conditions where growth stimulation is apparent, Tamoxifen reducess TGF-alpha expression. A similar discordinance was observed in Ishikawa cell xenograft growth in nude mice. In Tamoxifen treated mice the tumours were larger and had lower TGF-alpha mRNA levels than in estradiol treated mice (Gong et al., 1994).

Estrogen increased TGF-alpha expression several fold in human breast cancer cell lines (Bates et al., 1988), and Tamoxifen treatment inhibits endogenous expression of TGF-alpha (Bates et al., 1988; Murphy and Totzlaw, 1989). Furthermore, exogenously added TGF-alpha partially reverses the growth inhibitory effects of antiestrogens (Arteaga et al., 1988a). Although such evidence provides support for a mechanistic role of TGF-alpha in the estrogen/antiestrogen proliferative activities, not all data are consistent with this hypothesis. TGF-alpha alone probably does not have an essential role in estrogen induce proliferation of breast cancer cells. However, the data do not eliminate some less essential role of a TGF-alpha autocrine loop in estrogen action nor intracrine mechanisms as has been suggested for platelet-derived growth factor (Keating and Williams, 1988). Overexpression of TGF-alpha in MCF-7 cells via stable transfection experiments, however, does not result in estrogen independence nor Tamoxifen resistance (Clarke et al., 1989), although increased expression of TGF-alpha in human breast cancers *in vivo*, has been correlated with endocrine insensitivity (Nicholson et al., 1994). Such data suggest that TGF-alpha expression in breast cancer cells may contribute to estrogen-antiestrogen growth regulation but is alone unlikely to be a major component of estrogen action in mammary cancer.

EGF is expressed in some breast cancer cell lines and normal mammary epithelium (Murphy et al., 1988b). Antiestrogens have little if any effect on EGF expression in human breast cancer cells and progestins tend to be the major regulator of expression (Murphy et al., 1988b). Of course, the ability of cells to respond to EGF/TGF-alpha ligands irrespective of whether autocrine or paracrine mechanisms are involved, depends on the availability of the EGF-receptor. The EGF-receptor is expressed by both normal and neoplastic breast epithelial cells and can be regulated by several agents including estradiol and Tamoxifen in breast cancer cells (Berthois et al., 1989). Overexpression of either EGF-receptor or other members of this family e.g. HER-2/erb-B2/neu, in hormone dependent breast cancer cell lines is, however, often associated with estrogen independence and Tamoxifen resistance (Valverius et al., 1990; van Agthoven et al., 1992). Furthermore, the expression of the EGF-receptor of HER-2/erb-B2/neu in human breast cancer is inversely related to the expression of the estrogen receptor and elevated levels of either of these receptor-tyrosine kinases are associated with progression and hormone independence in breast cancer (Fitzpatrick et al., 1994; Sainsbury et al., 1987).

The effects of Tamoxifen on the transforming growth factor-β system

The TGF-ßs are a group of homodimeric proteins of approximately 25,000 dalton. TGF-ß$_1$, the most ubiquitious TGF-ß, is expressed in normal human endometrium and endometrial cancer cells and human breast cancer cells. TGF-ß$_1$ is derived from a larger biological inactive precursor molecule by proteolytic digestion. Plasmin is able to activate TGF-ß$_1$ *in vitro* and plasmin or an enzyme with similar specificity may be important in the activation of this growth factor *in vivo*. The TGF-ßs are usually inhibitory to normal epithelial cells and a reduced sensitivity to the inhibitory effects of this agent is associated with an extremely malignant phenotype.

Although there is little evidence of steroid hormone regulation of TGF-ß expression *in vivo*, it is possible to demonstrate estrogen and Tamoxifen regulation is a variety of cell lines including human breast and endometrial adenocarcinoma cells. Estradiol reduced TGF-ß$_1$ expression in some but not all endometrial cancer cell lines (Gong et al., 1991; Gong et al., 1992). In addition, estrogens have been found to decrease the expression of some members of the TGF-ß family in human breast cancer cells (Knabbe et al., 1987; Arteaga et al., 1988b, Arrick et al., 1990) and growth inhibition induced by antiestrogens has in some cases been accompanied by increased expression of TGF-ß. TGF-ß expression was found to be no longer responsive to antiestrogens in an antiestrogen resistant breast cancer cell line (Knabbe et al., 1987) and paradoxically increased expression and overexpression of members of the TGF-ß family have been associated with the development of estrogen independence in some human breast cancer cell lines (Dickson et al., 1987; Daly and Darbre, 1990; Arteaga et al., 1993). However, since some ER positive breast cancer cells respond to antiestrogen but not to exogenous TGF-ß (Arteaga et al., 1988) it would seem that factors other than increased TGF-ß alone are also involved in antiestrogen action.

Interaction of estrogen receptor pathways with growth factor pathways

Although there are reports that antiestrogens are unable to inhibit growth factor-stimulated growth in MCF-7 cells (Koga and Sutherland, 1987; Koga et al., 1989; Cormier and Jordan, 1989), several other studies suggest that antiestrogens can have antigrowth factor activity in the absence of detectable levels of estrogen (Vigon et al., 1987; Wakeling et al., 1989, Freiss et al., 1990). It was originally shown that antiestrogens could partially inhibit the proliferative effects of insulin, IGF-I and EGF on estrogen (Vigon et al., 1987). This activity may be mediated by the antiestrogen-altering expression of the growth factor receptor and/or other mechanisms. Interestingly, a considerable amount of data suggests that estrogen can sensitize breast cancer cells to particular growth factor activity (Stewart et al., 1990; Stewart et al., 1992). Although altered growth factor receptor levels due to estrogen are involved in sensitization in some cases, the mechanism by which this is achieved in other cases is unclear since no measurable effects on the level of expression of receptors for these particular growth factors have been demonstrated. Other data suggest that estrogen/antiestrogen regulation of membrane protein tyrosine phosphatase activity may play a role in the modulation of growth factor pathways (Freiss and Vignon, 1994).

Recently, data have been published which support the idea that some growth factors e.g. EGF, heregulin and IGF-I, via their membrane receptor, can activate the nuclear estrogen independently of estrogen, both *in vitro* and *in vivo* (Ignar-Trowbridge et al., 1992; Ignar-Trowbridge et al., 1993; Aronica and Katzenellenbogen, 1993; Pietras et al., 1995).

This likely occurs via a phosphorylation mechanism and results in growth factor-activating estrogen-dependent specific gene expression. Antiestrogens can inhibit this growth factor ligand-independent ER-mediated activity by binding to and inactivating the ER (Aronica and Katzenellenbogen, 1993). It has been suggested that antiestrogens are primarily anti-mitogenic agents serving to inactivate ER which has been activated in the absence of estrogen via some cross-talk mechanism or alternatively, the ER may simply serve to enhance intracellular concentrations of antiestrogens which may then interfer with polypeptide growth factor signalling via non-ER mediated mechanisms (which amongst others may include interactions with calmodulin or protein kinase C or phospholipase D, Lam, 1984; O'Brian et al., 1985; Brandes and Bogdanovic, 1986; Powers et al., 1991; Reddy et al., 1992; Kiss, 1994). Whether such interactions may involve ER-like molecules detected in cell membranes remains unclear (Watson et al., 1995).

Cross-talk and interactions between internal signalling pathways are another intriguing possibility. As discussed above there is compelling evidence that EGF can mimick estrogen action by activating the estrogen receptor even in the absence of estrogens. Ignar-Trowbridge and colleagues (1992, 1993) showed that antibodies to the EGF receptor or antiestrogen treatment inhibited this activity. Furthermore, the EGF activity was dependent on the TAF-1 region of the ER, while estrogen activation of the ERE-CAT reporter gene in this system was dependent on the TAF-2 region of the ER. Heregulin, via the HER-2/*neu* receptor, can also activate the ER in a ligand-independent fashion in MCF-7 human breast cancer cells (Pietras et al., 1995).

Conclusions and future directions

The data reviewed above indicate that the modulation of growth factor pathways by Tamoxifen may explain, at least in part, its growth modulatory activity. Most of the data are derived from *in vitro* cell culture models and do not take into account potential effects of Tamoxifen on hormonal systems. Recent evidence suggests that these effects may be important to Tamoxifen efficacy in the treatment of human breast cancer. Further insights into Tamoxifen modulation of growth factor expression may lead to the development of alternative novel treatment strategies in malignant and non-malignant breast and uterine disease. Furthermore, the altered expression of one or several of these factors may be one mechanism by which breast cancer cells develop resistance to Tamoxifen and alternatively may be involved in the development of endometrial neoplasia in Tamoxifen treated women.

REFERENCES

Aronica SM, Katzenellenbogen BS (1993): Stimulation of estrogen receptor-mediated transcription and alteration in the phosphorylation state of the rate uterine estrogen recetor by estrogen, cyclic adenosine monophosphate and insulin-like growth factors. *J Mol Endocrinol* 7:743-752

Arrick BA, Korc M, Derynck R (1990): Differential regulation of the expression of three transforming growth factor ß species in human breast cancer cell lines by estradiol. *Cancer Res* 50:229-303

Arteaga CL, Carty-Dugger T, Moses HL, Hurd SD, Pietenpol JA (1993): Transforming growth factor ß1 can induce estrogen-independent tumorigenicity of human breast cancer cells in athymic mice. *Cell Growth Diff* 4:193-201

Arteaga CL, Coronado E, Osborne CK (1988a): Blockade of the epidermal growth factor receptor inhibits transforming growth factor-alpha induced but not estrogen-induced growth of hormone-dependent human breast cancer. *J Mol Endocrinol* 2:1064-1069

Arteaga CL, Tandon AK, Von Hoff, DD, Osborne CK (1988b): Transforming growth factor ß: potential autocrine growth inhibitor of estrogen receptor-negative human breast cancer cells. *Cancer Res* 48:3898-3904

Bates SE, Davidson NE, Valverius EM, Freter CE, Dickson RB, Tam JP, Kudlow JE, Lippman ME, Salomon DS (1988): Expression of transforming growth factor alpha and its messenger ribonucleic acid in human breast cancer: its regulation by estrogen and its possible functional significance. *J Mol Endocrinol* 2:543-555

Berry M, Nunez A-M, Chambon P (1989): Estrogen-responsive element of the human pS2 gene is an imperfect palindromic sequence. *Proc Natl Acad Sci USA* 86:1218-1222

Berthois Y, Dong XF, Martin PM (1989): Regulation of epidermal growth factor receptor by estrogen and antiestrogen in the human breast cancer cell line MCF-7. *Biochem Biophys Res Commun* 159:126-131

Brandes LJ, Bogdanovic RP (1986): New evidence that the antiestrogen binding site may be a novel growth promoting histamine receptor which mediates the antiestrogenic and antiproliferative effects of tamoxifen. *Biochem Biophys Res Commun* 134:601-608

Brunner N, Yee D, Kern FG, Spang-Thomsen M, Lippman ME, Cullen KJ (1993): Effect of endocrine therapy on growth of T61 human breast cancer xenografts is directly correlated to a specific down regulation of insulin-like growth factor II (IGF-II). *Eur J Cancer* 29:562-569

Clarke R, Brunner N, Katz D, Glanz P, Dickson RB, Lippman ME, Kern FG
    (1989): The effects of a constitutive expression of transforming growth
    factor-alpha on the growth of MCF-7 human breast cancer cells *in vitro*
    and *in vivo*. *J Mol Endocrinol* 3:372-380
Clemmons DR, Camacho-Hubner C, Coronado E, Osborne CK (1990): Insulin-
    like growth factor binding protein secretion by breast carcinoma cell lines:
    correlation with estrogen receptor status. *Endocrinol* 127:2697-2686
Cohen P, Lamson G, Ikajima T, Rosenfeld RG (1993): Transfection of the
    human insulin-like growth factor-3 gene into Balb/c fibroblasts inhibits
    cellular growth. *J Mol Endocrinol* 7:380-386
Colletti RB, Roberts JD, Devlin JT, Copeland KC (1989): Effect of tamoxifen
    on plasma insulin-like growth factor-1 in patients with breast cancer.
    Cancer Res 49:1881-1884
Cormier EM, Jordan VC (1989): Contrasting ability of antiestrogens to inhibit
    MCF-7 growth stimulated by estradiol or epidermal growth factor. *Eur J
    Cancer Clin Oncol* 25:57-63
Cullen KJ, Lippman ME, Chow D, Hill S, Rosen N, Zwiebel JA (1992):
    Insulin-like growth factor-II overexpression in MCF-7 cells induces
    phenotypic changes associated with malignant progression. *J Mol
    Endocrinol* 6:91-199
Daly RJ, Darbre (1990): Cellular and molecular events in loss of estrogen
    sensitivity in ZR-75-1 and T-47D human breast cancer cells. *Cancer Res*
    50:5868-5875
DiAugustine RP, Petrusz P, Bell GI, Brown CF, Korach KS, McLachlan JA,
    Tebg CT (1988): Influence of estrogens on mouse uterine epidermal
    growth factor precursor protein and messenger ribonucleic acid.
    Endocrinol 122:2355-2363
Dickson RB, Kasid A, Huff KK, Bates SE, Knabbe C, Bronzert D, Gelman EP,
    Lippman ME (1987): Activation of growth factor secretion in tumorigenic
    states of breast cancer induced by 17b-estradiol or v-Ha-ras oncogene.
    Proc Natl Acad Sci USA 84:837-841
Derynck R (1988): Transforming growth factor-alpha. *Cell* 54:593-597
El-Ashry D, Danielson M, Lippman ME, Kern FG (1991): Human transforming
    growth factor-alpha contains an estrogen responsive element comprising
    of two imperfect palindromes. Proc 73rd Ann Meeting of the Endocrine
    Society, Abstract 950
Fitzpatrick SL, Brightwell J, Wittliff JL, Barrows GH, Schultz GS (1984):
    Epidermal growth factor binding by breast tumor biopsies and relationship
    to estrogen receptor and progestin receptor levels. *Cancer Res* 44:3448-
    3453
Freiss G, Prebois C, Rochefort H, Vignon F (1990): Anti-steroidal and anti-
    growth factor activities of antiestrogens. *J Steroid Biochem Molec Biol*
    37:777-781

Freiss G, Vignon F (1994): Antiestrogens increase protein tyrosine phosphatase activity in human breast cancer cells. *J Mol Endocrinol* 8:1389-1396

Gong Y, Anzai Y, Murphy LC, Ballejo G, Holinka CF, Gurpride E, Murphy LJ (1991):   Transforming growth factor gene expression in human endometrial adenocarcinoma cells: Regulation by progestins. *Cancer Res* 51:5476-5481

Gong Y, Ballejo G, Murphy LC (1992): Differential effects of estrogen and antiestrogen on transforming growth factor gene expression in endometrial adenocarcinoma cells. *Cancer Res* 52:1704-1710

Gong Y, Murphy LC, Murphy LJ (1994): Hormonal regulation of proliferation and transforming growth factors gene expression in human endometrial adenocarcinoma xenograft. *J Steroid Biochem Mol Biol* 50:13-19

Hana V, Murphy LJ (1994a): Interdependence of epidermal growth factor and insulin like growth factor-I expression in mouse uterus. *Endocrinol* 135:107-122

Hana V, Murphy LJ (1994b): Expression of insulin like growth factors and their binding proteins in the estrogen responsive Ishikawa human endometrial cancer cell line. *Endocrinol* 135:2511-2526

Holinka CF, Hata H, Kuramoto H, Gurpide E (1986): Effects of steroid hormones and antisteroids on alkaline phosphatase activity in human endometrial cancer cells (Ishikawa line). *Cancer Res* 46:2771-2774

Huff KK, Kaufman D, Gabbay KH, Spencer EM, Lippman ME, Dickson RB (1986): Secretion of an insulin-like growth factor-1-related protein in human breast cancer cells. *Cancer Res* 46:4613-4619

Ignar-Trowbridge DM, Nelson KG, Bidwell MC, Curtis SW, Washburn TF, McLachlan JA, Korach KS (1992): Coupling of dual signalling pathways: epidermal growth factor action involves the estrogen receptor. *Proc Natl Acad Sci USA* 89:4658-4662

Ignar-Trowbridge D, Teng C, Ross K. Parker M, Korach K, McLachlan J (1993):   Peptide growth factors elicit estrogen receptor dependent transcription of ERE. *J Mol Endocrinol* 7:992-993

Keating MT, Williams LT, (1988): Autocrine stimulation of intracellular PDGF receptors in V-sis transformed cells. *Science* 239:914-916

Kiss Z (1994): Tamoxifen stimulates phospholipase D activity by an estrogen independent mechanism. *FEBS Lett* 28:173-177

Knabbe C, Lippma ME, Wakefield LM, Flanders KC, Kasid A, Derynck R, Dickson RB (1987): Evidence that transforming growth factor-ß is a hormonally regulated negative growth factor in human breast cancer cells. *Cell* 48:417-428

Koga M, Musgrove EA, Sutherland RL (1989): Modulation of the growth inhibitory effects of progestins and antiestrogens on human breast cancer cells by epidermal growth factor and insulin. *Cancer Res* 49:112-116

Koga M, Sutherland RL (1987): Epidermal growth factor partially reverses the inhibitory effects of antiestrogens on T-47D human breast cancer cell growth. *Biochem Biophys Res Commun* 146:739-745

Lam H-Y P (1984): Tamoxifen is a calmodulin antagonist in the activation of a cAMP phosphodiesterase. *Biochem Biophys Res Commun* 118:27-32

Lien EA, Johannessen DC, Aakvaag A, Lonning PE (1992): Influence of tamoxifen, aminoglutethimide and goserelin on human plasma IGF-I levels in breast cancer patients. *J Steroid Biochem Mol Biol* 41:541-543

Lippman ME, Dickson RB (1989): Mechanisms of growth control in normal and malignant breast epithelium. *Rec Prog Horm Res* 45:383-440

Malet C, Gompel A, Spritzer P, Bricout N, Yaneva H, Mowszowicz I, Kuttenn F, Mauvais-Jarvis P (1988): Tamoxifen and hydroxytamoxifen isomers versus estradiol effects on normal human breast cells in culture. *Cancer Res* 48:7193-7199

Meyer M-E, Gronemeyer H, Turcotte B, Bocquel MT, Tasset D, Chambon P (1989): Steroid hormone receptors competes for factors that mediate their enhancer function. *Cell* 57:433-439

Molnar P, Murphy LJ (1994): Effects of oestrogen on rat uterine expression of insulin-like growth factor binding proteins. *J Mol Endocrinol* 13:59-67

Murphy LC, Dotzlaw H (1989): Regulation of transforming growth factor alpha and transforming growth factor beta mRNA abundance in T-47D human breast cancer cells. *J Mol Endocrinol* 3:611-617

Murphy LJ, Friesen HG (1988): Differential effects of estrogen and growth hormone on uterine and hepatic insulin-like growth factor-I gene expression in the ovariectomized, hypophysectomized rat. *Endocrinol* 122:325-332

Murphy LJ, Ghahary A (1990): Uterine insulin-like growth factor-I: Regulation of expression and its role in estrogen-induced uterine proliferation. *Endocr Rev* 11:443-453

Murphy LJ, Murphy LC, Friesen HG (1988a): Estrogen induces insulin-like growth factor-I expression in the rat uterus. *J Mol Endocrinol* 1:445-450

Murphy LC, Murphy LJ, Dubik D, Bell GI, Shiu (1988a): Epidermal growth factor gene expression in human breast cancer cells: regulation of expression by progestins. *Cancer Res* 48:4555-4560

Nelson KG, Takahashi T, Bossert NL, Walmer DK, McLachlan JA (1990): Epidermal growth factor replaces estrogen in the stimulation of female genital-tract growth and differentiation. *Proc Natl Acad Sci USA* 88:21-25

Nicholson RI, McClelland RA, Gee JM, Manning DL, Cannon P, Robertson JF, Ellis IO, Blamey RW (1994): Transforming growth factor-alpha and endocrine sensitivity in breast cancer. *Cancer Res* 54:1684-1689

O'Brian CA, Liskamp RM, Solomon DH, Weinstein IB (1985): Inhibition of protein kinase C by tamoxifen. *Cancer Res* 45:2462-2465

Oh Y, Muller HL, Lamson G, Rosenfeld RG (1993): Insulin-like growth factor (IGF)-indepdent action of IGF-binding protein-3 in Hs578T human breast cancer cells. *J Biol Chem* 268:14964-14971

Osborne CK, Coronado E, Allred DC, Wiebe VJ, DeGregorio MW (1991): Acquired tamoxifen resistance: correlation with reduced breast tumor levels of tamoxifen and isomerization of trans-4-hydroxytamixfen. *J Natl Cancer Inst* 83:1447-1482

Osborne CK, Coronado EB, Kitten LJ, Arteaga CL, Fuqua SAW, Ramasharma K, Marshall M, Li CH (1989): Insulin-lie growth factor II (IGF-II): a potential autocrine/paracrine growth factor for human breast cancer acting via the IGF-I receptor. *J Mol Endocrinol* 3:1701-1709

Peyrate JP, Bonneterre J, Hecquet B, Vennin P, Louchez MM, Fournier C, Lefebvre J, Demaille A (1993): Plasma insulin-like growth factor-1 (IGF-1) concentrations in human breast cancer. *Eur J Cancer* 29:492-497

Pietras R, Arboleda J, Reese D, Wongvipat N, Pegram M, Ramos L, Gorman C, Parker M, Sliwkowski M, Slamon D (1995): HER-2 tyrosine kinase pathway targets estrogen receptor and promotes independent growth in human breast cancer cells. *Oncogene* 10:2435-2446

Pollack M, Costantino J, Polychronakos C, Blauer SA, Guyda H, Redmond C, Fisher B, Margolese R (1990): Effects of tamoxifen on serum insulin-like growth factor I levels in stage I breast cancer patients. *J Natl Cancer Inst* 82:1693-1697

Powers RF, Mani SK, Codina J, Conneely OM, O'Malley BW (1991): Dopaminergic and ligand-independent activation of steroid hormone receptors. *Science* 254:1636-1641

Reddy KB, Mangold GL, Tandon AK, Yoneda T, Mundy GR, Zilberstein A, Osborne CK (1992): Inhibition of breast cancer cell growth *in vitro* by a tyrosine kinase inhibitor. *Cancer Res* 52:3636-3641

Sainsbury JRC, Needham GK, Malcolm A, Farndon JR, Harris AL (1987): Epidermal growth factor receptor status as a predictor of early recurrence of and death from breast cancer. *Lancet* i:1398-1399

Schule R, Muller M, Kaltschmidt C, Renkawitz R (1988): Many transcription factors interact synergistically with steroid receptors. *Science* 242:1418-1422

Shao ZM, Sheikh MS, Ordonez JV, Feng P, Kute T, Chen JC, Aisner S, Schnaper L, LeRoith D, Roberts CT, Fontana J (1993): IGFBP-3 gene expression and estrogen receptor status in human breast carcinoma. *Cancer Res* 52:5100-5103

Sheikh MS, Shao ZM, Hussain A, Chen JC, Roberts CT, LeRoith D, Fontana JA (1993): Retinoic acid and estrogen modulation of expression of insulin-like growth factor binding protein-4 gene expression and the estrogen receptor status of human breast cancer cells. *Biochem Biophys Res Comm* 193:1232-1238

Stewart AJ, Johnson MD, May FEB, Westley BR (1990): Role of insulin-like growth factors and the type-I insulin-like growth factor receptor in the estrogen-stimulated proliferation of human breast cancer. *J Biol Chem* 265:21172-21178

Stewart AJ, Westley BR, May FEB (1992): Modulation of the proliferative response of breast cancer cells to growth factors by oestrogen. *Br J Cancer* 66:640-648

Valverius EM, Velu T, Shankar V, Ciardiello F, Kim N, Salomon DS (1990): Overexpression of the epidermal growth factor receptor in human breast cancer cells fails to induce an estrogen-independent phenotype. *Int J Cancer* 46:712-718

van Agthoven T, van Agthoven TL, Protengen H, Foekens JA, Dorssers LC (1992): Ectopic expression of epidermal growth factor receptors induces hormone independence in ZR-75-1 human breast cancer cells. *Cancer Res* 52:5082-5088

van der Burg B, van Selm-Miltenburg A, deLaat S, van Zoelen EJ (1989): Direct effects of estrogen on c-fos and c-myc protooncogene expression and cellular proliferation in human breast cancer cells. *J Mol Cell Endocrinol* 64:223-228

Vignon F, Bouton MM, Rochefort H, (1987): Antiestrogens inhibit mitogenic effect of growth factors on breast cancer cells in the total absence of estrogens. *Biochem Biophys Res Commun* 146:1502-1508

Wakeling A, Newboult E, Peters SW (1989): Effects of antiestrogens on the proliferation of MCF-7 human breast cancer cells. *J Mol Endocrinol* 2:225-234

Watson CS, Pappas TC, Gametchu B (1995): Membrane estrogen receptors-molecular size and mechanistic interaction with thyrotropin releasing hormone. Proc. 77th Annual Meeting Endocrine Society, Abstract PI-420, p217

Webb P, Lopez GN, Uht RM, Kushner PJ (1995): Tamoxifen activation of the estrogen receptor/AP-1 pathway: potential origin for the cell-specific estrogen-like effects of antiestrogens. *J Mol Endocrinol* 9:443-456

Weisz A, Bresciani F (188): Estrogen induces expression of c-fos and c-mys protoncogenes in rat uterus. *J Mol Endocrinol* 9:443-446

Wiltschke C, Fuqua SAW (1995): Clinical relevance of estrogen receptor variants in breast cancer. *Trends Endocrinol Metab* 6:77-82

Yee D, Cullen KJ, Paik S, Perdue JF, Hampton B, Schwartz A, Lippman ME, Rosen N (1988): Insulin-like growth factor II mRNA expression in human breast cancer. *Cancer Res* 48:6691-6696

Yee D, Favoni RE, Lippman ME, Powell DR (1991): The pattern of insulin-like growth factor binding protein (IGFBP) expression in breast cancer cells suggest a strategy for their use as IGF inhibitors. *Breast Cancer Res Treat* 19:211-214

Yee D, Paik S, Lebovic G, Marcus R, Favoni R, Cullen K, Lippman ME, Rosen
    N (1989): Analysis of IGF-I gene expression in malignancy-evidence for
    a paracrine role in human breast cancer. *J Mol Endocrinol* 3:509-517

13. TAMOXIFEN AND DRUG-METABOLIZING ENZYMES

Markku Ahotupa

"Drug-metabolizing enzymes" is a general term for a heterogenous group of enzymes catalyzing the biotransformation of many endogenous as well as innumerable exogenous (such as drugs, chemical carcinogens, environmental pollutants) lipophilic compounds into more water-soluble derivatives. These enzyme systems are present to some degree virtually in all tissues of the body; yet, quantitatively the liver is by far the most important tissue with respect to biotransformation.

The biotransformation reactions have been traditionally divided into two phases. In phase I (catalyzed by cytochrome P450 -mediated monooxygenases) a polar group is introduced into the molecule. In phase II an endogenous molecule (most commonly glucuronic acid, sulfate, or glutathione) is conjugated with the polar group in the parent compound. Without the biotransformation reactions, highly lipid-soluble foreign compounds would remain indefinitely in the body. Therefore, biotransformation of xenobiotics is regarded as detoxification (Williams, 1959). Later it has become evident that, due to formation of reactive chemical species, biotransformation of a foreign compound may in some cases increase its toxicity (Pelkonen and Nebert, 1982).

Many of the phase I and phase II drug-metabolizing enzymes are today known to exist in multiple forms with slightly differing molecular structures, catalytic specificities, and regulation. Individual enzyme families and subfamilies, and their implications in the metabolism and toxicity of drugs and other xenobiotics is at present under active research. Characteristic for the drug-metabolizing enzymes is their inducibility by a great variety of chemicals: more than 300 chemicals have been described that induce their own metabolism or the metabolism of structurally related compounds (Conney, 1967). As a consequence of induction of drug-metabolizing enzymes, the action of drugs and other xenobiotics, as well as the metabolism and action of endogenous substrates (e.g. steroid hormones, lipid-soluble vitamins, prostaglandins), may be altered (Conney, 1982).

In all animal species investigated, Tamoxifen is extensively metabolized after oral administration. Early studies by Fromson and coworkers revealed that hydroxylation is a significant metabolic pathway for Tamoxifen, and most of Tamoxifen is excreted as glucuronides and other conjugates (Fromson et al., 1973). N-Desmethyltamoxifen and 4-hydroxytamoxifen are quantitatively the most significant metabolites of Tamoxifen, but several other metabolites have been identified (Fig. 1) (Jordan, 1984; Poon et al., 1993).

With increased knowledge on polymorphism of drug-metabolizing enzymes, more detailed information concerning interactions between Tamoxifen and drug-metabolizing enzymes has become available. The aim of this review is to present a synthesis of recent results on the role of individual drug-metabolizing enzymes in the biotransformation of Tamoxifen and the effects of Tamoxifen on expression of various drug-metabolizing enzymes. Based on this data, possible implications of interactions between Tamoxifen and drug-metabolizing enzymes will be discussed.

Drug-metabolizing enzymes

The microsomal, multisubstrate mixed function monooxygenase system catalyzes a number of oxidative as well as reductive phase I biotransformation reactions (e.g. Wislocki et al., 1980). These enzyme systems consist of three essential components: cytochrome P450 (CYP), NADPH-cytochrome P450 reductase, and phospholipid. The hemoprotein CYP, which serves as the terminal oxidase and substrate binding site of the monooxygenase system, primarily determines the substrate specificity of the enzyme (Lu and Lewin, 1974). In mammals, the CYPs form a superfamily of enzymes which can be generally divided into two classes: six families involved in biosynthesis of steroids and bile acids; four families mainly responsible for metabolism of foreign compounds (Table 1). Typically, many of the CYPs, particularly those in the CYP2 family, exhibit a large degree of inter- and intra-species variation with respect to

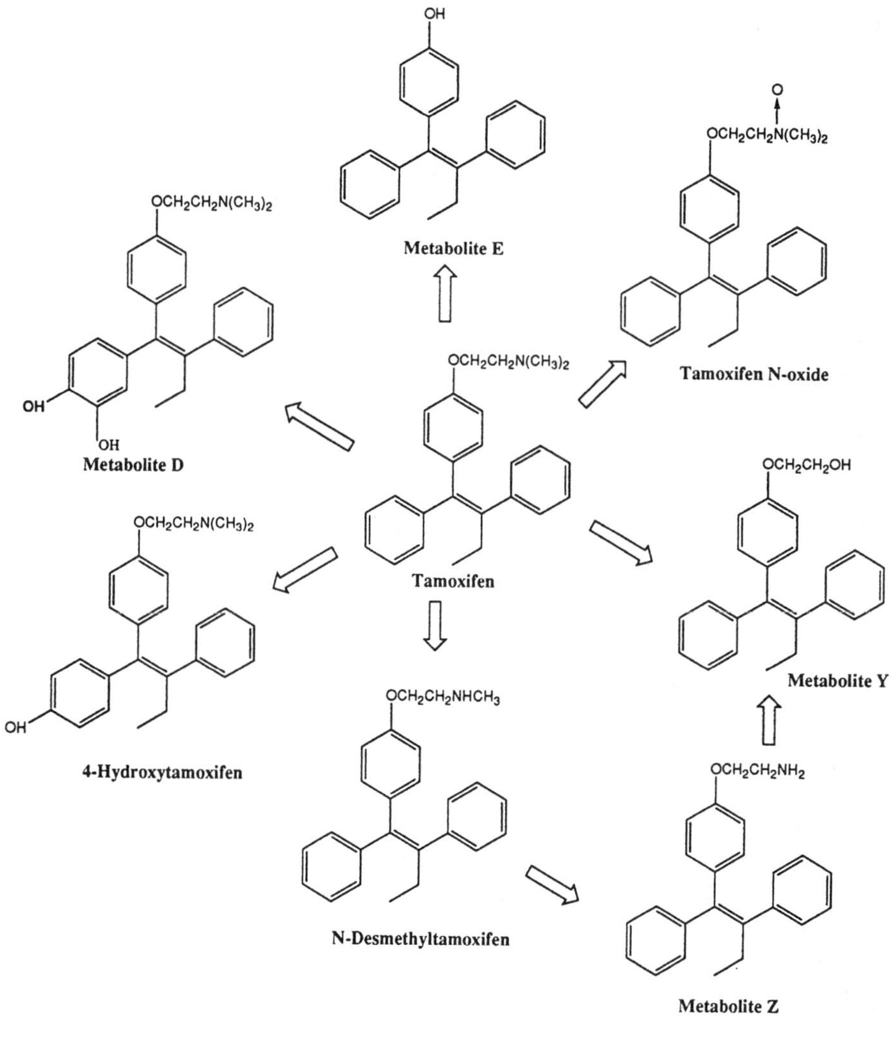

Figure 1. Metabolism of Tamoxifen

regulation and catalytic activities. Recent development in research on CYP enzymes in extensively reviewed (e.g. Gonzales, 1989; Gonzales 1992; Pelkonen and Breimer, 1994).

Table 1. Mammalian CYP families

CYP Family	No. of subfamilies	Function
CYP1	1	Xenobiotic metabolism
CYP2	8	Xenobiotic and steroid metabolism
CYP3	2	Xenobiotic and steroid metabolism
CYP4	2	Fatty acid hydroxylations
CYP5	1	Thromboxane synthesis
CYP7	1	Cholesterol 7α-hydroxylase
CYP11	2	Steroid 11β-hydroxylase
CYP17	1	Steroid 17α-hydroxylase
CYP19	1	Steroid aromatase
CYP21	1	Steroid 21-hydroxylase
CYP27	1	Cholesterol 27-hydroxylase

Adapted from Gonzales (1992), Raunio et al., 1995.

CYP- mediated metabolism may result in formation of epoxides which are highly reactive molecules capable of forming adducts e.g. with proteins and DNA. Epoxides may be further metabolized in enzymatic or nonenzymatic reactions with water or glutathione. Epoxide hydrolase catalyzes the reaction of epoxides with water. There seems to exist at least two microsomal and one cytosolic epoxide hydrolases, representing different forms of the enzyme (Levin et al., 1983).

The most significant phase II enzymes UDP-glucuronosyltransferase and glutathione S-transferase catalyze conjugation of a variety of endogenous and exogenous compounds with glucuronic acid and glutathione, respectively (Aitio, 1978). The UDP-glucuronosyltransferases are membrane proteins encoded by multiple genes of at least two gene families; at present, more than 30 UDP-glucuronosyltransferase isoforms have been identified (Clarke and Burchell, 1994). In case of the mammalian glutathione S-transferases, there are four major cytosolic families and at least one microsomal form of the enzyme (e.g. Beckett and Hayes, 1993).

Drug-metabolizing enzymes in the metabolism of Tamoxifen

Most of the data on the role of various drug-metabolizing enzymes in the metabolism of Tamoxifen comes from *in vitro* studies with microsomal preparations of either rat or human liver. Competing substrates or antibodies to individual enzymes have been used as tools, as well as reconstituted enzyme systems. Even though phase II reactions, too, are important metabolic pathways for Tamoxifen (Fromson et al., 1973; Poon et al., 1993), detailed studies on enzymes involved are lacking. The metabolism of Tamoxifen by CYP enzymes from either rat or human liver proceeds *in vitro* qualitatively by large in similar ways with respect to production of metabolites by the various isoenzymes. Yet, rat liver microsomes seem to be more active in metabolizing Tamoxifen *in vitro* than microsomes from human liver (Mani et al., 1993a; Lim et al., 1994). Apart from the liver, little is known about enzymes involved in biotransformation of Tamoxifen in extrahepatic tissues. (For a synopsis on drug-metabolizing enzymes implicated in the metabolism/toxicity of Tamoxifen, see Table 2).

Recent studies strongly suggest that in rat and human liver the CYP3A subfamily plays a major role in the main metabolic pathway of Tamoxifen, the formation of the N-desmethyl derivative. The metabolic rates for Tamoxifen N-demethylation by human liver microsomes correlated strongly with CYP3A content and testosterone 6β-hydroxylase and erythromycin N-demethylase activities, both known to be associated with CYP3A (Jacolot et al., 1991). Moreover, Tamoxifen N-demethylation was inhibited *in vitro* by alternate substrates for CYP3A, such as erythromycin, cyclosporin, nifedipine, and diltiazem (Jacolot et al., 1991). Treatment of rats with CYP inducers phenobarbital (PB), pregnenolone-16α-carbonitrile (PCN) and methylcholanthrene (MC) enhanced N-demethylation of Tamoxifen, suggesting potential involvement of multiple CYPs (Mani et al., 1993a). Antibodies to CYP3A1 inhibited N-demethylation in PB- and PCN-microsomes, while antibodies against CYP2B1/B2 did not (Mani et al., 1993a). Thus, enhanced Tamoxifen N-demethylation by microsomes from PB- or PCN-treated rats was likely due to induction of the CYP3A subfamily.

Inhibition studies with alternate substrates, as well as studies with reconstituted enzyme systems, indicated that enhanced Tamoxifen N-demethylation after MC treatment was due to increased CYP1A1/1A2 levels. Yet, antibodies against CYP1A1 did not inhibit N-demethylation of Tamoxifen in MC microsomes, and antibodies against CYP1A1/1A2 brought about only partial inhibition (Mani et al., 1993a). Thus, it seems that in MC microsomes CYP1A1 does not catalyze the reaction. In addition to CYP3A and CYP1A, also CYP2C11 and/or CYP 2C6 may catalyze Tamoxifen N-demethylation, as indicated by inhibition of the reaction by the monoclonal antibody anti-CYP2C11/2C6 (Mani et al., 1993a).

The other important pathway of Tamoxifen's metabolism, 4-hydroxylation, was not affected by common CYP inducers, indicating that this reaction is preferentially catalyzed in rat liver by constitutive CYPs (Mani et al., 1993a). Antibodies against CYP2B1/B2, 2C11/2C6, 2E1 and 3A1 failed to inhibit Tamoxifen 4-hydroxylation, and reconstituted CYP1A1 and CYP2B1 activities did not catalyze the reaction (Mani et al., 1993a). Tamoxifen hydroxylation was inhibited by estradiol in rat, but not in human liver microsomes, suggesting the contribution by CYP1A2 (Mani et al., 1993a). In avian liver, Tamoxifen 4-hydroxylation induced by 2,3,7,8-tetrachloro-p-dioxin(TCDD) and β-naphthoflavone is catalyzed by CYP "TCDD$_{AA}$" which is, if not identical, very closely related to CYP1A2 (Kupfer et al., 1994). In PB-

Table 2. Hepatic drug-metabolizing enzymes implicated formation of the main metabolites and toxic effects of Tamoxifen

Metabolite	Enzymes responsible	Reference
N-Desmethyltamoxifen	Human CYP3A	Jacolot et al., 1991
	"	Mani et al., 1993a
	Rat CYP1A, 2C, 3A	Mani et al., 1993a
4-Hydroxytamoxifen	Human and rat constitutive CYPs	Mani et al., 1993a
	Rat CYP 1A?	Mani et al., 1993a
	Avian CYP TCDD$_{AA}$	Kupfer et al., 1994
	Avian CYP2H1/H2	Kupfer et al., 1994
Tamoxifen N-oxide	Human and mouse FMO	Mani et al., 1993b

Toxic effect	Enzymes responsible	Reference
Protein binding	Human CYP2B6, 3A4	White et al., 1995
	Rat CYP3A1	Mani et al., 1994
	Rat FMO	Mani and Kupfer, 1991
	Peroxidases	Davies et al., 1995
Micronucleus formation	Human CYP2E1, 3A4 and 2D6	Styles et al., 1994

treated avian livers, CYP2H1/H2 had the highest, Tamoxifen 4-hydroxylase activity (Kupfer et al., 1994).

While antibodies to NADPH-cytochrome P450 reductase inhibited N-demethylation and 4-hydroxylation of Tamoxifen, the N-oxidation reaction was not affected. Purified mouse liver microsomal flavin-containing monooxygenase (FMO), on the other hand, converted Tamoxifen into the N-oxide and inhibitors of FMO inhibited Tamoxifen N-oxide formation by human liver microsomes, providing evidence for involvement of FMO. Enzymes responsible for the formation of other metabolites of Tamoxifen, including the recently identified epoxide metabolites (3,4-epoxytamoxifen, 3',4'-epoxytamoxifen and their hydrolysed derivatives; Lim et al., 1994) have not been identified.

Toremifene, another triphenylethylene anticancer drug, has a chemical structure which closely resembles that of Tamoxifen: the only difference is a chlorine atom substitution for a hydrogen atom on the ethylene alkyl side chain of Tamoxifen. The major metabolites of Toremifene are structurally similar to those of Tamoxifen (Berthou and Dreano, 1993) and, like in case of Tamoxifen, CYP3A plays a key role in catalyzing main metabolic pathways (Berthou et al., 1994).

In addition to the phase I biotransformation, CYP enzymes are involved in the interconversion of *trans*- and *cis*-4-hydroxytamoxifen (Williams et al., 1994). The hormonal effects of *trans* and *cis* forms of Tamoxifen are distinctly different (Wolf et al., 1993) and, hence, the CYP catalyzed isomerization may affect the therapeutic potency of Tamoxifen.

Drug-metabolizing enzymes and toxicity of Tamoxifen

Tamoxifen is reported to have a variety of toxic effects ranging from covalent binding to hepatic microsomes and DNA (Mani and Kupfer, 1991; Han and Liehr, 1992; White et al., 1992; Mani et al., 1994; Montandon and Williams, 1994; Potter et al., 1994; Randerath et al., 1994; Carthew et al., 1995; Davies et al., 1995; Hemminki et al., 1995; Pathak et al., 1995; White et al., 1995) to genotoxic effects in different test systems (Metzler and Schiffmann, 1991; Han and Liehr, 1992; White et al., 1992). Tamoxifen has also turned out to be a potent hepatocarcinogen in the rat, and there is evidence to suggest that Tamoxifen may produce carcinoma of the endometrium in humans (see review by Sasco, this book).

Studies by Mani and Kupfer (1991) showed that the *in vitro* binding of Tamoxifen to proteins in rat and human liver microsomes is CYP-dependent: the reaction required NADPH and oxygen, was inhibited by CO, CYP inhibitors and antibodies to NADPH-cytochrome P450 reductase. In comparison between various species, microsomal proteins of mouse liver were much more active than those of the rat or human liver in binding Tamoxifen (White et al., 1995).

The binding of Tamoxifen to microsomal proteins is markedly increased by PB treatment suggesting the involvement of inducible CYPs (Mani and Kupfer, 1991). In addition to PB, also PCN-treated rats showed enhanced binding of Tamoxifen to liver microsomes; MC-treatment, on the contrary, had no effect (Mani et al., 1994). In human liver microsomes, the binding of Tamoxifen correlated positively with CYP3A4 and CYP2B6 content (White et al., 1995). In PB- and PCN-induced rat liver microsomes, Tamoxifen binding was inhibited by alternate substrates of CYP3A. Moreover, antibodies against rat CYP3A1 inhibited effectively the binding of Tamoxifen in induced microsomes, whereas antibodies to CYP2B1/2B2 did not (Mani et al., 1994). Taken together, these results indicate involvement of CYP3A in binding of Tamoxifen to microsomal proteins in rat and human liver. In addition, CYP 2B6 may contribute to protein binding of Tamoxifen in human liver.

Incubations performed at different temperatures and pH, as well as studies with alternate substrates, revealed that in addition to CYP enzymes FMO may also be implicated in reactions leading to covalent binding of Tamoxifen to microsomal protein (Mani and Kupfer, 1991). Moreover, horseradish peroxidase and to a lesser extent lactoperoxidase and prostaglandin synthase were shown to catalyze binding of Tamoxifen to bovine serum albumin *in vitro* (Davies et al., 1995).

Tamoxifen-induced DNA damage has been demonstrated by use of the ^{32}P-postlabelling technique in rodent tissues *in vivo* (Han and Liehr, 1992; White et al., 1992; Montandon and Williams, 1994; Randerath et al., 1994; Carthew et al., 1995; Hemminki et al., 1995; Parthek et al., 1995), in incubations of pure DNA with Tamoxifen and activating systems *in vitro* (Davies et al., 1995; Hemminki et al., 1995; Parthak et al., 1995), and also in cultured human lymphocytes (Hemminki et al., 1995). In experimental animals the nature of DNA adducts formed seems to depend on the route of administration of Tamoxifen (Randerath et al., 1994). Contrary to what is seen in case of the protein binding, DNA adduct formation after Tamoxifen dosing is more abundant in rat than in mouse liver (White et al., 1992; Randerath et al., 1994). In a recent study with a small number of subjects Tamoxifen-induced DNA-adducts were not detected in liver obtained from women treated with the drug (Martin et al., 1995). In rat liver the amount of DNA adducts increases cumulatively with time during long-term Tamoxifen administration, and various rat strains differ from each other with respect to accumulation of hepatic DNA adducts (Carthew et al., 1995). Species and strain differences in formation of Tamoxifen-induced DNA adducts are in accordance with differential susceptibilities to Tamoxifen-inducible liver tumors (Tucker et al., 1984; Carthew et al., 1995). In accordance, the structurally related triphenylethylene derivative Toremifene, which unlike Tamoxifen is not hepatocarcinogenic to rats (Hard et al., 1993; Hirsimäki et al., 1993; Williams et al., 1993) is far less active than Tamoxifen in producing DNA damage in various test systems (White et al., 1992; Hard et al., 1993; Montandon and Williams, 1994; Hemminki et al., 1995).

It has been postulated that Tamoxifen-induced formation of DNA adducts is due to generation of electrophilic alkylating agents from Tamoxifen via α-hydroxylation in conjunction with 4-hydroxylation or secondary metabolic conjugation (Potter et al., 1994). The role of CYP-mediated metabolism in DNA adduct formation has not been confirmed, not to mention the involvement of individual CYP isoforms. DNA adducts are formed during incubation of pure DNA with Tamoxifen, rat liver microsomes and NADPH, suggesting possible involvement of CYP-dependent catalysis (Pathak and Bodell, 1994; Pathak et al., 1995). Somewhat more efficient adduct formation is seen when cumene hydroperoxide is used instead of NADPH as the cofactor for microsomal activation of Tamoxifen (Pathak et al., 1995). Horseradish peroxidase-catalyzed activation of 4-OH-Tamoxifen was also shown to lead to formation of adducted DNA (Pathak et al., 1995).

The contribution of individual CYP isoforms to genotoxicity of Tamoxifen was investigated in more detail in a study where clastogenic effects were measured by formation of micronuclei in human lymphoblastoid cell lines, each expressing increased enzyme activity associated with a specific CYP. CYP Activities which most actively catalyzed reactions leading to micronucleus formation were in the order CYP2E1 >CYP3A4 >CYP2D6 (Styles et al., 1994).

In addition to the protein and DNA binding of Tamoxifen, toxicity may result from the ability of Tamoxifen to increase the cellular production of reactive oxygen species. Due to the influence of PB-pretreatment, Tamoxifen-induced production of reactive oxygen species was suggested to be CYP-dependent (Turner III et al., 1991).

Effects of Tamoxifen on expression of drug-metabolizing enzymes

Effects of Tamoxifen on expression of various drug-metabolizing enzymes has been studied by measuring catalytic activities and levels of enzyme proteins and mRNA in the liver of Tamoxifen-treated experimental animals (Table 3). In general, while hepatic drug-metabolizing enzyme systems are readily affected by Tamoxifen treatment, only small effects are seen in mouse liver (White et al., 1993). Early studies showed that Tamoxifen treatment decreased CYP dependent enzyme activities in tissues of male rats, while corresponding activities in female rats were unaffected (Al-Turk et al., 1981; Melzer et al., 1984). More recently, White et al. (1993) reported 30- to 60-fold increases in benzyloxy- and pentoxyresorufin deethylase activities in the liver of Tamoxifen-treated rats. Smaller increases were also seen in ethoxyresorufin deethylation, 6β- and 16α-hydroxylation of testosterone, suggesting induction pattern with a significant PB-like component. Studies with antibodies showed that Tamoxifen-treatment induced 2- to 3-fold increases in CYP2B1, CYP2B2 and CYP3A1 proteins (White et al., 1993). Similar patterns of induction were also seen after treatment of rats with Toremifene or Droloxifene (3-hydroxytamoxifen). Studies by Nuwaysir et al. (1995) have further confirmed that Tamoxifen administration results in a PB-type induction of drug-metabolizing enzymes in rat liver. In accordance with White et al. (1993), they reported increased mRNA and protein levels of CYP2B1, CYP2B2, CYP3A and epoxide hydrolase in male and female F344 rat liver after Tamoxifen administration. The expression of CYP1A1 and CYP1A2 was not affected. Due to differences in induction profiles between Tamoxifen and PB, and also in the sex-related sensitivity to induction, it was suggested that the molecular mechanisms by which Tamoxifen and PB produce enzyme induction are not identical (Nuwaysir et al., 1995). Compared to PB, the potency of Tamoxifen as an inducer of drug-metabolizing enzymes was found weak. Yet, on a mg/kg basis, the dose women receive for disease management is comparable to the dose level at which Tamoxifen induced expression of drug-metabolizing enzymes in rat liver (Nuwaysir et al., 1995).

Confirming the studies by White et al. (1993), ethoxyresorufin and ethoxycoumarin O-deethylase activities were found to be slightly induced in rat liver during long-term treatment with either Tamoxifen of Toremifene (Ahotupa et al., 1994). Enhancement of the catalytic activities was stronger by Tamoxifen. The ethoxyresorufin O-deethylase activity was elevated at all time points studied (from 5 weeks to 1 year) and, interestingly, still elevated 13 weeks after withdrawal of the drug. A most striking observation was the strong inhibition of NADPH production by the hexose monophosphate shunt (HMS) by both Tamoxifen and Toremifene, which in case of the Toremifene treatment lasted through the experiment (Ahotupa et al., 1994). In this long-term study Tamoxifen, at a dose level (45 mg/kg daily) that produced liver tumors to rats, enhanced the activity of glutathione S-transferase at all time points studied and also HMS activity at the two last time points of the study; both enzyme activities were found further elevated in Tamoxifen-induced liver tumors. Toremifene, which did not induce liver tumors, had no such effects on these enzyme activities (Ahotupa et al., 1994). It is worth noticing that glutathione S-transferase as well as glucose 6-phosphate dehydrogenase (a major component of the HMS) activities are both known to be elevated in preneoplastic nodules of the liver (Farber, 1984). The different hepatocarcinogenic potential of

Table 3. Effects of Tamoxifen treatment on drug-metabolizing enzymes in rat liver

Enzyme	Sex	Effect	Reference
Arylhydrocarbon hydroxylase(c)	male	decrease	Al-Turk et al., 1981
	female	no effect	Al-Turk et al., 1981
Aniline hydroxylase(c)	female	no effect	Meltzer et al., 1984
Ethoxycoumarin deethylase(c)	male	decrease	Al-Turk et al., 1981
	female	no effect	Al-Turk et al., 1981
	female	increase	Ahotupa et al., 1994
Ethoxyresorufin deethylase(c)	female	increase	White et al., 1993
	female	increase	Ahotupa et al., 1994
Benzyloxyresorufin dealkylase(c)	female	increase	White et al., 1993
Pentoxyresorufin deethylase(c)	female	increase	White et al., 1993
Testosterone 6β-hydroxylase(c)	female	increase	White et al., 1993
Testosterone 16α-hydroxylase(c)	female	increase	White et al., 1993
CYP2B1(p)	female	increase	White et al., 1993
CYP2B1(p,m)	both sexes	increase	Nuwaysir et al., 1995
CYP2B2(p)	female	increase	White et al., 1993
CYP2B2(p,m)	both sexes	increase	Nuwaysir et al., 1995
CYP1A1 and CYP1A2(p,m)	both sexes	no effect	Nuwaysir et al., 1995
Epoxide hydrolase(p,m)	both sexes	increase	Nuwaysir et al., 1995
Glutathione S-transferase(c)	female	increase	Ahotupa et al., 1994

c, catalytic activity; p, amount of enzyme protein; m, amount of mRNA

Tamoxifen and the structurally related Toremifene was thus reflected in differential effects on enzymatic markers of liver preneoplasia. Yet, these studies did not reveal whether drug-metabolizing enzymes played any role in the development of Tamoxifen-induced liver tumors in the rat.

Possible implications of interactions between Tamoxifen and drug-metabolizing enzymes

The increased knowledge on the role of individual CYP isoforms in the metabolism and toxicity of Tamoxifen, together with the better understanding of factors affecting expression of the CYP enzymes, has enabled estimation of possible influence of various affectors of CYP function (competing substrates, CYP inducing drugs, tobacco smoke, alcohol, diseases, etc.) on metabolism, therapeutic effectiveness and toxicity of Tamoxifen. Similarly, possible influences of Tamoxifen treatment on CYP-dependent metabolism of other drugs or endogenous compounds may be predicted. As an example, a life threatening interaction between Tamoxifen and warfarin has been described (Lodwick et al., 1987; Tenni et al., 1989): Tamoxifen and warfarin are both metabolized by CYP3A (see Raunio et al., 1995) and it is therefore possible that the drastically decreased elimination of warfarin, which was noted after initiation of Tamoxifen therapy in patients undergoing warfarin anticoagulant treatment, was due to competition between these drugs in binding to same CYP isoforms. In accordance, it is possible that Tamoxifen treatment affects biotransformation and thus the therapeutic potency of a number of cardiovascular drugs (quinidine, nifedipine, diltiazem, lidocaine, lovastatin), antibiotics (erythromycin, troleandomycin), CNS drugs (triazolam, midazolam) and steroids, whose metabolism is known to be CYP3A-dependent in man (see Raunio et al., 1995).

Knowing the central role that CYP3A-mediated catalysis plays in the biotransformation of Tamoxifen, it is possible that common CYP3A inducers (e.g. barbiturates, rifampicin, dexamethasone, triacetyloleandomycin; see Pelkonen and Breimer, 1994) may enhance the metabolism, increase toxic effects, and alter therapeutic potency of Tamoxifen. Tamoxifen treatment itself also induces CYP activities (Table 3) that are responsible for its own metabolism (Table 2). Induction of CYP and other drug-metabolizing enzymes may result in altered accumulation of Tamoxifen, which was shown to accompany the development of Tamoxifen resistance (Osborne et al., 1991). Further, as

CYP2E1 seems to be implicated in toxicity of Tamoxifen, inducing factors such as alcohol, isoniazid treatment, and diabetes (see Pelkonen and Breimer, 1994) may increase toxicity of Tamoxifen.

Another way by which Tamoxifen may potentially alter the metabolism of drugs and also endogenous compounds is inhibition of NADPH production by HMS (Ahotupa et al., 1994): as an important cofactor, the availability of NADPH is known to affect reactions catalyzed by the drug-metabolizing enzymes (Wu et al., 1986). In addition to drug metabolism and several biosynthetic reactions, NADPH is essential for function of the intracellular glutathione redox cycle, i.e. reduction of oxidized glutathione by glutathione reductase. There seems to be an apparent interdependence between HMS activity and the level of reduced glutathione in the liver of rats treated with Tamoxifen (Ahotupa et al., 1994).

Conclusions

Recent studies on Tamoxifen and drug-metabolizing enzymes have set forth individual CYP isoforms responsible for the catalysis of main metabolic pathways of Tamoxifen. Toxicity of Tamoxifen results from the CYP and FMO mediated metabolism, and the contribution by individual CYPs has been studied. Similarly, the pattern of CYP isoenzymes induced by Tamoxifen in rodent liver has been clarified, and resembles the PB-type of induction. Long-term Tamoxifen treatment produces in rat liver alterations in enzyme activities similar to those seen in preneoplastic nodules of the liver. Apart from the CYP enzymes, much less is known about enzymes catalyzing the 2nd phase in biotransformation of Tamoxifen, and effects of Tamoxifen treatment in extrahepatic rodent tissues and in humans are not known. Based on the present knowledge, it is possible to estimate which factors (most importantly other drugs), through their effects on critical CYP enzymes, might have influence on metabolism, therapeutic effectiveness and toxicity of Tamoxifen. Similarly, it is possible to estimate how Tamoxifen, by affecting the CYP-dependent metabolism, might alter CYP-dependent metabolism of other drugs and endogenous compounds. In addition to acting directly at the CYP level, Tamoxifen may potentially affect the metabolism of drugs and endogenous compounds, and also several biosynthetic reactions, by altering the cellular production of the cofactor NADPH.

REFERENCES

Ahotupa M, Hirsimäki P, Pärssinen R, Mäntylä E (1994): Alterations of drug metabolizing and antioxidant enzyme activities during tamoxifen-induced hepatocarcinogenesis in the rat. *Carcinogenesis* 15:863-868

Aitio A, ed. (1978): Conjugation Reactions in Drug Biotransformation. New York: Elsevier North Holland Biomedical Press

Al-Turk WA, Stohs SJ, Roche EB (1981): Effect of tamoxifen treatment on liver, lung and intestinal mixed-function oxidases in male and female rats. *Drug Metab Dispos* 9:327-330

Beckett GJ, Hayes JD (1993): Glutathione S-transferases: biomedical applications. *Advan Clin Chem* 30:281-380

Berthou F, Dreano Y (1993): High-performance liquid chromatographic analysis of tamoxifen, toremifene and their major human metabolites. *J Chromatogr* 616:117-127

Berthou F, Dreano Y, Belloc C, Kangas L, Gautier J-C, Beaune P (1994): Involvement of cytochrome P450 3A enzyme family in the major metabolic pathways of toremifene in human liver microsomes. *Biochem Pharmacol* 47:1883-1895

Carthew P, Rich KJ, Martin EA, deMatteis F, Lim CK, Manson MM, Festing MFW, White INH, Smith LL (1995): DNA damage as assessed by P-postlabelling in three rat strains exposed to dietary tamoxifen: the relationship between cell proliferation and liver tumour formation. *Carcinogenesis* 16:1299-1304

Clarke DJ, Burchell B (1994): The uridine diphosphate glucuronosyltransferase multigene family: function and regulation. *Handbook of Exp Pharm* 112:3-43

Conney AH (1967): Pharmacological implications of microsomal enzyme induction. *Pharmacol Rev* 19:317-366

Conney AH (1982): Induction of microsomal enzymes by foreign chemicals and carcinogenesis by polycyclic aromatic hydrocarbons: GHA Clowes memorial lecture. *Cancer Res* 42:4875-4917

Davies AM, Martin EA, Jones RM, Lim CK, Smith LL, White INH (1995): Peroxidase activation of tamoxifen resulting in DNA damage and covalently bound protein adducts. *Carcinogenesis* 16:539-545

Farber E (1984): Cellular biochemistry of the stepwise development of cancer with chemicals: GHA Clowes memorial lecture. *Cancer Res* 44:5463-5474

Fromson JM, Pearson S, Bramah S (1973): The metabolism of tamoxifen (I.C.I. 46,474). Part I: In laboratory animals. *Xenobiotica* 3:693-709

Gonzales FJ (1989): The molecular biology of cytochrome P450s. *Pharmacol Rev* 40:243-288

Gonzales FJ (1992): Human cytochromes P450: problems and prospects. *TiPS* 13:346-352

Han X, Liehr JG (1992): Induction of covalent DNA adducts in rodents by tamoxifen. *Cancer Res* 52:1360-1363

Hard GC, Iatropoulos MJ, Jordan K, Radi L, Kaltenberg OP, Imondi AR, Williams GM (1993): Major difference in the hepatocarcinogenicity and DNA adduct forming ability between toremifene and tamoxifen in female Crl:CD(BR) rats. *Cancer Res* 53:4534-4541

Hemminki K, Widlak P, Hou, S-M (1995): DNA adducts caused by tamoxifen and toremifene in human microsomal system and lymphocytes in vitro. *Carcinogenesis* 16:1661-1664

Hirsimäki P, Hirsimäki Y, Nieminen L, Payne BJ (1993): Tamoxifen induces hepatocellular carcinoma in rat liver: a 1-year study with two antiestrogens. *Arch Toxicol* 67:49-54

Jacolot F, Simon I, Dreano Y, Beaune P, Riche C, Berthou F (1991): Indentification of the cytochrome P450IIIA family as the enzymes involved in the N-demethylation of tamoxifen in human liver microsomes. *Biochem Pharmacol* 41:1911-1919

Jordan VC (1984): Biochemical pharmacology of antiestrogen action. *Pharmacol Rev* 36:245-276

Kupfer D, Mani C, Lee CA, Rifkind AB (1994): Induction of tamoxifen-4-hydroxylation by 2,3,7,8-tetrachlorodibenzo-p-dioxin (TCDD), b-naphthoflavone (bNF), and phenobarbital (PB) in avian liver: identification of P450 TCDD$_{AA}$ as catalyst of 4-hydroxylation induced by TCDD and bNF. *Cancer Res* 54:3140-3144

Levin W, Michaud DP, Thomas PE, Jerina DM (1983): Distinct rat hepatic microsomal epoxide hydrolases catalyze the hydration of cholesterol 5,6-oxide and certain xenobiotic alkene and arene oxides. *Arch Biochem Biophys* 220:485-494

Lim CK, Yuan Z-X, Lamb JH, White INH, DeMatteis F, Smith LL (1994): A comparative study of tamoxifen metabolism in female rat, mouse and human liver microsomes. *Carcinogenesis* 15:589-593

Lodwick R, McKonkey B, Brown AM, Beeley L (1987): Life threatening interaction between tamoxifen and warfarin. *Br Med J* 295:1141

Lu AYH, Levin W (1974): The resolution and reconstitution of the liver microsomal hydroxylation system. *Biochem Biophys Acta* 344:205-240

Mani C, Kupfer D (1991): Cytochrome P450-mediated activation and irreversible binding of the antiestrogen tamoxifen to proteins in rat and human liver: possible involvement of flavin-containing monooxygenases in tamoxifen activation. *Cancer Res* 51:6052-6058

Mani C, Gelboin HV, Park SS, Pearce R, Parkinson A, Kupfer D (1993a): Metabolism of the antimammary cancer antiestrogenic agent tamoxifen. I. Cytochrome P450-catalyzed N-demethylation and 4-hydroxylation. *Drug Metab Dispos* 21:645-656

Mani C, Hodgson E, Kupfer D (1993b): Metabolism of the antimammary cancer antiestrogenic agent tamoxifen. II. Flavin-containing monooxygenase-mediated N-oxidation. *Drug Metab Dispos* 21:657-661

Mani C, Pearce R, Parkinson A, Kupfer D (1994): Involvement of cytochrome P4503A in catalysis of tamoxifen activation and covalent binding to rat and human liver microsomes. *Carcinogenesis* 15:2715-2720

Martin EA, Rich KJ, White INH, Woods KL, Powles TJ, Smith LL (1995): P-Postlabelled DNA adducts in liver obtained from women treated with tamoxifen. *Carcinogenesis* 16:1651-1654

Meltzer NM, Stang P, Sternson LA (1984): Influence of tamoxifen and its N-desmethyl and 4-hydroxy metabolites on rat liver microsomal enzymes. *Biochem Pharmacol* 33:115-123

Metzler M, Schiffmann D (1991): Structural requirements for the *in vitro* transformation of Syrian hamster embryo cells by stilbene estrogens and triphenylethylene-type antiestrogens. *Am J Clin Oncol* 14:30-35

Montandon F, Williams GM (1994): Comparison of DNA reactivity of the polyphenylethylene hormonal agents diethylstilbestrol, tamoxifen and toremifene in rat and hamster liver. *Arch Toxicol* 68:272-275

Nuwaysir EF, Dragan YP, Jefcoate CR, Jordan VC, Pitot HC (1995): Effects of tamoxifen administration on the expression of xenobiotic metabolizing enzymes in rat liver. *Cancer Res* 55:1780-1786

Osborne CK, Coronaro E, Allred DC, Wiebe V, deGregorio M (1991): Acquired tamoxifen resistance: correlation with reduced breast tumor levels of tamoxifen and isomerization of trans-4-hydroxytamoxifen. *J Natl Cancer Inst* 83:1477-148

Pathak DN, Bodell WJ (1994): DNA adduct formation by tamoxifen with rat and human liver microsomal activation systems. *Carcinogenesis* 15:529-532

Pathak DN, Pongracz K, Bodell WJ (1995): Microsomal and peroxidase activation of 4-hydroxytamoxifen to form DNA adducts: comparison with DNA adducts formed in Sprague-Dawley rats treated with tamoxifen. *Carcinogenesis* 16:11-15

Pelkonen O, Breimer DD (1994): Role of environmental factors in the pharmacokinetics of drugs: considerations with respect to animal models, P-450 enzymes, and probe drugs. In: Handbook of Experimental Pharmacology, vol. 110, Welling PG, Balant LP, eds. Heidelberg: Springer-Verlag

Pelkonen O, Nebert DW (1982): Metabolism of polycyclic aromatic hydrocarbons: etiologic role in carcinogenesis. *Pharmacol Rev* 34:189-222

Poon GK, Chui YC, McCague R, Lonning PE, Feng R, Rowlands MG, Jarman M (1993): Analysis of phase I and phase II metabolites of tamoxifen in breast cancer patients. *Drug Metab Dispos* 21:1119-1124

Potter GA, McCague R, Jarman M (1994): A mechanistic hypothesis for DNA adduct formation following hepatic oxidative metabolism. *Carcinogenesis* 15:439-442

Randerath K, Moorthy B, Mabon N, Sriram P (1994): Tamoxifen: evidence by P-postlabeling and use of metabolic inhibitors for two distinct pathways leading to mouse hepatic DNA adduct formation and identification of 4-hydroxytamoxifen as a proximate metabolite. *Carcinogenesis* 15:2087-2094

Raunio H, Pasanen M, Mäenpää J, Hakkola J, Pelkonen O (1995): Expression of extrahepatic cytochrome P450 in humans. In: Advances in Drug Metabolism in Man, Pacifici GM, Fracchia GN, eds. Luxembourg: European Comission, Office for Official Publications of the European Communities

Styles JA, Davies A, Lim CK, deMatteis F, Stanley LA, White INH, Yuan Z-X, Smith LL (1994): Genotoxicity of tamoxifen, tamoxifen epoxide and toremifene in human lymphoblastoid cells containing human cytochrome P450s. *Carcinogenesis* 15:5-9

Tenni P, Lalich DL, Byrne MJ (1989): Life threatening interaction between tamoxifen and warfarin. *Br Med J* 298:93

Tucker MJ, Adam HJ, Patterson JS (1984): Tamoxifen. In: Safety Testing of New Drugs, Laurence DR, McLean AEM, Weatherall M, eds. New York: Academic Press

Turner III MJ, Fields CE, Everman DB (1991): Evidence for superoxide formation during hepatic metabolism of tamoxifen. *Biochem Pharmacol* 41:1701-1705

White INH, de Matteis F, Davies A, Smith LL, Crofton-Sleigh C, Venitt S, Hewer A, Phillips DH (1992): Genotoxic potential of tamoxifen and analogues in female Fischer F344/n rats, DBA/2 and C57BL/6 mice and in human MCL-5 cells. *Carcinogenesis* 13:2197-2203

White INH, Davies A, Smith LL, Dawson S, DeMatteis F (1993): Induction of CYP2B1 and 3A1, and associated monooxygenase activities by tamoxifen and certain analogues in the livers of female rats and mice. *Biochem Pharmacol* 45:21-30

White INH, deMatteis F, Gibbs AH, Lim CK, Wolf CR, Henderson C, Smith LL (1995): Species differences in the covalent binding of (C)tamoxifen to liver microsomes and the forms of cytochrome P450 involved. *Biochem Pharmacol* 49:1035-1042

Williams RT (1959): Detoxication Mechanisms. London: Chapman & Hall

Williams GM, Iatropoulos MJ, Djordjevic MV, Kaltenberg OP (1993): The triphenylethylene drug tamoxifen is a strong liver carcinogen in the rat. *Carcinogenesis* 14:315-317

Williams ML, Lennard MS, Martin IJ, Tucker GT (1994): Interindividual variation in the isomerization of 4-hydroxytamoxifen by human liver microsomes: involvement of cytochromes P450. *Carcinogenesis* 15:2733-2738

Wislocki PG, Miwa GT, Lu AYH (1980): Reactions catalyzed by the cytochrome P450 system. In: Enzymatic Basis of Detoxication Vol 1, Jacoby WB, ed. New York: Academic Press

Wolf DM, Langan-Fahay SM, Parker CJ, McCague R, Jordan VC (1993): Investigation of the mechanism of tamoxifen-stimulated breast tumor growth with nonisomerizable analogues of tamoxifen and metabolites. *J Natl Cancer Inst* 85:806-812

Wu Y-R, Conway JG, Kauffman FC, Thurman RG (1986): Stimulation of mixed-function oxidation by NADPH in perfused mouse livers. Studies with saponin-permeabilized tissue. *Biochem Pharmacol* 35:3607-3612

14. MEMBRANE ANTIOXIDANT-MEDIATED CARDIOPROTECTIVE ANTICARCINOGENIC ACTIONS OF TAMOXIFEN

Helen Wiseman

In order to understand the possible importance of the reported membrane antioxidant action of Tamoxifen to its cardioprotective and anticarcinogenic effects, the basics of membrane and lipoprotein composition and structure and how these are influences by free radical-mediated oxidative stress need to be appreciated and these will now be briefly explored (see Figure 1 for an overview).

Membranes

Membranes are of great importance to cell structure and function. The cell is surrounded by a plasma membrane and other membranes form a continuous intracellular surface (endoplastic reticulum) and form the structural basis of intracellular organelles such as mitochondria (Gurr and Harwood, 1991). The main lipids in animal cell membranes are phospholipids based on glycerol such as phosphatidylserine, phosphatidyelthanolamine, phostphatidylcholine and phosphatidylinositol, each with variable fatty acid side chains. The basic structure of all membranes is the phospholipid bilayer and the presence of a wide range of different proteins confers on membranes a great diversity of function. Plasma membranes contain cholesterol in large amounts (often equimolar with the phospholipid) whereas endoplasmic reticulum, mitochondrial and nuclear membranes have a low cholesterol content (Gurr and Harwood, 1991). In the contemporary basic model for membrane structure,

Figure 1. An overview of the membrane antioxidant-mediated cardioprotective and anticarcinomgenic anctions of Tamoxifen

TAMOXIFEN
↓
MEMBRANE ANTIOXIDANT ACTION
↓   ↓

PROTECTION OF LDL	PROTECTION OF NUCLEAR
AND CARDIAC MEMBRANES	MEMBRANES AGAINST LIPID
AGAINST OXIDATIVE DAMAGE	PEROXIDATION

↓   ↓

CONTRIBUTES TOGETHER WITH	CONTRIBUTES TOGETHER
LOWERING OF CHOLESTEROL,	WITH PREVENTION OF
HOMOCYSTEINE AND LIPO-	HYDROGEN PEROXIDE
PROTEIN(a) LEVELS TO THE	RELEASE TO THE
PREVENTION OF	PREVENTION OF DNA
ATHEROSCLEROSIS	DAMAGE

↓   ↓

CARDIOPROTECTIVE ACTION   ANTICARCINOGENIC ACTION

extrinsic proteins are loosely adsorbed to the lipid bilayer, while the intrinsic proteins are imbedded in the bilayer and can transverse the whole bilayer (Gurr and Harwood, 1991; Peck, 1994). Lipid and protein molecules can rapidly diffuse laterally in each half of the lipid bilayer, whereas migration from one bilayer to another (flip-flop) is rare and slow and this preserves the asymmetry of natural membranes (Zachowski, 1993; Williamson and Schlegel, 1994). This lateral diffusion possibility is denoted by the term membrane fluidity and is dependent of the presence of unsaturated and polyunsaturated fatty acid side chains in the membrane lipids, which lowers the melting or phase transition temperature of the system (Gurr and Harwood, 1991; New, 1992). Increasing the cholesterol and the saturated fatty acid content of a membrane both result in a decrease in membrane fluidity. Cholesterol has a rigidifying effect on the membrane by inhibiting the overall flexing motion of the acyl (hydrocarbon) chains. Membrane fluidity has an important influence on important membrane functions including the conformation and therefore the activity of membrane associated enzymes and receptors, which are involved in a wide range of functions from cell signalling to nutrient uptake (Peck, 1994).

Lipoprotein particles

The phospholipid monolayer of lipoprotein particles makes them of related interest to membranes. It is the LDL (low density lipoprotein) particle that is of particular interest in relation to its susceptibility to undergo the oxidative damage implicated in atherosclerosis (see below). Its structure is a large central core of cholesteryl ester and triglycerides surrounded by a monolayer of phospholipid molecules and free cholesterol, with the apoprotein B embedded in this outer layer (Rice-Evans and Bruckdorfer, 1992).

Free radicals

Free radicals are any species capable of an independent existence that contains one or more unpaired electron (Halliwell and Gutteridge, 1989; Halliwell, 1993, 1994). Reactive oxygen species (ROS) is a collective term and refers to not only oxygen-centred radicals such as superoxide ($O_2^{\cdot-}$) and the hydroxyl radical ($OH^{\cdot}$) but also to hydrogen peroxide (H_2O_2), singlet oxygen ($^1O_2$), hypochlorous acid (HOCl) and ozone (O_3). ROS thus include some potentially dangerous, non-radical derivatives of oxygen. Reactive nitrogen species (RNS) (Darley-Usmar et al., 1995) can be derived from nitric oxide (NO) and include the damaging species peroxynitrite ($ONOO^-$) (Darley-Usmar et al., 1995).

Free radicals are produced as the by-products of normal metabolism, $O_2^{\cdot-}$, $OH^{\cdot}$ and $NO^{\cdot}$ and ROS such as H_2O_2 are all formed *in vivo*. Indeed, $O_2^{\cdot-}$ and H_2O_2 are continuously produced e.g. by activated phagocytes and endothelium cells by a plasma membrane enzyme, by NADPH oxidase (role in pathogen killing). The production of superoxide as a by-product of metabolism can be considered to be a chemical accident and results from auto-oxidation reactions and the leakage of electrons from electron transport chains onto oxygen (Halliwel and Gutteridge, 1989); Halliwell, 1993, 1994).

Phagocytes make $NO^{\cdot}$ in response to pathogens and it is also made by neutrophils at sites of inflammation and by vascular endothelial cells. Vascular endothelial cells make $NO^{\cdot}$ from the oxidation of arginine by nitric oxide synthase (NOS) and use it through signal transduction mechanisms to achieve the relaxation of vascular smooth muscle. Macrophages produce large amounts of $NO^{\cdot}$ in response to bacterial endotoxins, or cytokines. The hydroxyl radical is produced in living organisms by 2 mechanisms: 1) splitting of covalent bonds in water by background ionizing radiation, 2) reaction of transition metal ions with H_2O_2, Cu (I) and Fe (II) to reduce H_2O_2 to OH^- (Halliwell and Gutteridge, 1989; Halliwell 1993, 1994).

However, iron is handled carefully *in vivo* e.g. transported as transferin and stored as ferritin and haemosiderin, which mimizes "free" iron in cells and extracellular fluids. The same is true for copper, which is sequestered as caeruloplasmin. Sequestration restricts iron availability to bacteria and contributes to antioxidant defences (Halliwell and Gutteridge, 1989: Halliwell, 1993, 1994). ROS/RNS in excess can facilitate iron release e.g. O_2^- mobilizes iron from ferritin, NO^- releases iron from iron-sulphur proteins. Intracellular iron is also released on cell lysis and can lead to tissue damage (Halliwell and Gutteridge, 1989; Halliwell, 1993, 1994).

Oxidative damage

Possible free radical damage to cellular target sites, includes oxidative damage to membranes (lipids and proteins), DNA and other proteins. Lipid peroxidation is a free radical-mediated chain-reaction, which can be initiated by OH^- and attacks polyunsaturated fatty acids in membranes and plasma lipoprotein particles resulting in oxidative damage (Halliwell and Gutteridge, 1989: Halliwell, 1993, 1994). Lipid peroxidation will also damage membrane proteins directly through free radical attack (Neuzil et al., 1993; Dean et al., 1993; Stadtman, 1993). In addition, lipid hydroperoxides are readily decomposed by traces of transition metal ions to produce the free radical intermediates of lipid peroxidation capable of propagating the chain reaction. Oxidative DNA damage include OH^--mediated modification of DNA bases. Protein modifications include oxidation of thiol groups and the formation of nitrosothiols and nitrotyrosine residues as a result of RNS attack (Darley-Usmar et al., 1995).

An antioxidant is "any substance that, when present at low concentrations compared to those of an oxidizable substrate, significantly delays or prevents oxidation of that substrate" (Halliwell, 1990). "Oxidizable substrates" include the DNA, lipids, proteins (including of membranes and lipoproteins) and carbohydrates. Physiological antioxidants include proteins such as superoxide dismutase also glutathione peroxidase, catalase and caeruloplasmin. Vitamin E (including alpha-tocopherol), vitamin C (ascorbic acid or ascorbate), glutathione, selenium, ß-carotene, albumin, uric acid, oestrogens, flavonoids, isoflavonoid type phyto-oestrogens and coenzyme Q (ubiquinone) are also antioxidants that may be important (Halliwell, 1990; Halliwell and Gutteridge, 1994; Gey, 1995).

In healthy individuals the generation of ROS (and RNS) should be in balance with antioxidant defences. However, a slow genral accumulation of oxidative damage contributes to the ageing process and age related diseases such as cancer (Ames, 1989). When imbalance occurs this is referred to as oxidative stress. Oxidative stress can be caused by 1) depletion of antioxidant levels e.g. malnutrition lowers antioxidant vitamin and glutathione levels 2) increased ROS formation e.g. by toxic chemicals, some drugs and at sites of inflammation. Free radicals have been implicated in over 100 diseases including cardiovascular disease and cancer (Gutteridge, 1993). However, in many cases they are not the major cause of disease but rather a consequence and complicating component of the underlying disease pathology leading to lipid peroxidation as a consequence rather than a cause of cell injury (Gutteridge, 1993).

An increased formation of ROS accompanies tissue injury in most if not all human diseases and although some may be caused by oxidative stress e.g. ionizing radiation leading to OH^{-}-mediated damage, Keshan disease arising from a lack of selenium and neurological disorders arising from a lack of vitamin E, in others e.g. rheumatoid arthritis, myocardial stunning (depression of contractile function) and inflammatory bowel disease the increased production of ROS is likely to be secondary though still important. In cancer, ROS/RNS-mediated damage to DNA bases is implicated in mutation and tumourigenesis, (Cerutti, 1994; Wiseman and Halliwell, 1995) and oxidative damage to low-density lipoproteins is implicated in atherosclerosis (Witzum, 1994: see below).

A wide range of drugs and dietary components have been reported to protect human LDL against oxidative modification. This may be of importance because oxidative damage to LDL (particularly to the apoprotein B molecule) is considered to be an important stage in the development of atherosclerosis: it is a prerequisite for macrophage uptake and cellular accumulation of cholesterol leading to the formation of the atheromal fatty streak (Witzum, 1994; Parathasarathy and Santanan, 1994). Lipid peroxidation is thought to start in the polyunsaturated fatty acids of the phospholipids on the surface of LDL and then propagate to core lipids resulting in modification of the cholesterol, phospholipids and the apolipoprotein B molecule, in addition to the polyunsaturated fatty acids (Witzum, 1994; Parathasarathy and

Santanam, 1994). This oxidative hypothesis of atherosclerosis and the likely effectiveness of dietary antioxidants is supported by recent evidence from clinical trials (Witzum, 1994; Parathasarathy and Santanam, 1994; Gey, 1995; Frei, 1995).

Study and measurement of oxidative membrane damage

In many studies of oxidative membrane damage, liver microsomes can be used and membrane susceptibility to lipid peroxidation induced e.g. by Fe(III)/ascorbate is measured and correlated with different diets. Microsomes are a heterogenous mixture of vesicles derived from both endoplasmic reticulum and plasma membranes and are used as an *in vitro* test system to assess the ability of a wide range of drugs and dietary components to protect against membrane lipid peroxidation (Halliwell and Gutteridge, 1989). Liposomes are used extensively as a model membrane system for studying the influence of drugs and dietary components membrane lipid peroxidation *in vitro* (Chatterjee and Agarwal, 1988). Liposomes are artificial lipid structures, made by shaking or sonicating phospholipids in aqueous suspension (New, 1992). In studies investigating drug and dietary influences on membrane susceptibility to oxidative damage in humans, erythrocytes are often isolated from subjects and the production of lipid peroxidation products following hydrogen peroxide induced oxidative stress is frequently measured as TBARS (thiobarbituric acid reactive substances) (Girelli et al., 1994).

In most studies on the action of drugs and dietary components on oxidative damage to LDL, human LDL is stimulated to undergo lipid peroxidation by the addition of Cu(II) ions: a widely used experimental system that is relevant to events occurring within the atherosclerotic lesion (Smith et al., 1992) and appears to involve pre-existing lipid hydroperoxidases (Thomas et al., 1994).

Membrane and lipoprotein lipid peroxidation can be measured by a number of different methods each with its own merits and drawbacks (Halliwell and Chirico, 1993). The most extensively used method is probably the TBA (thiobarbituric acid) test. The test sample is heated with TBA at low pH and the absorbance of a pink chromogen presumed to be a $(TBA)_2$-malondialdehyde adduct (although the term TBARS is frequently used) is measured at 532 nm. Although the TBA test is adequate for measuring lipid peroxidation in defined membrane systems such as microsomes and liposomes, its application to body fluids has many problems relating to its lack of specificity (Halliwell and Chirico,

1993). A modified TBA test has been developed that avoids many of the artefacts resulting from the reaction of TBA with other body-fluid constituents to give different chromogens and uses HPLC to separate the authentic $(TBA)_2$-MDA adduct from other chromogens absorbing at 532 nm (Halliwell and Chirico, 1993).

Membrane antioxidant action of Tamoxifen

Tamoxifen, its derivatives and 17 ß-oestradiol (structures shown in Figure 2) have been found to be good inhibitors of lipid peroxidation in microsomal and pre-formed liposomal systems (Wiseman et al., 1990a, 1992, 1993a; Wiseman, 1994a,b,c,d; Wiseman, 1995). 4-Hydroxytamoxifen was found to be a better inhibitor of microsomal lipid peroxidation in both the Fe(III)-ascorbate and Fe (III)-ADP/NADPH systems and of liposomal peroxidation, than Tamoxifen, 3-hydroxytamoxifen (droloxifene) or 17 ß-oestradiol (see Tables 1 and 2).

Time course studies have showed that Tamoxifen, related compounds and 17 ß-oestradiol all inhibited microsomal and liposomal lipid peroxidation throughout the incubation period. There was no clear evidence of a lag period followed by an acceleration of peroxidation to the control rate (Wiseman et al., 1990a, 1992, 1993a; Wiseman, 1994a,b,c,d; Wiseman, 1995). This suggests that these compounds are unlikely to be classical chain-breaking antioxidants, even though hydroxy groups with potentially donatable hydrogen atoms are present in many of these compounds (Tamoxifen itself being an exception). It has been suggested that these compounds act in part or in whole by stabilising membranes against peroxidation, in a manner similar to cholesterol, *via* a decrease in membrane fluidity (Wiseman et al., 1990a, 1992, 1993a; 1994; Wiseman and Halliwell, 1993; Wiseman, 1994a,b,c,d,;Wiseman, 1995). Indeed, such an ability to decrease membrane fluidity has been demonstrated for Tamoxifen and related compounds (Wiseman et al., 1993b; Wiseman and Quinn, 1994).

Tamoxifen and 4-hydroxytamoxifen have both been reported to be inhibitors of Fe(III)-dependent lipid peroxidation in rat cardiac microsomes (Wiseman et al., 1993a). Tamoxifen was also a good inhibitor of lipid peroxidation in cardiovascular injury and the development of atherosclerosis; therefore, some of the cardioprotective effect of Tamoxifen may be related to its ability to inhibit membrane lipid peroxidation.

Figure 2. Structures of Tamoxifen and related compounds

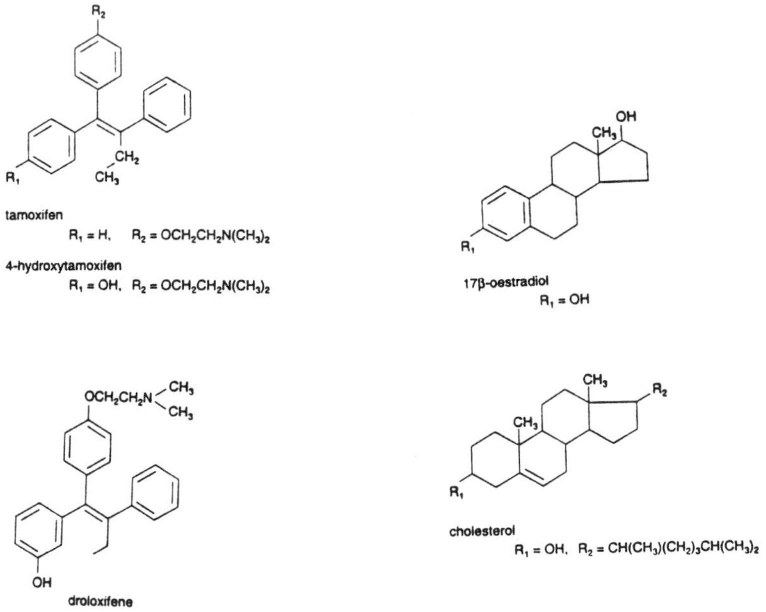
R2
R1
CH2
CH3
tamoxifen
R1 = H, R2 = OCH2CH2N(CH3)2
4-hydroxytamoxifen
R1 = OH, R2 = OCH2CH2N(CH3)2
OH
CH3
R1
17β-oestradiol
R1 = OH
OCH2CH2N
CH3
CH3
OH
droloxifene
CH3
R2
CH3
R1
cholesterol
R1 = OH, R2 = CH(CH3)(CH2)3CH(CH3)2

When introduced into liposomes during their preparation (Wiseman et al., 1990b; Wiseman, 1994a,b,c,d,; Wiseman, 1995), Tamoxifen inhibited lipid peroxidation to a greater extent than cholesterol. Cholesterol cannot enter pre-formed liposomal membranes and thus has no effect in that system. 4-Hydroxytamoxifen and 17 ß-oestradiol were of similar effectiveness and both were more effective than Tamoxifen (see Table 3).

Antioxidant-mediated cardioprotective action of Tamoxifen

There is considerable interest in the possible cardioprotective action of Tamoxifen. Although hormonally related cancers such as breast cancer are the most common causes of mortality in women aged 40-60 years old, in women over the age of 60 cardiovascular disease becomes the leading cause of death. This makes consideration of the long-term effects of Tamoxifen therapy particularly important. The potential benefits of

Table 1. Inhibition of microsomal lipid peroxidation by Tamoxifen and related compounds

Compound/drug	IC_{50} values (micromole)	
	Fe(III)-ascorbate system	Fe(III)-ADP/NADPH system
Tamoxifen	11	18
4-Hydroxytamoxifen	3	3
N-Desmethyltamoxifen	18	25
cis-Tamoxifen	16	23
3-Hydroxytamoxifen citrate	13	11
Tamoxifen citrate	17	19
17ß-Oestradiol	11	9
Ergosterol	NR	NR
Cholesterol	NR	R

(NR = 50% inhibition of lipid peroxidation not reached)

Table 2. Inhibition of liposomal lipid peroxidation in the preformed liposome system by Tamoxifen and related compounds

Compound/drug	IC_{50} values for preformed liposomal system (micromole)
Tamoxifen	63
17ß-Oestradiol	11
4-Hydroxytamoxifen	9
3-Hydroxytamoxifen citrate	38
Tamoxifen citrate	62
Ergosterol	NR
Cholesterol	NR

Table 3. Inhibition of liposomal lipid peroxidation by Tamoxifen and related compounds when introduced into liposomes during preparation

Compound/drug	IC_{50} values for introduced into liposomal system (microgam)
Tamoxifen	50
4-Hydroxytamoxifen	3.6
17ß-Oestradiol	4
Ergosterol	53
Cholesterol	720

prophylactic Tamoxifen therapy including protection against coronary heart disease and osteoporosis, in addition to decreasing the risk of breast cancer should outweigh the risk of deleterious side-effects. Retrospective studies on the two randomised arms of Scottish adjuvant Tamoxifen trial showed a significant decrease in the incidence of fatal myocardial infarction in breast cancer patients treated with Tamoxifen (McDonald and Stewart, 1991). Furthermore, the Stockholm randomised trial of adjuvant Tamoxifen therapy in post-menopausal women with early-stage breast cancer showed that even short-term Tamoxifen therapy significantly decreased occurrence of coronary heart disease (Rutqvist and Mattsson, 1993).

Protection of low density lipoproteins against oxidative damage

Tamoxifen and in particular 4-hydroxytamoxifen have been found to protect isolated human LDL against oxidative modification (Wiseman et al., 1993c; Wiseman, 1994a,b,c,d; Wiseman, 1995). When isolated human LDL was stimulated to undergo lipid peroxidation by the addition of CU(II) ions, 4-hydroxytamoxifen was found to be a more potent inhibitor of Cu(II) ion-dependent lipid peroxidation than both Tamoxifen and 17 ß-oestradiol (see Table 4).

4-Hydroxytamoxifen also effectively   prevented peroxidation-induced modifications in the surface charge of the LDL, whereas Tamoxifen did not. Alterations in the surface charge of LDL are associated with its recognition and uptake by macrophages in atherosclerotic lesions.

The protective ability of the 4-hydroxy metabolite of Tamoxifen could contribute to the observed beneficial cardiovascular effects of

Tamoxifen therapy. The lack of effectiveness of Tamoxifen itself in preventing alteration of the surface charge of LDL may be because it is a much less effective inhibitor of lipid peroxidation than 4-hydroxytamoxifen.

Tamoxifen and its derivatives are all highly lipophilic compounds that may accumulate in atheromal plaques to achieve the protective concentrations reported (Wiseman et al., 1993c). Tamoxifen (and 4-hydroxytamoxifen) may stabilise LDL against lipid peroxidation by interactions between their hydrophobic rings and the polyunsaturated residues of the phospholipid layer of LDL. This suggestion is supported by the inhibition of lipid peroxidation arising from similar interactions in liposomal membranes (Wiseman et al., 1993b).

Comparison with oestrogen

Tamoxifen shows structural similarity to sterols including oestrogen (see Figure 2). Although often described as an antioestrogen anticancer drug, it can also be a partial or full oestrogen agonist depending on the target organ or tissue. The similar cardioprotective actions observed for both Tamoxifen and oestrogens suggests that Tamoxifen acts as an oestrogen mimetic cardioprotectant.

The ability of oestrogen to protect LDL against oxidative damage could contribute to the cardiovascular benefits observed on oestrogen administration in postmenopausal women (Stampfer et al., 1991; Miller, 1994). 17 ß-Oestradiol inhibits the oxidation of human LDL both *in vitro* (Huber et al., 1990; Rifici and Khachadurian, 1992; Wiseman et al., 1993c) and when administered to postmenopausal women prior to LDL isolation (Sack et al., 1994). Acute intra-arterial infusion of 17 ß-oestradiol increased serum oestradiol levels from typical postmenopausal levels to physiological concentrations for reproductive-aged woman at mid-cycle and significantly prolonged the lag time of LDL compared to baseline levels and indicates a decrease in susceptibility to oxidation (Sack et al., 1994). However, oestrogen hormonal replacement therapy has been indicated to carry similar risks of endometrial cancer to Tamoxifen prophylaxis and therefore, requires careful monitoring (Gelety and Judd, 1992). Clinical investigations similar to the studies on 17 ß-oestradiol are now required to explore the *in vivo* effects of Tamoxifen on LDL oxidation. If clinical evidence for the inhibition of LDL oxidation by Tamoxifen could be obtained than this would be an important addition to the debate on the use of Tamoxifen to prevent breast cancer in postmenopausal women (Wiseman, 1994a,b,c,d; Wiseman, 1995).

Table 4. Inhibition of low density lipoprotein peroxidation by Tamoxifen and related compounds

Compound/drug	IC_{50} values (micromole)
Tamoxifen	29.3
4-Hydroxytamoxifen	1.9
17ß-Oestradiol	3.1

Other cardioprotective effects of Tamoxifen: influence on cholesterol and lipoprotein and homocysteine levels

Treatment with Tamoxifen as an adjuvant in a group of 124 women with stage I and II breast cancer produced a significant decrease in serum cholesterol levels compared with a control group of 81 women with stage I and II breast cancer who were not taking a hormonal treatment or supplement (Schapira et al., 1990). In the Wisconsin Tamoxifen Study (randomised placebo-controlled double-blind study in disease-free women) Tamoxifen treatment was found to lower total cholesterol levels by 26 mg/dl and LDL cholesterol levels by 20% after three months of treatment (Love et al., 1991, 1994). Similarly the Royal Marsden Hospital preventative feasibility trial, again in disease-free women, reported a decrease of 15% in serum cholesterol levels (Powles et al., 1990; Jones and Powles, 1992). The Wisconsin Tamoxifen Study reported also that fibrinogen levels decreased by 52 mg/dl after six months and this may be associated with a decreased risk of arterial thrombosis (Love et al., 1992, 1994). Furthermore, the Royal Marsden Hospital pilot trial reported no adverse effect of Tamoxifen on coagulation (fibrinogen/antithrombin III ratio) (Powles et al., 1990; Jones and Powles, 1992).

Plasma levels of the lipoprotein (a) have been suggested to account for much of the previously unattributable risk for coronary heart disease (Hayden and Reidy, 1995). Lipoprotein (a) levels are not influenced by the dietary changes that can lower many of the other risk factors for coronary heart disease. The reasons for the extreme atherogenicity of lipoprotein (a) are not yet clear but upon oxidative modification it may promote macrophage transformation to foam cells and it may do this even more effectively than oxidised LDL (Witzum, 1994) (see above). Lipoprotein (a) may also directly promote the growth of atherosclerotic plaques. It is of great interest, therefore, that Tamoxifen has been reported to decrease the circulating levels of lipoprotein a in postmenopausal women and in breast cancer patients (Shewmon et al., 1994a,b).

Elevated plasma levels of homocysteine is another risk factor for cardiovascular disease (Ueland et al., 1992) and can induce oxidative damage to LDL (Hirano et al., 1994). Tamoxifen has been reported to decrease plasma levels of homocysteine (Anker et al., 1995). In a study of 31 postmenopausal women with breast cancer, the plasma homocysteine level was decreased by a mean value of 30% after 9-12 months of Tamoxifen treatment (Anker et al., 1995).

Antioxidant-mediated anticarcinogenic action of Tamoxifen

Oxidative DNA damage may be involved in the development of breast cancer. Increased steady-state levels of DNA base damage, with a pattern characteristic of hydroxyl radical attack, have been reported in DNA from invasive ductal carcinoma (IDC) (Malins and Haimanot, 1991; Malins et al., 1993). One study found a 9-fold increase in 8-OHG, 8-hydroxyadenine and 2,6-diamino-4-hydroxy-5-formamidopyrimidine in DNA from IDC compared to control tissue (Malins and Haimanot, 1991). It is not clear though whether this is due to decreased DNA repair and/or increased oxidative DNA damage. DNA damage by ROS is also implicated in inflammatory breast disease (Wiseman and Halliwell, 1995), where malignant progression can occur.

Tamoxifen has been reported to suppress formation of the ROS H_2O_2 by human neutrophils (Lim et al., 1992; Wei and Frenkel, 1993). Hydrogen peroxide is capable of the malignant transformation of cells and tumour promotion, and it can also react with transition metal ions that are is close proximity with nuclear DNA to produce the hydroxyl radical. Tamoxifen could therefore act as an anticarcinogenic agent by suppressing hydrogen peroxide production by neutrophils, thus also preventing hydroxyl radical-mediated DNA damage.

Another possible mutagenic effect of the ROS involves their attack on membrane lipids, to initiate lipid peroxidation. The lipid peroxides formed can subsequently decompose to mutagenic carbonyl products. For example, 4-hydroxynonenal is genotoxic to lymphocytes and hepatocytes and also disrupts gap-junction communications in cultured endothelial cells (Esterbauer, 1993). Lipid peroxidation has been suggested to have a role in human breast cancer risk: urinary excretion of the mutagen malondialdehyde has been shown to be approximately double in women with mammographic displasia (high risk) than in women without these changes (Boyd and McGuire, 1991).

Tamoxifen may also play an anticarcinogenic role by inhibiting formation of the reactive intermediates and products arising from lipid peroxidation in the nuclear membrane that could otherwise damage nuclear DNA. The Tamoxifen metabolite, 4-hydroxytamoxifen was a more powerful inhibitor of lipid peroxidation than Tamoxifen in nuclear membranes (Wiseman and Halliwell, 1994). These anticarcinogenic actions of Tamoxifen could contribute to its prophylactic use against breast cancer.

Future importance of the antioxidant-mediated anticarcinogenic and cardioprotective actions of Tamoxifen

Potential alternatives to Tamoxifen for breast cancer treatment include the Tamoxifen derivative droloxifene (Bruning, 1992; Hasmann et al., 1994) and the pure oestrogen antagonists (derived from 17 ß-oestradiol) such as ICI 164 384 and ICI 182 780 (structures shown in Figure 3). Droloxifene has several advantages over Tamoxifen, including a shorter terminal elimination half-life, lower accumulation, improved drug tolerability and decreased occurrence of resistant cancer cells and a decreased risk of endometrial cancer (Bruning, 1992; Hasmann et al., 1994). Furthermore, it is an effective antioxidant (Wiseman et al., 1992).

ICI 182 780 is being investigated for use with breast cancer patients (De Friend et al., 1994) in particular those who have suffered a relapse following development of resistance to Tamoxifen therapy (Wakeling, 1993; Dowsett et al., 1995). Although the cardioprotective plasma cholesterol-lowering action of Tamoxifen arises from its partial oestrogen antagonist action, pure antioestrogens may still achieve a cardioprotective

Figure 3. Structures of pure oestrogen antagonists

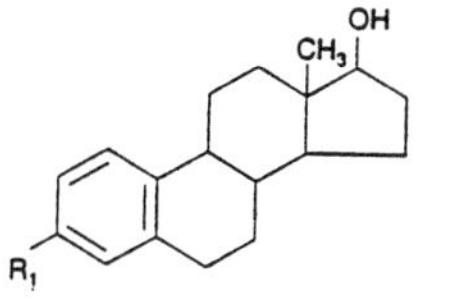

17β-oestradiol

R₁ = OH

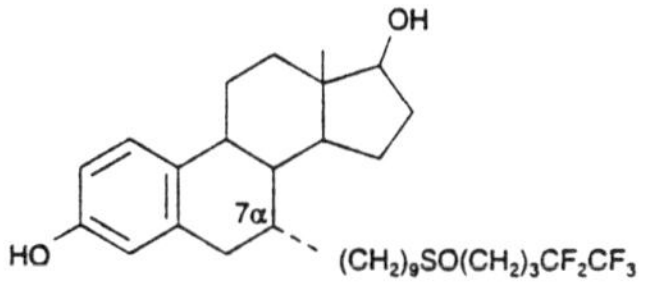

ICI182780

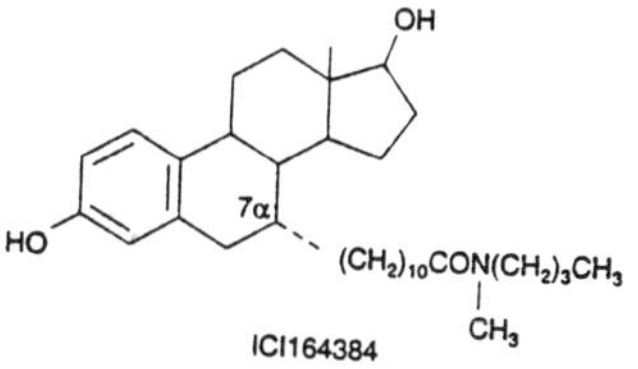

ICI164384

action similar to that of Tamoxifen even in the absence of cholesterol lowering abilities providing they are potent antioxidants and can protect LDL against oxidative modification.

Protection of LDL against oxidative damage is likely to be an important component of the cardioprotective action of Tamoxifen. ICI 164 384 has been reported to be a good inhibitor of lipid peroxidation in both microsomal and liposomal systems and was overall of comparable effectiveness with Tamoxifen although not as effective as 4-hydroxytamoxifen and 17 ß-oestradiol (Wiseman, 1994c). The ability of these new pure oestrogen antagonists to protect LDL against oxidative damage also requires urgent investigation to provide a more relevant indicator of possible antioxidant and cardioprotective action.

The justification for the routine use of Tamoxifen as a protective agent against breast cancer in healthy women could depend not only on its effectiveness as a prophylactic agent but also on its other beneficial health effects such as its possible antioxidant-mediated cardioprotective action. The results of the large prophylactic Tamoxifen trials are thus awaited with interest to see if Tamoxifen is successful as an anticarcinogenic agent and whether significant cardioprotection is observed (Wiseman, 1994a, 1995).

REFERENCES

Ames BN (1989): Endogenous oxidative DNA damage, aging and cancer. *Free Rad Res Communs* 7:121-128

Anker G, Lonning PE, Ueland PM, Refsum H and Lein EA (1995): Plasma levels of the atherogenic amino acid homocysteine in post-menopausal women with breast cancer treated with tamoxifen. *Int J Cancer* 60:365-368

Bruning PE (1992): Droloxifene, a new anti-oestrogen in postmenopausal advanced breast cancer: preliminary results of a double-blind dose-finding study phase II trial. *Eur J Cancer* 28A:1404-1407

Boyd NF and McGuire V (1991): The possible role of lipid peroxidation in breast cancer risk. *Free Rad Biol Med* 10:185-190

Cerutti P (1994): Oxy-radicals and cancer. *Lancet* 344:862-863

Chatterjee SN and Agarwal S (1988): Liposomes as a membrane model for study of lipid peroxidation. *Free Rad Biol Med* 4:51-72

Darley-Usmar V, Wiseman H and Halliwell (1995): Nitric oxide and oxygen radicals: A question of balance. *FEBS Lett* (in press)

Dean RT, Gieseg S and Davies MJ (1993): Reactive species and their accumulation on radical-damaged proteins. *Trends Biochem Sci* 18:437-441

De Friend DJ, Howell A, Nicholson RI, Anderson E, Dowsett M, Mansel RE, Blamey RW, Bundred NJ, Robertson JF, Saunders C, Baum M, Walton P, Sutcliffe F and Wakeling AE (1994): Investigation of a new pure antioestrogen (ICI 182 780) in women with primary breast cancer. *Cancer Res* 54:408-414

Dowsett M, Johnston SRD, Iveson TJ and Smith IE (1995): Response to specific anti-oestrogen (ICI 182 780) in tamoxifen-resistant breast cancer. *Lancet* 345:525

Esterbauer H (1993): Cytotoxicity and genotoxicity of lipid-oxidation products. *Am J Clin Nutr* (suppl) 57:779s-786s

Esterbauer H, Gebicki J, Puhl H and Jurgens G (1992): The role of lipid peroxidation and antioxidants in oxidative modification of LDL. *Free Rad Biol Med* 13:341-390

Frei B (1995): Cardiovascular disease and nutrient antioxidants: Role of low-density lipoprotein oxidation. *Critical Reviews in Food Science and Nutrition* 35:83-98

Gelety TJ and Judd HL (1992): Menopause: new indications and management strategies. *Curr Opin Obstet Gynecol* 4:346-353

Gey KF (1995): Ten-year retrospective on the antioxidant hypothesis of arteriosclerosis: Threshold plasma levels of antioxidant micronutrients related to minimum cardiovascular risk. *J Nutr Biochem* 6:206-236

Girelli D, Olivieri O, Stanzial AM, Guarini P, Trevisan MT, Bassi A and Corrocher R (1994): Factors affecting the thiobarbituric acid test as index of red blood cell suspectibility to lipid peroxidation: A multivariate analysis. *Clin Chim Acta* 227:45-57

Gurr MI and Harwood JL (1991): Lipid Biochemistry: An Introduction. 4th ed. London: Chapman and Hall

Gutteridge JMC (1993): Free radicals in disease processes: A complication of cause and consequence. *Free Rad Res Communs* 19:141-158

Gutteridge JMC and Halliwell B (1994): Antioxidants in Nutrition, Health and Disease. Oxford: Oxford University Press

Halliwell B (1990): How to characterize a biological antioxidant. *Free Rad Res Commun* 9:1-32

Halliwell B (1993): The role of oxygen radicals in human disease, with particular reference to the vascular system. *Haemostasis* (suppl) 23:118-126

Halliwell B (1994): Free radicals and antioxidants: a personal view. *Nutrition Reviews* 52:253-265

Halliwell B and Chirico S (1993): Lipid peroxidation: Its mechanism, measurement and significance. *Am J Clin Nutr* 57:15S-25S

Halliwell B and Gutteridge JMC (1989): Free Radical Biology and Medicine 2nd edition. Oxford: Clarendon Press

Hasmann M, Rattel B and Loser (1994): Preclinical data for droloxifene. *Cancer Lett* 84:101-116

Hayden MR and Reidy M (1995): Many roads lead to atheroma. *Nature Med* 1:22-23

Hirano K, Ogihara T, Miki M, Yauda H, Tamai H, Kawamura N and Mino M (1994): Homocysteine induces iron-catalysed lipid peroxidation of low-density lipoprotein that is prevented by alpha-tocopherol. *Free Rad Res* 21:267-276

Jones AL and Powles TJ (1992): The development of cancer chemoprevention trials. In: Introducing New Treatments for Cancer Practical, Ethical and Legal Problems. Williams CJ, ed. Chichester: John Wiley & Sons

Lim JS, Frenkel K and Toll W (1992): Tamoxifen supresses tumour promoter-induced hydrogen peroxide formation by human neutrophils. *Cancer Res* 52:4969-4972

Love RR, Wiebe DA, Feyzi JM, Newcombe PA and Chappell RJ (1994): Effects of tamoxifen on cardiovascular risk factors in postmenopausal women after 5 years of treatment. *J Natl Cancer Institute* 86:1534-1537

Love RR, Surawicz TS and Williams EC (1992): Antithrombin III level, fibrinogen level, and platelet count changes with adjuvant tamoxifen therapy. *Arch Int Med* 152:317-320

Love RR, Wiebe DA, Newcombe PA, Cameron L, Leventhal H, Jordan VC, Feyzi J and DeMets DL (1991): Effects of tamoxifen on cardiovascular risk factors in postmenopausal women. *Ann Intern Med* 15:860-864

Malins DC, and Haimanot R (1991): Major alterations in the nucleotide structure of DNA in cancer of the female breast. *Cancer Res* 51:5430-5432

Malins DC, Holmes EH, Polissar NL and Gunselman SJ (1993): The etiology of breast cancer: Characteristic alterations in hydroxyl radical-induced DNA base lesions during oncogenesis with potential for evaluating incidence of risk. *Cancer* 71:3036-3043

McDonald CC and Stewart HJ (1991): Fatal myocardial infarction in the Scottish adjuvant tamoxifen trial. *Br Med J* 303:435-437

Miller VT (1994): Lipids, lipoproteins, women and cardiovascular disease. *Atherosclerosis* (suppl)108:S73-S82

Neuzil J, Gebicki JM and Stocker R (1993): Radical-induced chain oxidation of proteins and its inhibition by chain-breaking antioxidants. *Biochem J* 293:601-606

New RRC (1992): Liposomes: A practical approach. Oxford: IRL Press

Parthasarathy S and Santanam N (1994): Mechanism of oxidation, antioxidants and atherosclerosis. *Curr Opin Lipodol* 5:371-375

Peck MD (1994): Interactions of lipids with immune function I: Biochemical effects of dietary lipids on plasma membranes. *J Nutr Biochem* 5:466-478

Powles TJ, Tillyer CR, Jones AL, Treleavan J, Davey JB, McKinna JA (1990): Prevention of breast cancer with tamoxifen: An update of the Royal Marsden Hospital pilot programme. *Eur J Cancer* 6:680-684

Rice-Evans CA and Bruckdorfer KR (1992): Free radicals, lipoproteins and cardiovascular dysfunction. *Molec Aspects Med* 13:1-111

Rifici VA and Khachadurian AK (1992): The inhibition of low-density lipoprotein oxidation by 17 ß-estradiol. *Metabolism* 41:1110-1114

Rutqvist LE and Mattsson A (1993): Cardiac and thromboembolic morbidity among postmenopausal women with early-stage breast cancer in a randomized trial of adjuvant tamoxifen. The Stockhom Breast Cancer Study Group. *J Natl Cancer Inst* 85:1398-1406

Sack MN, Rader DJ and Cannon RO (1994): Oesterogen and inhibition of oxidation of low-density lipoproteins in postmenopausal women. *Lancet* 343:269-270

Schapira DV, Kumar NB and Lyman GH (1990): Serum cholesterol reduction with tamoxifen. *Breast Cancer Res Treat* 17:3-7

Shewmon DA, Stoch JL, Abusamra LC, Kristan MA, Baker S and Heiniluoma KM (1994): Tamoxifen decreased lipoprotein(a) in patients with breast cancer. *Metabolism* 43:531-532

Shewmon DA, Stock JL, Rosen CJ, Heiniluoma KM, Hogue MM, Morrison A, Doyle EM, Ukena T, Weale V and Baker S (1994): Tamoxifen and estrogen lower circulating lipoprotein(a) concentrations in healthy postmenopausal women. *Arterioscler Thromb* 14:1586-1593

Smith C, Mitchinson M, Aruoma OI and Halliwell B (1992): Stimulation of lipid peroxidation and hydroxyl radical generation by the contents of human atherosclerotic lesions. *Biochem J* 286:901-905

Stadtman ER (1993): Oxidation of free amino acids and amino acid residues in proteins by radiolysis and by metal-catalysed reactions. *Ann Rev Biochem* 62:797-821

Stampfer MJ, Colditz GA, Willett WC, Manson JE, Rosner B, Speizer FE and Hennekens CH (1991): Postmenopausal estrogen therapy and cardiovascular disease: Ten-year follow-up from the nurses' health study. *New Engl J Med* 325:756-762

Thomas JP, Kalyanaraman B and Girotti AW (1994): Involvement of pre-existing lipid hydroperoxides in Cu^{2+}-stimulated oxidation of low-density lipoprotein. *Arch Biochem Biophys* 315:244-254

Ueland PM, Refsum H and Brattstrom L (1992): Atherosclerotic cardiovascular disease, hemostasis and endothelial function. In: Plasma Homocysteine and Cardiovascular Disease. Francis RB ed. New York: Marcel Dekker Inc.

Wakeling AE (1993): The future of new pure antioestrogens in clinical breast cancer. *Breast Cancer Res Treat* 25:1-10

Wei H and Frenkel K (1993): Relationship of oxidative events and DNA oxidation in SENCAR mice to *in vivo* promoting activity of phorbol ester-type tumour promoters. *Carcinogenesis* 14:195-201

Williamson P and Schegel RA (1994): Back and forth: the regulation and function of transbilayer phospholipid movement in eukaryotic cells. *Molec Membrane Biol* 11:199-216

Wiseman H (1994a): Tamoxifen: Molecular Basis of Use in Cancer Treatment and Prevention. Chichester: John Wiley & Sons

Wiseman H (1994b): Tamoxifen: new membrane-mediated mechanisms of action and therapeutic advances. *Trends Pharmacol Sci* 15:83-89

Wiseman H (1994c): The antioxidant action of a pure antiestrogen: Ability to inhibit lipid peroxidation compared to tamoxifen and 17ß-oestradiol and relevance to its anticancer potential. *Biochem Pharmacol* 47:493-498

Wiseman H (1994d): Tamoxifen and estrogens as membrane antioxidants: Comparison with cholesterol. *Methods in Enzymology Vol. 234 Oxygen Radicals in Biological Systems Part D* Packer L ed. San Diego: Academic Press

Wiseman H (1995): Tamoxifen as an antioxidant and cardioprotectant. In: Biochemical Society Symposium 61, Free radicals and oxidative stress: environment drugs and food additives, Rice-Evans C and Halliwell B eds. Lond: ortland Press

Wiseman H and Halliwell B (1993): Carcinogenic antioxidants: Diethylstilboestrol, hexoestrol and 17 alpha-ethynyloestradiol. *FEBS Lett* 332:159-163

Wiseman H and Halliwell B (1994): Tamoxifen and related compounds protect against lipid peroxidation in isolated nuclei: Relevance to the potential anticarcinogenic benefits of breast cancer prevention and therapy with tamoxifen. *Free Rad Biol Med* 17:485-488

Wiseman H and Halliwell B (1995): Damage to DNA by reactive oxygen and nitrogen species: Role in inflammatory disease and progression to cancer. *Biochem J* (in press)

Wiseman H and Quinn P (1994): The antioxidant action of synthetic oestrogens involves decreased membrane fluidity: Relevance to their potential use as anticancer and cardioprotective agents compared to tamoxifen. *Free Rad Res* 21:187-194

Wiseman H, Arnstein HRV, Cannon M and Halliwell B (1990b): Mechanism of inhibition of lipid peroxidation by tamoxifen and 4-hydroxytamoxifen introduced into lipsomes: Similarity to cholesterol and ergosterol. *FEBS Lett* 274:107-110

Wiseman H, Cannon M, Arnstein HRV and Halliwell B (1993a): Tamoxifen inhibits peroxidation in cardiac microsomes: Comparison with liver microsomes and potential relevance to the cardiovascular benefits associated with cancer prevention and treatment by tamoxifen. *Biochem Pharmacol* 45:1851-1855

Wiseman H, Laughton MJ, Arnstein HRV, Cannon M and Halliwell B (1990a): The antioxidant action of tamoxifen and its metabolites. Inhibition of lipid peroxidation. *FEBS Lett* 263:192-194

Wiseman H, Smith C, Halliwell B, Cannon M, Arnstein HRV and Lennard MS (1992): Droloxifene (3-hydroxytamoxifen) has membrane antioxidant ability: Potential relevance to its mechanism of therapeutic action in breast cancer. *Cancer Lett* 66:61-68

Wiseman H, Paganga G, Rice-Evans C, Halliwell B (1993c): Protective actions of tamoxifen and 4-hydroxytamoxifen against oxidative damage to human low-density lipoproteins. A mechanism accounting for the cardioprotective action of tamoxifen? *Biochem J* 292:635-638

Wiseman H, Quinn P, and Halliwell B (1993b): Tamoxifen and related compounds decrease membrane fluidity in liposomes. Mechanism for the antioxidant action of tamoxifen and relevance to its anticancer and cardioprotective actions? *FEBS Lett* 330:53-56

Witzum JL (1994):   The oxidation hypothesis of atherosclerosis.   *Lancet*
    344:792-795
Zachowski A (1993):   Phospholipids in animal eukaryotic membranes:
    transverse asymmetry and movement. *Biochem J* 294:1-14

15. ANTIESTROGEN REGULATION OF *erb*B2 EXPRESSION IN HUMAN BREAST CANCER CELLS

Anni M.Wärri and Pirkko L. Härkönen

> *"Genes are thicker*
> *than water."*
> *(Meredith Small)*

The *erb*B2 protein is supposed to have important functions as a growth factor receptor during growth and differentiation as well as in normal function of the mammary epithelium. It can be activated to a transforming oncogene and in human breast cancer, the amplification and/or overexpression of *erb*B2 gene is associated with aggressive growth of the tumor and poor prognosis of the patient. The expression of *erb*B2 is regulated by estrogen and the antiestrogens Tamoxifen and Toremifene which are both used in the treatment of breast cancer. The knowledge of the role and mechanisms of the antiestrogen regulation of this important growth factor receptor and potential oncogene would provide important information of the biology and therapeutic possibilities of human breast cancer.

The erbB2 protein is a growth factor receptor

The *erb*B2 protein belongs to the receptor tyrosine kinases which mediate the effects of polypeptide growth factors on cell growth and differentiation. The *erb*B2 gene (also called HER-2 or *neu* according to the rat homologue) encodes a transmembrane glycoprotein of 185 kD with a tyrosine kinase activity. It is closely related to the genes encoding EGF receptor as well as *erb*B3 and *erb*B4 proteins which belong to the class I receptor subfamily of the receptor tyrosine kinases (Ullrich and Schlessinger, 1990; Peles and Yarden, 1993). Binding of specific ligands to the extracellular domains of these receptors leads to stimulation of their intrinsic tyrosine kinase activity and activation of the intracellular signal transduction pathways. Under experimental conditions, aberrant activation of the receptor tyrosine kinases leads to malignant transformation and growth stimulation of several cell types (Peles and Yarden, 1993). Activation of the genes for the EGF and *erb*B receptor family by amplification or other mechanisms frequently observed in human malignancies are supposed to be associated with tumorigenesis and/or progression of tumor growth. Amplification and/or overexpression of *erb*B2 gene have been particularly associated with aggressive growth and poor prognosis of human breast cancer (Slamon et al., 1987; 1989; Perren, 1991).

So far, no specific ligand has been found for *erb*B2 protein although several polypeptide factors are known to indirectly stimulate its tyrosine kinase activity. They do so by binding specifically to other members of the EGF receptor subfamily (EGFR, *erb*B3, *erb*B4) which form heterodimers with *erb*B2 protein (Peles and Yarden, 1993; Carraway and Cantley, 1994; Plowman et al., 1994). The *erb*B2 protein can thus be autophosphorylated and indirectly activated at least by EGF and TGFalpha which are ligands for EGF receptor. The same is true for the heregulins which are specific ligands for *erb*B3 and *erb*B4. The heregulins (also called neuregulin, *neu* differentiation factor, ARIA = acetylcholinereceptor- inducing activity, glial growth factor) are products of a single heregulin gene formed by alternative splicing of the primary transcript (Marchionni et al., 1993; Peles and Yarden, 1993).

Although it is possible that there is a specific ligand and distinct, as yet unknown function for *erb*B2 it is evident in any case that this receptor protein definitely plays an important role as a modulator of the functions of the other *erb*B receptor tyrosine kinases and the EGF receptor by forming heterodimers with them. It is possible that each combination of the receptor heterodimers initiates and specifies a distinct signal transduction pathway. This could explain the diversity of functions associated with *erb*B2 protein in different cell types such as mammary epithelial and breast cancer cells, neural cells and differentiating myotubes.

In the absence of a specific ligand, various indirect approaches have been used to analyse the signal transduction pathways of *erb*B2. They have included use of a chimeric receptor formed by EGF receptor ectodomain fused to the transmembrane and intracellular domains of *erb*B2 (Lehväslaiho et al., 1989) or the constitutively activated, mutated *erb*B2. Also, monoclonal antibodies (such as 4D5) against *erb*B2 which stimulate autophosphorylation and kinase activity of the protein have been used to mimic the function of a putative specific ligand (Dougall et al., 1994). The studies with EGF receptor/*erb*B2 chimeras demonstrated activation of several early response genes as well as the genes involved in transcriptional activation or cell-cycle progression. The stimulation was very similar to that seen in case of the EGF receptor-mediated activation (Koskinen et al., 1990). In studies on the signal transduction pathways initiated by *erb*B2, phosphorylation and activation of different cytosolic signal transducers has been observed (Dougall et al., 1994; Stein et al., 1994). It is possible that the *erb*B2 activation leading to stimulation of cell proliferation is coupled to the MAP kinase pathways whereas other mechanisms may be involved in differentiative signalling (Peles and Yarden, 1993) but the significance of different mediators in the physiological or oncogenic actions of *erb*B2 is poorly understood.

The function of normal *erb*B2 is not known but it has been associated both with growth, development and expression of the differentiated phenotype of the mammary gland and other tissues and cells. The *erb*B2 protein and other *erb*B receptors are expressed mainly in epithelial and neural tissues but also in several other cell types during embryonal development and in adult organisms (Kraus et al., 1989; Prigent and Lemoine, 1992). In the fetal mammary gland they are expressed in developing epithelia of the growing and branching ductal tree. During pregnancy, *erb*B2 expression is associated with tubular morphogenesis and it is also high during the lobulo-alveolar development of the glandular tree towards the end of pregnancy (Meyer and Birchmeier, 1994). The expression of the *erb*B receptors is associated with the expression of various forms of neuregulin in the surrounding mesenchyme. This suggests an important role for the *erb*B receptors in mediation of inductive signals of mesenchymal origin on the differentiation of the mammary gland.

Besides the phases of rapid growth and differentiation, elevated *erb*B2 protein levels have also been reported in the fully differentiated, lactating mammary gland of the rat (Dati et al., 1990). Accordingly, stimulation of *erb*B2/*neu* autophosphorylation by heregulins and other candidate ligands was observed to mainly promote differentiation in several mammary epithelial and breast cancer cell lines (Taverna et al., 1991; Bacus et al., 1992; Marte et al., 1995). It is obvious that a specific combination of a particular ligand (one of the heregulins, EGF or TGFalpha) and a particular form of heterodimer with another class I receptor tyrosine kinase eventually determines whether the biological effect of *erb*B2 in a given situation is growth or differentiation promoting (Peles and Yarden, 1993; Marte et al., 1995). The complex pattern of the ligands and receptors involved may thus largely explain why previous results concerning the function of *erb*B2 seemed rather conflicting. However, the obvious importance of *erb*B2 in the biology of clinical breast cancer emphasises its particular role in the network of class I receptor tyrosine kinase interactions.

The activated erbB2 is a transforming oncogene

The oncogenic potential of *erb*B2 has been demonstrated by experimental studies *in vitro* and *in vivo*. A point mutation in the transmembrane domain of the rat *neu* protein leads to constitutively increased tyrosine kinase activity and converts rat *neu* into a transforming oncogene (Hung et al., 1986; Bargmann and Weinberg, 1988; Stern et al., 1988). In transgenic mice, overexpression of mutated (Müller at al., 1988; Bouchard et al., 1989) as well as unactivated (Guy et al., 1992) rat *neu* coupled to a mammary specific MMTV (mouse mammary tumor virus) LTR-promoter resulted in the development of mammary adenocarcinomas.

No mutations of human *erb*B2 gene have been found, however, in clinical human breast cancers in which the activation and expression of high level of *erb*B2 protein appears to occur through amplification and/or overexpression of the gene. It has been experimentally shown, however, that overexpression of transfected non-mutated human *erb*B2 in mouse fibroblasts (Hudziak et al., 1987; DiFiore et al., 1987) as well as in immortalized human mammary epithelial cells (Pierce et al., 1991) led to their malignant transformation and tumor growth in atymic mice.

The erbB2 is overexpressed in a large proportion of in human breast cancers

The *erb*B2 gene is overexpressed in about 20-25% of human breast cancers (van de Vijver and Nusse, 1991; Ciocca et al., 1992). A role for *erb*B2 in human breast cancer has been proposed on the basis of studies correlating the *erb*B2 amplification and/or high protein levels with aggressive growth of the tumors and poor prognosis of the patients

(Slamon et al., 1987; 1989; Gullick et la., 1991; Kallioniemi et al., 1991). The high incidence of the *erb*B2 gene amplification in non-invasive breast tumors as well as staining of most if not all of malignant cells within a tumor suggest that the activation of this oncogene is one of the earliest and most common genetic lesions in human breast cancer (Liu et al., 1992; Kallioniemi et al., 1992).

Overexpression of *erb*B2 without gene amplification has been detected in a considerable proportion of human breast cancer patients with tumors expressing high levels of *erb*B2 protein associated with a poor clinical outcome (Kraus et al., 1987; Slamon et al., 1987; 1989). This suggests that other mechanisms than amplification can also lead to enhanced expression and, probably, to oncogenic activation of *erb*B2 in human breast cancers. In addition, the high level of *erb*B2 protein expression in human breast cancers has been found to strongly correlate with the absence of estrogen and progesterone receptors (Borg et al., 1991; Perren, 1991; Gasparini et al., 1993) which leads to the question of possible steroid regulation of *erb*B2.

The mechanisms of regulation of normal and amplified *erb*B2 expression thus seem to be of great importance when considering the possibilities of controlling growth and progression of breast cancer cells. This is especiallly true for possible regulation by Tamoxifen and Toremifene which are widely used in the treatment of breast cancer (Jordan and Murphy, 1990). Both substances (Kallio et al., 1986) are potent antiestrogens but they have also shown to have antitumor effects which are mediated by other mechanisms (Kangas et al., 1986; Jordan and Murphy, 1990). In the following we will discuss possible mechanisms of *erb*B2 regulation by Tamoxifen and Toremifene.

The antiestrogens Tamoxifen and Toremifene regulate erbB2 expression

The expression of *erb*B2 mRNA and protein has been shown to be under hormone and growth factor regulation in several human breast cancer cell lines which contain a single copy of the gene (Dati et al., 1990, Read et al., 1990; Wärri et al., 1991; Taverna et al., 1994). In the presence of estrogen, *erb*B2 expression is strongly suppressed. In contrast, it is induced upon withdrawal of estrogen or treatment of breast cancer cells with the antiestrogens Toremifene (Wärri et al., 1991; Wärri, 1993) or Tamoxifen (Dati et al., 1990, Read et al., 1990; Wärri et al, 1991, Taverna 1994). These results were also confirmed *in vivo* in nude mouse tumors of human MCF-7 or ZR 75-1 breast cancer cells in which *erb*B2

mRNA was rapidly induced by treatment of the mice with Tamoxifen or
Toremifene (Wärri et al., 1991). It is notable that in these breast cancer
cell lines which are all stimulated to proliferate actively in the presence
of estrogen the high growth rate was associated with suppression of
erbB2 expression both *in vivo* and *in vitro*. Also, progesterone (Taverna
et al., 1994) as well as retinoic acid and prolactin (unpublished results)
which all have differentiating effects seemed to increase erbB2 mRNA
levels in human breast cancer cells. The levels of erbB2 mRNA were
also high in nonproliferating, confluent cultures (Taverna et al., 1994).

*Mechanisms of estrogen and antiestrogen regulation of erbB2 mRNA
expression are different*

The analysis of estrogen suppression of erbB2 mRNA expression showed
that the synthesis of new proteins was not required (Wärri, 1993). This
could be explained by direct effect of estrogen on erbB2 transcription
which conclusion is also supported by the decreased erbB2 promoter
activity as demonstrated in transient transfection assays (Taverna et al.,
1994). The analysis of erbB2 promoter structure has demonstrated both
positive and negative regulatory elements (Chen and Gill, 1994) but no
estrogen or steroid responsive elements have been found (Hudson et al.,
1990). The deletion analysis of 5' upstream sequences of the rat
neu/erbB2 promoter has demonstrated, however, a 140 bp fragment which
was able to confer suppressive effect of estrogen on a heterologous
promoter (Russell and Hung, 1992). These observations could be
explained by the interaction of the ligand-activated estrogen receptor with
another transcription factor which interaction would lead to suppression
of erbB2 transcription.

There are recent data on estrogen regulation of target gene
transcription by the interaction of the ligand-activated estrogen receptor
with specific promoter sequences via binding to intervening transcription
factors instead of directly binding to estrogen responsive elements
(Philips et al., 1993; Webb et al., 1995). The characteristics of the
factors and sequences involved in the mediation of estrogen effect by
protein-protein interactions are not fully understood but it is probable that
erbB2 is one of the target genes regulated by this type of mechanism.

The induction of erbB2 after Tamoxifen or Toremifene addition
or estrogen withdrawal was observed after 12 h but expression of erbB2
mRNA returned to the level of hormone-depleted controls only after 3
days (Wärri et al., 1991; Wärri, 1993). The interval required led to

anticipate that the mechanisms of antiestrogen induction are probably indirect. This was also suggested by the experiments using the inhibitors of RNA and protein synthesis which showed that the *de novo* protein synthesis is required for Toremifene induction of *erb*B2 mRNA expression. This was in contrast to estrogen suppression of *erb*B2 mRNA expression which was not dependent on the *de novo* protein synthesis. The results suggest, however, that synthesis of additional transcription factor(s) was required for Toremifene induction of *erb*B2 mRNA expression.   Hollywood and Hurst (1993) recently described a DNA-binding protein, called OB2-1 which might be responsible for enhanced *erb*B2 expression irrespective of the amplification of the gene. It is not yet known, however, whether Tamoxifen or Toremifene-activated estrogen receptor would be able to interfere with the expression or binding activity of this transcription factor.

Another mechanism of increasing the steady-state level of a specific mRNA is to slow down the rate of its degradation. Experiments with the inhibitors of RNA synthesis suggested that the half-life of *erb*B2 mRNA in various breast cancer cell lines was relatively long (9-12 h). Comparable estimations have recently been reported both for a single-copy (Hollywood and Hurst, 1993) and amplified *erb*B2 (Pasleau et al., 1993) in cancer cells as well as in non-malignant HBL-100 mammary epithelial cells (Hollywood and Hurst, 1993). They indicate that prolonged mRNA half-life does not contribute to the enhanced *erb*B2 expression in breast cancer cells in comparison to nontransformed mammary cells. The addition of Toremifene to the culture medium of ZR-75-1 or MCF-7 human breast cancer cells did, however, clearly increase the half-life of *erb*B2 mRNA in comparison to the cells grown without the antiestrogen and in the absence of estrogen (Wärri, 1993). This indicates that in addition to induction of *erb*B2 gene transcription which is likely to occur by Toremifene inhibition of estrogen interaction with its receptor (Kallio et al., 1986), Toremifene separately affects the rate of mRNA turnover. Both transcriptional and posttranscriptional mechanisms thus contribute to the high level of *erb*B2 mRNA expression observed during Tamoxifen and Toremifene treatment of breast cancer cells.

Amplification of erbB2 gene is associated with loss of Tamoxifen and Toremifene responsiveness

The regulation of *erb*B2 gene by estrogen and antiestrogens is clearly different in human breast cancer cells in which *erb*B2 is amplified (Wärri et al., 1994; 1995). In BT-474 human breast cancer cells the expression of amplified *erb*B2 could be only transiently decreased by estrogen and in the prolonged treatment, no effect on *erb*B2 expression was observed although proliferation of the cells was still stimulated by estrogen. The relative refractoriness to estrogen was associated with total resistance to Tamoxifen and Toremifene which could not affect either proliferation or *erb*B2 expression in these cells (Wärri et al., 1994).

The responses of the BT-474 cells are reminiscent of the situation in clinical breast tumors in which *erb*B2 is amplified and the level of functional estrogen receptors low or undetectable (Wright et al., 1989; Kallioniemi et al., 1991). Clinically most *erb*B2 amplified tumors which are estrogen receptor-positive are resistant to Tamoxifen treatment (Wright et al., 1992; Borg et al., 1993). A corresponding result was also obtained experimentally in MCF-7 cells which became Tamoxifen-resistant after transfection with and overexpression of *erb*B2 gene although their growth rate was still stimulated by estrogen (Benz et al., 1992). The observation demonstrates that Tamoxifen responsiveness is not determined only by the presence of functional estrogen receptors. It also suggests that the function of normal, unactivated *erb*B2 protein may have an important role in Tamoxifen and Toremifene responsiveness of human breast cancer cells.

Shedding of the ectodomain of erbB2 protein provides an additional level of antiestrogen regulation

The extracellular domain of *erb*B2 protein has been recently found in the serum samples of the patients with breast cancers which overexpress *erb*B2 (Leitzel et al., 1991; Breuer et al., 1993; Isola et al., 1993). It has also been detected in the sera of tumor-bearing nude mice as well as in the cell culture media of human breast cancer cells (Alper et al., 1991; Lin and Clinton, 1991; Zabrecky et al., 1991). The size of the shedded fragment (approximately 105-130 kD) is close to the predicted size (118 kD) of the extracellular domain of unfragmented 185 kD *erb*B2 protein.

We found that the concentration of extracellular domain was substantially increased *in vitro* in the culture medium of the BT-474 human breast cancer cells which were grown in the presence of Toremifene (Wärri et al., 1995). The effect was concentration dependent. It greatly exceeded the slight increase observed when the cells were grown in the absence of estrogen in comparison to the cultures in the estrogen-containing medium. These data indicate that Toremifene may specifically contribute to the shedding of the extracellular domain of *erb*B2. This mechanism seems to concern, however, only the breast cancer cells which express *erb*B2 protein at a very high level. No extracellular domain could be detected in the analysis of the media conditioned by the breast cancer cell lines (MCF-7, ZR-75-1, T47D) expressing a single-copy *erb*B2 (Wärri et al., 1995).

The mechanisms of synthesis and cleavage of the soluble extracellular domain have not yet been settled. Gene rearrangement, alternative splicing, and proteolytic cleavage are all possible as shown for several other membrane-spanning receptors. Scott et al. (1993) have reported that a 2.3 kb mRNA, produced by alternative splicing of the *erb*B2 transcript, encodes a truncated *erb*B2 protein. This closely corresponds to the extracellular domain of about 100 kD found in the conditioned media of BT-474 and SK-BR-3 cells (Alper et al., 1990, Zabrecky et al., 1991). The 2.3 kb transcript was detectable in the analysis of BT-474 mRNA, but its level did not show any response to the treatment with Toremifene. Nor did the levels of cellular *erb*B2 protein change (Wärri et al., 1994). The remaining possibility of Toremifene induction or stimulation of the proteolytic cleavage of *erb*B2 protein required to produce the extracellular domain observed has not yet been studied. It is most likely, however, that posttranscriptional or posttranslational mechanisms are involved in the production of the soluble extracellular domain during the treatment with the antiestrogens Tamoxifen and Toremifene.

The regulation of the level of soluble extracellular domain of *erb*B2 protein might provide an extra level of antiestrogen control of the function of *erb*B2 protein in breast cancer cells. In case of the breast cancer cells which contained activated, amplified *erb*B2 this might also be the only mechanism by which the antiestrogens are able to influence the level and function of *erb*B2 protein. By competing for a cognate ligand, if any exists, or by heterodimerisation with the extracellular parts of the EGF-receptor and other *erb*B receptors, the soluble extracellular *erb*B2 domain might greatly influence the function of the receptor family (Scott et al., 1993). The significance of the shedding and antiestrogen regulation of the *erb*B2 extracellular domain remains, however, to be explored.

Possible role of erbB2 in response of human breast cancer to antiestrogens

Clinically the overexpression of *erb*B2 seems to be mostly associated with therapeutic resistance to Tamoxifen or Toremifene (Perren, 1991; Benz et al., 1992; Borg et al., 1994). This seems to be true also in the cases in which tumors are still estrogen receptor-positive. This observation is important when therapeutic possibilities are considered.

The role of *erb*B2 in growth regression of Tamoxifen or Toremifene responsive breast cancers is not known. There is, however, one report which shows that short Tamoxifen treatment of breast cancer patients leads to a marked increase in the cytoplasmic *erb*B2 immunoreactivity in estrogen receptor-positive tumors (Johnston et al., 1993). Much less increase of cytoplasmic staining was observed in estrogen receptor-negative tumors. In addition, Tamoxifen response of *erb*B2 immunoreactivity seemed to be associated with the tumors in which the level of membrane-located *erb*B2 protein was low as would be the case in the cells expressing normal, nonamplified *erb*B2. It is not known whether cytoplasmic *erb*B2 immunoreactivity represents the receptor form which has been endocytosed or the protein which is being synthesised but the observation strogly suggests that changes of normal, nonamplified *erb*B2 expression may occur and be of importance in the antiestrogen response of breast cancer cells.

In breast cancer tissue the expression and function of *erb*B2 is coupled to other receptor tyrosine kinases and heregulins or other putative ligands. They are known to be expressed in tumor tissues but their role in tumorigenesis and progression is not yet known. Their antihormone regulation is not known either, but it is evident that *in vivo*, the functional outcome of changes in *erb*B2 expression is also dependent on them.

Summary

The antiestrogens tamoxifen and toremifene induce the expression of normal *erb*B2 which is supposed to be an important regulator of growth and differentiation of breast cancer cells. The induction occurs both at transcriptional and posttranscriptional levels. Antiestrogen stimulation of *erb*B2 expression is associated with cessation of growth of breast cancer cells. The antiestrogen regulation of *erb*B2 expression is lost in breast cancer cells which contain the amplified and activated *erb*B2 gene. This is often accompanied by resistance of cell growth to the antiestrogens.

Tamoxifen and Toremifene are, however, able to increase the cleavage and shedding of the *erb*B2 protein ectodomain in these cells and possibly affect growth regulation by amplified *erb*B2.

REFERENCES

Alper Ö, Yamaguchi K, Hitomi J, Honda S, Matsiushima T, Abe K (1991): The presence of c-*erb*B-2 gene product-related protein in culture medium conditioned by breast cancer cell line SK-BR-3. *Cell Growth Different* 1:591-599

Bacus SS, Huberman E, Chin D, Kiguchi K, Simpson S, Lippman M, Lupu R (1992): A ligand for the *erb*B-2 oncogene product (gp 30) induces differentiation of human breast cancer cells. *Cell Growth Different* 3:401-411

Bargmann CI, Weinberg RA (1988): Increased tyrosine kinase activity associated with the protein encoded by the activated *neu* oncogene. *Proc Natl Acad Sci USA* 85:5394-5398

Benz CC, Scott GK, Sarup JC, Johnson RM, Tripathy D, Coronado E, Shepard HM, Osborne CK (1992): Estrogen-dependent, tamoxifen-resistant tumorigenic growth of MCF-7 cells transfected with HER2/*neu*. *Breast Cancer Res Treat* 244:85-95

Borg Å, Baldetorp B, Fernö M, Killander D, Olsson H, Sigurdsson H (1991): *ERB*B2 amplification in breast cancer with a high rate of proliferation. *Oncogene* 6:137-143

Borg Å, Baldetorp B, Fernö M, Killander D, Olsson H, Rydén S, Sigurdsson H (1994): *ERB*B2 amplification is associated with tamoxifen resistence in steroid receptor positive breast cancer. *Cancer Lett* 81:137-144

Bouchard L, Lamarre L, Tremblay PL, Jolicoeur P (1989): Stochastic appearance of mammary tumors in transgenic mice carrying the MMTV/c-*neu* oncogene. *Cell* 57:931-936

Breuer B, Luo J-C, DeVivo I, Pincus M, Tatum AH, Daucher J, Minick R, Osborne M, Miller D, Nowak E, Code H, Carney WP, Brandt-Rauf PW (1993): Detection of elevated c-*erb*B-2 oncoprotein in the serum and tissue in breast cancer. *Med Sci Res* 21:383-384

Carraway III KL, Cantley LC (1994): A new aquaintance for *erb*B3 and *erb*B4: A role for receptor heterodimerization in growth signaling. *Cell* 78:5-8

Chen Y, Gill GN (1994): Positive and negative regulatory elements in the human *erb*B-2 gene promoter. *Oncogene* 9:2269-2276

Ciocca DR, Fujimura FK, Tandon AK, Clark GM, Mark C, Lee-Chen G-J, Pounds GW, Vendely P, Owens MA, Pandian MR, McGuire WL (1992): Correlation of HER2/*neu* amplification with expression and with other prognostic factors in 1103 breast cancers. *J Natl Cancer Inst* 84:1279-1282

Dati C, Antoniotti S, Taverna D, Perroteau I, De Bortoli M (1990): Inhibition of c-*erb*B-2 oncogene expression by estrogens in human breast cancer cells. *Oncogene* 5:1001-1006

Di Fiore PP, Pierce JH, Kraus MH, Segatto O, King CR, Aaronson SA (1987): *erb*B-2 is a potent oncogene when overexpressed in NIH/3T3 cells. *Science* 237:178-182

Dougall WC, Qian X, Peterson NC, Miller M, Samanta A, Greene MI (1994): The *neu*-oncogene: signal transduction pathways, transformation mechanisms and evolving therapies. *Oncogene* 9:2109-2123

Gasparini G, Pozza F, Harris AL (1993): Evaluating the potential usefulness of new prognostic and predictive indicators in node-negative breast cancer patients. *J Natl Cancer Inst* 85:1206-1219

Gullick WJ, Love SB, Wright C, Barnes DM, Gusterson B, Harris AL, Altman DG (1991): c-*erb*B-2 protein overexpression in breast cancer is a risk factor in patients with involved and uninvolved lymph nodes. *Br J Cancer* 63:434-438

Guy CT, Webster MA, Schaller M, Parsons TJ, Cardiff RD, Muller WJ (1992): Expression of the *neu* proto-oncogene in the mammary epithelium of transgenic mice induces metastatic disease. *Proc Natl Acad Sci USA* 89:10578-10582

Hollywood DP, Hurst HC (1993): A novel transcription factor, OB2-1, is required for overexpression of the proto-oncogene c-*erb*B-2 in mammary tumour lines. *EMBO J* 12:2369-2375

Hudson LG, Ertl AP, Gill GN (1990): Structure and inducible regulation of the human c-*erb*B2/*neu* promoter. *J Biol Chem* 265:4389-4393

Hudziak RM, Schlessinger J, Ullrich A (1987): Increased expression of the putative growth factor receptor p185[HER2] causes transformation and tumorigenesis of NIH 3T3 cells. *Proc Natl Acad Sci USA* 84:7159-7163

Hung M-C, Schechter AL, Chevray P-YM, Stern DF, Weinberg RA (1986): Molecular cloning of the *neu* gene: Absence of gross structural alteration in oncogenic alleles. *Proc Natl Acad Sci USA* 83:261-264

Isola JJ, Holli K, Oksa H, Teramoto Y, Kallioniemi O-P (1994): Elevated *erb*B2 oncoprotein levels in pre-operative and follow-up serum samples define breast cancer patients with aggressive disease course. *Cancer* 3:652-658

Johnston SRD, McLennan KA, Salter J, Sacks NM, McKinna JA, Baum M, Smith IE, Dowsett M (1993): Tamoxifen induces the expression of cytoplasmic c-*erb*B2 immunoreactivity in oestrogen-receptor positive breast carcinomas *in-vivo*. *The Breast* 2:93-99

Jordan VC, Murphy CS (1990): Endocrine pharmacology of antiestrogens as antitumor agents. *Endocr Rev* 11:578-610

Kallio S, Kangas L, Blanco G, Johansson R, Karjalainen A, Perilä M, Piippo I, Sundquist H, Södervall M, Toivola R (1986): A new triphenylethylene compound, Fc-1157a. I. Hormonal effects. *Cancer Chemother Pharmacol* 17:103-108

Kallioniemi O-P, Holli K, Visakorpi T, Koivula T, Helin HH and Isola JJ (1993): Association of c-*erb*B-2 protein overexpression with high rate of cell proliferation, increased risk of visceral metastasis and poor long-term survival in breast cancer. *Int J Cancer* 49:650-655

Kallioniemi O-P, Kallioniemi A, Kurisu W, Thor A, Chen L-C, Smith HS, Waldman, FM, Pinkel D, Gray, JW (1992): *ERBB2* amplification in breast cancer analyzed by fluorescence *in situ* hybridization. *Proc Natl Acad Sci USA* 89:5321-5325

Kangas L, Nieminen A-L, Blanco G, Grönroos M, Kallio S, Karjalainen A, Perilä M, Södervall M, Toivola R (1986): A new triphenylethylene compound, Fc-1157a. II. Antitumor effect. *Cancer Chemother Pharmacol* 17:109-113

Koskinen P, Lehväslaiho H, MacDonald-Bravo H, Alitalo K, Bravo R (1990): Similar early responses to ligand-activated EGFR and *neu* tyrosine kinases in NIH3T3 cells. *Oncogene* 5:615-618

Kraus MH, Fedi P, Starks V, Muraro R and Aaronson SA (1993): Demonstration of ligand-dependent signaling by the *erb*B-3 tyrosine kinase and its constitutive activation in human breast tumor cells. *Proc Natl Acad Sci USA* 90:2900-2904

Langton BC, Crenshaw MC, Chao LA, Stuart SG, Akita RW, Jackson JE (1991): An antigen immunologically related to the extracellular domain of gp185 in shed from nude mouse tumors over-expressing the c-*erb*B-2 (HER-2/*neu*) oncogene. *Cancer Res* 51:2593-2598

Lehväslaiho H, Lehtola L, Sistonen L, Alitalo KA (1989): Chimeric EGF-R/*neu* proto-oncogene allows to regulate neu tyrosine kinase and cell transformation. *EMBO J* 8:159-166

Leitzel K, Teramoto Y, Sampson EL, Wallingford GA, Weaver S, Domero L, Harvey H, Lipton A (1991): Elevated c-*erb*B-2 levels in the serum and tumor extracts of breast cancer patients. *Proc Am Assoc Cancer Res* 32:997-1005

Lin YJ and Clinton GM (1991): A soluble protein related to the HER-2 proto-oncogene product is released from human breast carcinoma cells. *Oncogene* 6:639-643

Marchionni MA, Goodearl ADJ, Che MS, Bermingham-McDonogh O, Kirk C, Hendricks M, Danehy F, Misumi D, Sudhalter J, Kovayashi K, Wroblewski D, Lynch C, Baldassare M, Hiles I, Davis JB, Hsuan JJ, Totty N, Otsu M, McBurney RN, Waterfield MD, Stroobant P, Gwynne D (1993): Glial growth factors are alternatively spliced *erb*B2 ligands expressed in the nervous system. *Nature* 362:312-318

Marte BM, Jeschke M, Graus-Porta D, Taverna D, Hofer P, Groner B, Yarden Y, Hynes NE (1995): *Neu* differentiation factor/heregulin modulates growth and differentiation of HC 11 mammary epithelial cells. *Mol Endocrinol* 9:14-23

Meyer D and Birchmeier C (1994): Distinct isoforms of neuregulin are expressed in mesenchymal and neuronal cells during mouse development. *Proc Natl Acad Sci USA* 91:1064-1068

Müller WJ, Sinn E, Pattengale PK, Wallace R, Leder P (1988): Single-step induction of mammary adenocarcinoma in transgenic mice bearing the activated c-*neu* oncogene. *Cell* 54:105-115

Pasleau F, Grooteclaes M, Gol-Winkler R (1993): Expression of the c-*erb*B2 gene in the Bt-474 human mammary tumor cell line: measurement of c-*erb*B2 mRNA half-life. *Oncogene* 8:849-85

Peles E and Yarden Y (1993): *Neu* and its ligands: from an oncogene to neural factors. *BioEssays* 15:815-824

Perren TJ (1991): c-*erb*B-2 oncogene as a prognostic marker in breast cancer. *Br J Cancer* 63:328-332

Philips A, Chalbos D, Rochefort H (1993): Estradiol increases and antiestrogens antagonize the growth factor-induced Activator Protein-1 activity in MCF-7 breast cancer cells without affecting c-*fos* and c-*jun* synthesis. *J Biol Chem* 268:14103-14108

Pierce JH, Arnheim P, DiMarco E, Artrip J, Kraus MH, Lonardo F (1991): Oncogenic potential of *erb*B2 in human mammary epithelial cells. *Oncogene* 6:1189-1194

Plowman GD, Culouscou J-M, Whitney GS, Green JM, Carlton GW, Foy L, Neubauer MG, Shoyab M (1993): Ligand-specific activation of HER-4/p180^{erbB4}, a fourth member of the epidermal growth factor receptor family. *Proc Natl Acad Sci USA* 90:1746-1750

Prigent SA, Lemoine NR (1992): The type 1 (EGFR-related) family of growth factor receptors and their ligands. *Progr Growth Factor Res* 4:1-24

Read LD, Keith D Jr, Slamon DJ, Katzenellenbogen BS (1990): Hormonal modulation of HER-2/*neu* proto-oncogene messenger ribonucleic acid and p185 protein expression in human breast cancer cell lines. *Cancer Res* 50:3947-3951

Russel KS, Hung M-C (1992): Transcriptional repression of the *neu* proto-oncogene by estrogen stimulated estrogen receptor. *Cancer Res* 52:6624-6629

Scott GK, Robels R, Park JW, Montgomery PA, Daniel J, Holmes WE, Keller GA, Li W-L, Fendly BM, Wood WI, Shepard M, Benz CC (1993): A truncated intracellular HER2/*neu* receptor produced by alternative RNA processing affects growth of human carcinoma cells. *Mol Cell Biol* 13:2247-2257

Slamon DJ, Clark GM, Wong SG, Levin WJ, Ullrich A, McGuire WL (1987): Human breast cancer, correlation of relapse and survival with amplification of the HER-2/*neu* oncogene. *Science* 235:177-182

Slamon DJ Godolphin W, Jones LA, Holt JA, Wong SG, Keith DE, Levin WJ, Stuart SG, Udove J, Ullrich A, Press MF (1989): Studies of the HER-2/*neu* proto-oncogene in human breast and ovarian cancer. *Science* 244:707-712

Stein D, Wu J, Fuqua SAW, Roonprapunt C, Yajnik V, D'Eustachio P, Moskow JJ, Buchberg AM, Osborne CK, Margolis B (1994): The SH2 domain protein GRB-7 is co-amplified, overexpressed and in a tight complex with HER2 in breast cancer. *EMBO J* 13:6:1331-1340

Stern DF, Kamps MP, Cao H (1988): Oncogenic activation of p185^{neu} stimulates tyrosine phosphorylation *in vivo*. *Mol Cell Biol* 8:3969-3973

Taverna D, Groner B, Hynes NE (1991): Epidermal growth factor receptor, platelet-derived growth factor receptor, and c-*erb*B-2 receptor activation all promote growth but have distinctive effects upon mouse mammary epithelial cell differentiation. *Cell Growth Different* 2:145-154

Taverna D, Antoniotti S, Maggiora P, Dati C, De Bortoli M, Hynes NE (1994): *erb*B-2 expression in estrogen-receptor-positive breast-tumor cells is regulated by growth-modulatory reagents. *Int J Cancer* 56:522-528

Ullrich A, Schlessinger J (1990): Signal transduction by receptors with tyrosine kinase activity. *Cell* 61:203-212

Van de Vijver MJ, Nusse R (1991): The molecular biology of breast cancer. *Biochim Biophys Acta* 1072:35-50

Wärri AM, Laine AM, Majasuo KE, Alitalo KK, Härkönen PL (1991): Estrogen suppression of *erb*B2 expression is associated with increased growth rate of ZR 75-1 human breast cancer cells *in vitro* and in nude mice. *Int J Cancer* 49:616-623

Wärri AM (1993): Toremifene-induced regression in breast cancer. Cellular and molecular mechanisms. Academic Dissertation. University of Turku, Turku, Finland

Wärri AM, Isola JJ, Härkönen PL (1994): Estrogen and antiestrogen regulation of amplified *erb*B2 gene expression in human cancer cells. In: Hormonal Carcinogenesis, 2nd Ed., J.J. Li, S. Nandi and S.A. Li (Eds) Springer-Verlag

Wärri AM, Isola JJ, Härkönen PL (1995): Antiestrogen stimulation of *erb*B2 ectodomain shedding from BT-474 human breast cancer cells with *erb*B2 gene amplification. *Eur J Cancer* (In Press)

Webb P, Lopez GN, Uht RM, Kushner PJ (1995): Tamoxifen activation of the
     estrogen receptor/AP-i pathway: Potential origin for the cell-specific
     estrogen-like effects of antiestrogens. *Mol Endocrinol* 9:443-456
Wright C, Nicholson S, Angus B, Sainsbury JRC, Farndon J, Cairns J, Harris
     AL, Horne CHW (1992): Relationship between c-*erb*B-2 protein
     product expression and response to endocrine therapy in advanced breast
     cancer. *Br J Cancer* 65:118-121
Zabrecky JR, Lam T, McKenzie SJ, Carney, W (1991): The extracellular
     domain of p185*neu* is released from the surface of human breast
     carcinoma cells, SK-BR-3. *J Biol Chem* 266:1716-1720

16. ENHANCEMENT OF THE ANTINEOPLASTIC EFFECTS OF TAMOXIFEN BY SOMATOSTATIN ANALOGUES

Michael Pollak

Tamoxifen is the most widely used compound in breast cancer treatment. The history of its development and introduction into clinical practice has been reviewed elsewhere (Lerner and Jordan, 1990). The first application of Tamoxifen in breast cancer management was in the palliative treatment of metastatic disease. In this setting, the drug clearly had an extremely favourable risk/benefit profile. Dramatic responses to Tamoxifen are not rare, and for many patients, long-term control of metastatic proliferation by Tamoxifen leads to major improvements in quality of life. The positive experience in the metastatic setting justified trials of the drug in post-surgical adjuvant treatment. This clinical research showed that patients in several important prognostic groups, improvements in disease-free survival and survival result from adjuvant Tamoxifen therapy. In general, the risk/benefit profile of the drug remains favourable when it is used as post-surgical adjuvant therapy, particularly for post-menopausal patients. There is a low incidence of uterine toxicity, particularly if the drug is given at higher than 20 mg/day. This risk is clearly outweighed by reduction in risk of breast cancer recurrence, and perhaps by favourable effects on serum lipid profiles and bone density. Adjuvant therapy accounts for the majority of Tamoxifen usage in the 1990's. The possibility that Tamoxifen will also be useful for breast cancer prevention in certain women at high risk is being addressed in ongoing clinical trials.

While data from clinical trials do not support the opinion that toxicity is a major problem, there remains a serious limitation to Tamoxifen therapy. The problem is the limited nature of its efficacy, even in patients with estrogen receptor positive tumors. Although responses to the drug in metastatic disease are common and clinically useful, such responses are rarely long-term. The development of Tamoxifen resistance and progression of metastatic disease while patients are receiving the drug is commonplace. Similarly, in the adjuvant setting, while it is clear that the risk of developing clinically obvious metastases is significantly decreased in many groups of patients by postoperative Tamoxifen treatment, such therapy by no means guarantees that progression of micrometastases will not occur, and the failure of adjuvant Tamoxifen therapy to prevent development of macrometastatic disease is frequently seen.

Thus, an important research goal is to develop ways to enhance Tamoxifen efficacy or delay the emergence of resistance. In this regard, recent preclinical data suggests that it may be beneficial to combine Tamoxifen with somatostatin analogues, and several large scale trials are now planned to determine the clinical relevance of these preclinical results. An example of another approach to this problem is the combination of retinoids with antiestrogens. Relative to other approaches that are immediately ready for clinical testing, the antiestrogen-somatostatin approach has the advantage of a favourable and documented long-term toxicity profile, and demonstrated improvement of efficacy over single-agent Tamoxifen in a preclinical model system. Other promising approaches suggested by recent laboratory work are not presently ready for clinical testing, because they involve novel compounds for which long-term toxicity information is unavailable. The long-term toxicity information is a particularly important issue with respect to proposed novel adjuvant therapies.

Mechanisms of antineoplastic activity of somatostatin analogues

Somatostatin was originally isolated as a hypothalamic factor that inhibited release of growth hormone by the pituitary gland. It is now recognized that somatostatin has many functions apart from the inhibition of growth hormone release and that somatostatin receptors are widely distributed beyond the pituitary. In general, the functions of somatostatin are inhibitory: inhibition of growth hormone release, inhibition of gastric acid secretion, inhibition of proliferation, etc. (reviewed in: Reichlin, 1983). Therapeutic use of native somatostatin is impractical because of its short term serum half-life (~ 1 minute). Several analogues such as octreotide (SMS 201-995) and RC-160 that have substantially longer serum half lives and retain bioactivity have been synthesized. It is now recognized that there are at least 5 distinct somatostatin receptor subtypes (Patel and Srikant, 1994). The specificity of action of various analogues in each type of receptor is the subject of ongoing investigation. Recent data suggest that at least some of the antiproliferative effects of somatostatin are mediated in large part by the type 2 somatostatin receptor (Buscail et al., 1995). Both octreotide and RC-160 bind to this receptor.

There is substantial literature demonstrating considerable antineoplastic activity of somatostatin analogues in many *in vitro* and *in vivo* experimental systems (reviewed in Schally, 1988; Weckbecker et al., 1993). Increasing information concerning mechanisms of action has emerged over the past decade. There are two proposed mechanisms, and it is important to emphasize that these mechanisms are not mutually exclusive.

Direct mechanism. The 'direct' mechanism of antineoplatic action referes to inhibition of proliferation and/or induction of apoptosis that arises as a consequence of a somatostatin analogue binding to a somatostatin receptor on the target neoplastic cell. Although somatostatin-receptor-negative cells clearly cannot be influenced by the direct mechanism, recent data show that a large proportion of breast cancers (and others) are in fact somatostatin receptor positive (van Eijck et al., 1994). Characterization of the molecular basis of the signal transduction pathways associated with each of the 5 somatostatin receptor subtypes is ongoing. There is evidence that one important signal transduction pathway involves upregulation of phosphotyrosine phosphatase activity following binding of somatostatin or a somatostatin analogue to somatostatin receptors (Buscail et al., 1994). This activity is the opposite of that associated with tyrosine kinase - type peptide growth factor receptors and therefore it is not unexpected that proliferation inhibition would be a consequence of upregulation of this activity.

Indirect mechanism. The 'indirect' mechanism of action refers to inhibition of proliferation that arises as a consequence of systemic effects of administration of somatostatin analogues, rather than binding of somatostatin analogues to neoplastic cells. Even somatostatin-receptor-negative neoplasms might be inhibited by indirect mechanisms. Several indirect antineoplastic actions of somatostatin analogues have been proposed. The indirect mechanism that has received the most attention to date concerns the effect of somatostatin analogues on systemic IGF-1 physiology. IGF-1 is an important mitogen for many neoplastic cell types (Macaulay, 1992; Pollack et al., 1987), and also inhibits apoptosis (Resnicoff et al., 1995) and encourages cell motility (Stacke et al., 1988). This indirect mechanisms of somatostatin analogue action may involve suppression of angiogenesis, as there is data to suggest that IGF-1 facilitates endothelial cell proliferation (Nako-Hayshi et al., 1992). It is well established that somatostatin analogues lower acromegalic growth hormone and IGF-1 levels towards normal. It also has been shown that these agents can lower normal GH and IGF-1 levels (Pollak et al., 1989). The dose-response characteristics here differ from the acromegalic situation, as a result of physiological efforts at counter-regulation, for example by increased growth hormone releasing hormone secretion. The concept proposed is that a modest growth hormone/IGF-1 deficiency in an adult might be associated with substantial inhibition of IGF-1 responsive neoplasms, with only minor symptoms for the patient. An implicit assumption is that reduction in serum IGF-1 level correlates with changes in tissue IGF-1 bioactivity. There are *in vivo* experimental systems in which a somatostatin analogue has been found to inhibit the growth of a somatostatin-receptor negative, IGF-1 receptor positive neoplasm (Reubi, 1985).

In the case of breast cancer, it has been suggested (Pollak et al., 1990; Stoll, 1992) that a rationale for reduction of IGF-1 level can be derived from the epidemiological evidence that breast cancer incidence is higher (deWaard et al., 1995; Vatten et al., 1992; Murata et al., 1982; Tretli, 1989; Vatten and Kvinnsland, 1990; Hunter and Willett, 1993) and prognosis worse (deWaard et al., 1995; Vatten et al., 1992; Tretli, 1989) in taller women, and that height is related in part to IGF-1 level, which varies considerably between normal individuals (Juul et al., 1995). It also has been shown that human breast cancer xenograft growth is reduced in mice that are genetically IGF-1 deficient relative to controls, despite equal estrogen supplementation (Yang et al., 1995). This line of reasoning is speculative, but does deserve study, particularly in the light of separate supportive data from skeletal morphometry studies (Mondina et al., 1992).

Rationale for coadministration of antiestrogens and somatostatin analogues

With respect to the proposed direct mechanism of action somatostatin analogues. It has been demonstrated in an early report (Setyono-Han et al., 1987), and since confirmed, that a direct antineoplatic effect of octreotide on estrogen-receptor positive breast cancer cells can be detected using *in vitro* tissue culture systems. Interestingly, the antiproliferative effect of octreotide was clearly maximized in the absence of estrogens (Setyono-Han et al., 1987). The molecular basis for the attenuation of the antiproliferative effect of octreotide by estrogens is uncharacterized, but this observation provides a rationale for coadministrating an antiestrogen with octreotide. Perhaps consistent with this result is the observation that the antineoplastic action of the somatostatin analogue RC-160 in the MXT breast tumor model is enhanced by coadministration of an LHRH analogue, which lowers estradiol levels (Szepeshazi et al., 1992).

With respect to the proposed indirect mechanism of action of somatostatin analogues. A recently characterized effect of antiestrogen therapy in both clinical (Pollak et al., 1990; Friedl et al., 1993) and laboratory (Pollak, 1993; Huynh et al., 1993) studies is a supression of IGF-1 gene expression and serum IGF-1 level. These were somewhat unexpected observations, as inhibition of IGF-1 gene expression was not obviously an "antiestrogenic" effect. There are now data that suggest that this inhibitory action is related in part to inhibition of pituitary growth hormone output (Tannenbaum et al., 1992; Malaab et al., 1992), and in part to direct inhibition of IGF-1 gene expression in various target organs for metastasis (Huynh et al., 1993).

It has been shown that octreotide and Tamoxifen combined suppress serum IGF-1 levels and IGF-1 gene expression more potently than either agents alone in short-term experiments carried out on rats (Huynh and Pollak, 1994). This demonstrates a potentially relevant biological interaction, and is compatible with an additive antineoplastic effect. Furthermore, recent clinical data demonstrate an enhanced suppression of IGF-1 serum level in patients receiving the combination of octreotide and Tamoxifen relative to those receiving Tamoxifen alone (Pollak et al., 1995). However, this result cannot be extrapolated to a conclusion regarding a benefit in terms of efficacy, as the hypothesis that decline in serum IGF-1 is a surrogate endpoint related to efficacy is unproven.

Preclinical results of combined somatostatin and antiestrogen therapy

Combined octreotide-Tamoxifen therapy has been studied using the DMBA-induced rat mammary tumor model (Weckbecker et al., 1994). Despite some limitations, this model has proven reliable in predicting clinical activity of hormonal therapies for breast cancer (Welsch, 1985). The model detects antineoplastic activity of Tamoxifen, which is greater than the activity of octreotide. However, the incidence and growth of DMBA-induced tumors is significantly reduced in animals co-treated with both agents relative to either agent alone. Furthermore, we were able to detect enhancement of the inhibitory effect of oophorectomy on growth of DMBA-induced tumors (Weckbecker et al., 1994). These neoplasms reproducibly regress following oophorectomy, but later regrow. This phenomenon may have features in common with certain forms of resistance to hormonal therapy seen clinically. When octreotide was administered post-oophorectomy, the incidence of re-growth of tumors resistant to endocrine treatment was greatly reduced.

In experimental systems, a consistent observation has been that the response to octreotide-containing regimens is greater in smaller neoplasms than larger neoplasms. The basis for this is unclear. It is consistent with the proposal that at least a part of the antineoplastic activity is an antiangiogenic one. It also is possible that with neoplastic progression, tumors become less dependent on exogenous IGF-1 and/or loose a somatostatin-receptor-positive phenotype, either or both of which would reduce responsivity to somatostatin analogues. This fact suggests that somatostatin analogues would be more effective in the adjuvant setting than in the management of macrometastatic disease.

Clinical results of combined somatostatin and antiestrogen therapy

Single agent activity of somatostatin analogues in advanced, heavily treated breast cancer is very low, despite some isolated reports of disease stabilization. There are no substantial data regarding the use of any somatostatin analogue as first-line therapy, and such trials are not anticipated because preclinical data do not suggest that somatostatin analogues as single agents have greater activity than currently used hormonal therapies. Rather, they support the hypothesis that the efficacy of antiestrogen therapy may be enhanced by coadministration of somatostatin analogues.

A recent trial at the Mayo Clinic attempted to compare the efficacies of octreotide, Tamoxifen, and the combination as first line therapy for metastatic breast cancer. There were no serious adverse effects among participants. Interim analysis of this trial suggested that single agent octreotide was inferior to the other two arms, and focused interest on the possibility of enhanced progression-free survival in the combination group over the Tamoxifen-alone group. However, this trial has recently been closed to further accural due to problems in accural rate. These arose because of practical considerations related to the inconvenient dosage formulation of octreotide used (multiple daily subcutaneous injections) and to the increased use of adjuvant Tamoxifen, which was in cases considered an exclusion criteria. Final outcome analysis of this trial is not yet available as patients remain on protocol treatment at this time. Analysis of blood samples obtained in a subset of participants in this trial, however, has demonstrated that the treatment-related decline in serum IGF-1 levels was significantly greater in the combination group than in the Tamoxifen-alone group (Pollak et al. 1995). This trial contributed to the justification for a new trial in metastatic disease that will be carried out in part in countries where adjuvant Tamoxifen therapy is less frequently used than in North America, and will use the more convenient monthly depot formulation.

Conclusion

There is a clear clinical need to improve the efficacy of antiestrogen therapy. Coadministration of a somatostain analogue is one of several approaches that have been suggested in this regard. The preclinical evidence of improved efficacy in the DMBA model is clear, and the development of a depot formulation of octreotide, together with the established long-term safety profile of this agent, make clinical trials feasible. In 1996, the US National Cancer Institute, through the NSABP trials group, intends to launch a major adjuvant trial for stage I breast cancer patients, and a similar adjuvant trial directed at stage I and stage II patients is planned by the National Cancer Institute of Canada. In addition, a multinational trial of this combination in previously untreated metastatic breast cancer is to begin. All of these trials will involve randomization to Tamoxifen vs. Tamoxifen plus octreotide. In addition to the standard clinical endpoints, these trials will have an important 'translational' research component that will generate data regarding, for example, the effect of each treatment arm on IGF-1 physiology, and the relationship of this to outcome.

REFERENCES

Buscail L, Delesque N, Esteve JP, Saint-Laurent N, Prats H, Clerc P, Robberecht P, Bell GI, Liebow C, Schally AV et al. (1994): Stimulation of tyrosine phosphatase and inhibition of cell proliferation by somatostatin analogues: medication by human somatostatin receptors subtypes SSTR1 and SSTR2. *Proc Natl Acad Sci USA* 91:2315-9

Buscail L, Esteve JP, Saint-Laurent N, Bertrand V, Reisine T, O'Carroll AM, Bell GI, Schally AV, Vaysse N, Susini C (1995): Inhibition of cell proliferation by the somatostatin analogue RC-160 is mediated by somatostatin receptor subtypes SSTR2 and SSTR5 through different mechanisms. *Proc Natl Acad Sci USA* 92:1580-4

deWaard F, Cornelis J, Aoki K, Yoshida M (1995): Breast cancer incidence according to weight and height in two cities of the Netherlands and Aichi prefecture, Japan. *Cancer* 40:1269-75

Friedl A, Jordan VC, Pollak M (1993): Suppression of serum IGF-1 levels in breast cancer patients during adjuvant tamoxifen therapy. *Eur J Cancer* 29A:1368-72

Hunter D, Willett W (1993): Diet, body size, and breast cancer. *Epidemiological Reviews* 15:110-32

Huynh HT, Tetenes E, Wallace L, Pollak M (1993): *In vivo* inhibition of insulin-like growth factor-I gene expression by tamoxifen. *Cancer Res* 53:1727-30

Huynh HT, Pollak M (1994): Enhancement of tamoxifen-induced suppression of insulin-like growth factor I gene expression and serum level by a somatostatin analogue. *Biochem Biophys Res Comm* 203:253-9

Juul A, Bang P, Hertel N et al. (1995): Serum insulin-like growth factor I in 1030 healthy children, adolescents, and adults: relation to age, sex, stage of puberty, testicular size, and body mass index. *J Clin Endocrinol Metab* 78:744-52

Lerner L, Jordan VC (1990): Development of antiestrogens and their use in breast cancer: eighth cain memorial award lecture. *Cancer Res* 50:4177-89

Macaulay VM (1992): Insulin-like growth factors and cancer. *Br J Cancer* 65:311-20

Malaab SA, Pollak M, Goodyer CG (1992): Direct effects of tamoxifen growth hormone secretion by pituitary cells *in vitro*. *Eur J Cancer* 28A:788-93

Mondina R, Borsellino G, Poma S, Baroni M, Di Nubila B, Sacchi P (1992): Breast carcinoma and skeletal formation. *Eur J Cancer* 28A:1068-70

Murata M, Kuno K, Sakamoto G (1982): Epidemiology of family predisposition for breast cancer in Japan. *JNCI* 69:1229-34

Nako-Hayshi J, Jto H, Kanayasu T, Morita I, Murota S (1992): Stimulatory effects of insulin and IGF-1 on migration and tube formation by vascular endothelial cells. *Atherogen* 92:141-9

Patel YC, Srikant CB (1994): Subtype selectivity of peptide analogs for all five cloned human somatostatin receptors (hsste 1-5). *Endocrinol* 135:2814-7

Pollak M, Perdue JF, Margolese RG, Baer K, Richard M (1987): Presence of somatomedin receptors on primary human breast and colon carcinomas. *Cancer Lett* 38:223-30

Pollak M, Polychronakos C, Guyda H (1989): IGF-1 levels in patients with neoplasms potentially dependent on IGF-1. *Anticancer Res* 9:889-92

Pollak M, Costantino J, Polychronakos C, Blauer S, Guyda H, Redmond C, Fisher B, Margolese R (1990): Effect of tamoxifen on serum insulin-like growth factor I levels in stage I breast cancer patients. *JNCI* 82:1693-7

Pollak M (1993): In: Effects of adjuvant tamoxifen therapy on growth hormone and insulin-like growth factor I (IGF-I) physiology. Salmon SE, ed. Adjuvant Therapy of Cancer VIL J.B. Lippincott Company

Pollak M, Ingle JN, Deroo B, Nickerson T (1995): Coadministration of octreotide enhances tamoxifen-induced suppression of serum IGF-1 levels in patients with metastatic breast cancer. Submitted for publication

Reichlin S (1983): Somatostatin *New Eng J Med* 309:1495-501

Resnicoff M, Abraham D, Yutanawiboonchai W, Rotman HL, Kajstura J, Rubin R, Zoltick P, Baserga R (1995): The Insulin-Like Growth Factor I Receptor Protects Tumor Cells from Apoptosis *in Vivo. Cancer Res* 55:2463-9

Reubi JC (1985): A somatostatin analogue inhibits chondrosarcoma and insulinoma tumour growth. *Acta Endo* 109:108-14

Schally AV (1988): Oncological applications of somatostatin analogues. *Cancer Res* 48:6877-85

Setyono-Han B, Henkelman MS, Foekens JA, Klijn GM (1987): Direct inhibitory effects of somatostatin (analogues) on the growth of human breast cancer cells. *Cancer Res* 47:1566-70

Stoll B (1992): Breast cancer risk in Japanese women with special reference to the growth hormone-insulin-like growth factor axis. *Jpn J Clin Oncol* 22:1-5

Stacke ML, Kohn EC, Aznavoorian SA, Wilson LL, Salomon D, Krutsch HC, Liotta LA, Schiffmann E (1988): Insulin-like growth factors stimulate chemotaxis in human melanoma cells. *Biochem Biophys Res Comm* 153:1076-83

Szepeshazi K, Milovanovic S, Lapis K, Groot K, Schally AV (1992): Growth inhibition of estrogen independent MXT mouse mammary carcinomas in mice treated with an agonist or antagonist of LH-RH, an analog of somatostatin, or a combination. *Breast Cancer Res Treat* 21:181-92

Tannenbaum GS, Gurd W, Lapointe M, Pollak M (1992): Tamoxifen attenuates pulsatile growth hormone secretion: mediation in part by somatostatin. *Endocrinol* 130:3395-401

Tretli S (1989): Height and weight in relation to breast cancer morbidity and mortality. A prospective study of 570,000 women in Norway. *Int J Cancer* 44:23-30

van Eijck CH, Krenning EP, Bootsma A, Lindemans J, Jeekel J, Reubi JC, Lamberts SW (1994): Somatostatin-receptor scintigraphy in primary breast cancer. *Lancet* 343:640-3

Vatten LJ, Kvinnsland S (1990): Body height and risk of breast cancer. A prospective study of 23,831 Norwegian women. *Br J Cancer* 61:881-5

Vatten L, Kvikstad A, Nymoen E (1992): Incidence and mortality of breast cancer related to body height and living conditions during childhood and adolescence. *Eur J Cancer* 28:128-31

Weckbecker G, Raulf F, Stolz B, Bruns C (1993): Somatostatin analogs for diagnosis and treatment of cancer (Review). *Pharmac Ther* 60:245-64

Weckbecker G, Tolcsvai L, Stolz B, Pollak M, Bruns C (1994): Somatostatin analogue octreotide enhances the antineoplastic effects of tamoxifen and ovariectomy on 7,12-dimethylbenz(a)anathracene-induced rat mammary carcinomas. *Cancer Res* 54:6334-7

Welsch CW (1985): Host factors affecting the growth of carcinogen-induced rat mammary carcinomas: A review and tribute to Charles Brenton Huggins. *Cancer Res* 45:3415-43

Yang X, Beamer W, Huynh HT, Pollak M (1995): Reduced growth of human breast cancer xenografts in hosts homozygous for the "lit" mutation. Submitted for publication

17. CONCLUSIONS

J.A. Kellen

> *"With high hope for the*
> *future, no prediction is*
> *ventured" (A. Lincoln)*

The cautious optimism of this quotation may well be applied to cancer research in general and the role of antiestrogens in particular. The fact that the malignant cell often retains some sensitivity to signals which control growth and function in their normal counterpart - allows us to hope. The instability and heterogeneity of any cancer cell population, with its inherent dynamics and ability to bypass apoptotic regulation, considerably weakens our ability to predict cause and effect.

Most researchers and clinicians must have accidentally encountered critical fragments of information, in the conscious pursuit of altogether different problems. In order to single out valid information, they had to make loose assumptions, which is not well accepted by our peers and leads to discouraging retreats. However, orthodoxy in thinking, together with the acceptance of dogms, is a comfortable and safe path to mediocrity: better be a half-step ahead and understood than a whole mile in front and ignored. The ancient dictum of Heraclitus: ...upon those who step into the same rivers, different and ever different waters flow... has retained its validity and message, for quite a while.

Survival strategies of tumours are highly differentiated, causing geno- and phenotypic instability; the natural history of each malignant growth is the result of a continuous interplay between various tumour compartments (or subpopulations) and various, often alternating systems of the host (Freitas and Baronzio, 1994).

Very soon after the introduction and wide acceptance of Tamoxifen as a therapeutic agent, primarily in breast cancer, its complex pharmaceutical behaviour was noticed. The apparent unpredictability of many Tamoxifen effects has stimulated an extraordinary number of seemingly unrelated data; the puzzle pieces are far from making sense as a coherent picture. One of the causes of unexpected behaviour of such an essentially simple substance is its potential for triggering point mutations in ligand-binding areas which, in turn, may alter responsiveness of receptors to both steroids and antisteroids (Mahfound et al., 1995). The mutagenicity of Tamoxifen (for ex. on the *hprt* locus in V79 cells, Rajah and Pento, 1995) is further evidence for its capacity for DNA adduct formation (Carthew et al., 1995). There is now consensus as to the possibility, under circumstances not completely known and beyond our control, that Tamoxifen can act as a carcinogen. At this time, the risk-benefit ratio, prior to its wide-spread administration, requires careful weighing and remains relevant (King, 1995).

To mention some not so recent, but probably useful observations: Tamoxifen exerts some control on the adhesive behaviour of some tumour cells; it is not clear whether this control is exercised through hormone-responsive structures, but there is no doubt as to the importance of this action on the modulation of cancer progression (Millon et al., 1989; Fernö et al., 1994). Membrane fluidity and its alterations are another less explored target of Tamoxifen which may affect cytotoxicity in the final outcome after exposure, independent on the receptor status (Clarke et al., 1990).

Multidrug resistance remains at present the single most significant factor limiting our success in cancer treatment, after an initial effective response. It remains a complex problem, mediated by more than one mechanism, some known and some not. Besides the "classical" P-glycoprotein overexpression, topoisomerase alterations and changes in xenobiotic detoxification, activation of proto-oncogens (counteracting apoptosis) has become the "dernier cri" (Mestdagh et al., 1995). The delicate interplay between mdr1, p53 as well as the Bcl2 genes, together with the effect of Tamoxifen (and other antiestrogens) on their altered expression is gaining deserved attention. To use a trivial expression: last but not least, this may well be one of the nonhormonal actions of these compounds and another explanation of their beneficial effect in the restoration of apoptosis.

Because of its good tolerance and paucity of side effects, Tamoxifen plays or should play a role in the reversal of MDR. It ranks among the calcium channel blockers, cyclosporines, calmodulin antagonists and antibiotics as a "steroid hormone-like" agent (albeit it obviously is not a steroid) and certainly exerts its welcome effect at high, but nevertheless relatively non-toxic levels (Kellen, 1994).

Another obviously underexploited facet of Tamoxifen action is its (estrogen-like) senzitizing effect on various, but not all, cancer cells; the effect does not appear to be estrogen receptor dependent. Target cell senzitization to the action of NK cells (a very desirable, "physiological" approach to combat cancer) by Tamoxifen involves active, complex metabolic participation of the treated cells in apoptosis, as documented by accelerated release of ^{3}H-thymidine after the cytotoxic insult by NK cells, resulting in immune cytolysis (Baral et al., 1996).

Of course, Tamoxifen is haunted by the same inoxerable spectres: treatment failure eventually occurs because tumours become insensitive to the drug, or alternatively, tumours even become stimulated rather than inhibited by Tamoxifen (Bogden et al., 1995). Following chronic Tamoxifen treatment, the response of tumour cell subpopulations is increasingly heterogeneous; some populations may even expand (Graham et al., 1992). The development of drug resistance to Tamoxifen, paired with its estrogenic properties, may support strategies of temporary(?) withdrawal of the drug (Howell et al., 1992) which may prove beneficial. On the other hand, it makes little biochemical sense to continue Tamoxifen administration after tumour recurrence - which is commonly the case, based on the assumption that Tamoxifen switches from being an adjuvant to a chemotherapeutic agent (Horwitz, 1995). This apparently irrational school of thinking may be reconsidered in the light of multiple other effects of Tamixofen, not related to its anti-hormone mode of action. Repeated responses after reintroduction of Tamoxifen in hosts who had previously acquired resistance have been reported (Shannon and Harnett, 1994).

The addition of Tamoxifen into various established or new combination protocols, in cancer other than of breast, makes interesting reading and shows some promise. The opposite is also true: combination of Tamoxifen with LH-RH analogues, such as goserelin and others, is expected to counteract "residual" estrogen action, especially in post-menopausal women and thus achieve a more complete estrogen blockade (Buzoni et al., 1995). However, the original postulate: no receptors - no antiestrogen effect, has long been abandoned; the detectable existence of a variety of ligand sites has complicated the problem (Marsigliante et al., 1994). Also, beneficial effects of Tamoxifen in conjunction with other drugs (compared to "standard" treatment programs) are notoriously difficult to isolate. Small differences (i.e. in survival) between treatment arms are known to pose statistical obstacles. On the other hand, failure to demonstrate an objective response does not necessarily mean ineffective treatment (Markman, 1993). A positive result of short duration may be a welcome improvement of life quality for an individual but may not be statistically meaningful.

A basic shortcoming of results obtained in cells or animals (which constitute the majority of data reported in this book) is the difficulty, if not impossibility, to extrapolate them into the human situation. Even the best models suffer from lack of reproducibility, obsolescence and are unable to mimic in detail human tumour characteristics, the natural course of the disease and variations in responses to therapy. Furthermore, we all suffer from (but are not likely to admit to) a general lack of understanding probability (Levy, 1994); this is particularly pertinent to the interpretation of trials which, with all their refinements and care in design, are often a false reflection of reality. There are hormone independent molecular pathologies leading to breast cancer, such as BRCA gene mutation(s); unless women participating in Tamoxifen prevention trails are tested for the presence (or absence) of such predisposing factors, the outcome and validity of such studies are questionable. A few weeks or even months statistically gained in prolonging an intolerable life may add to the scientific prestige of the therapeut, but means little to the suffering patient. These thoughts are not an expression of nihilism, but an effort to introduce some measure of perspective into the usefulness of our endeavours. To quote the stirring words of Richard Margolese (1994): "Think of the host; hope but do not hope too much..."

The magic bullet, lethal to cancer cells only, remains elusive, the promise of increasing success in cancer therapy lies, in the foreseeable future, in combinations of surgery, radiation, hormone-, chemo-, immuno- and gene-therapy. Their hierarchy and importance need to be individually orchestrated. Unfortunately, optimal treatment is often more a matter of opinion or empirical experience than based on fact. True, facts are at times difficult to sort out; we are overwhelmed by a tide of information, but we are basically ill-informed.

Tamoxifen must be recognized as more than just another antihormonal agent, but as a remarkable factor with wide range of action - a great deal more than expected, judging solely by its relatively simple structure. We hope to have set the stage for broader and imaginative thinking.

Complacency and feelings of accomplishment, based on the vast body of knowledge already acquired, are dangerous soporifics. The door has been opened - a little -, nothing more.
"The woods are lovely, dark and deep
But I have promises to keep
And miles to go before I sleep
And miles to go before I sleep..." (R. Frost).

REFERENCES

Baral E, Nagy E, Kangas L, Berczi I (1996): Immunotherapy of the SL2-5 murine lymphoma with natural killer cells and Tamoxifen or Toremifene. In press, *Cancer*

Bogden AE, Keyes SR, Grant W, Silver M, Batista LI, LePage D (1995): Estrogen Sensitivity and the Therapeutic Benefit of Lanreotide Tamoxifen Combination in the Treatment of Breast Tumors. *Proc AACR* 36:523

Buzoni R, Biganzoli L, Bajetta E, Celio L, Fornasiero A, Mariani L, Zilemno N, Di Bartolomeo M, Di Leo A, Arcangeli G, Aitini E, Farina G, Schieppati GH, Galuzzo D, Marinetti A (1995): Combination Goserelin and Tamoxifen Therapy in Premenopausal Advanced Breast Cancer: a Multicentre Study by the ITMO Group. *Brit J Cancer* 71:1111-1114

Carthew P, Rich KJ, Martin EA, DeMattheis F, Lim CK, Manson MM, Festing FW, White IHN, Smith LL (1995): DNA damage as assessed by ^{32}P-postlabelling in three rat strains exposed to dietary Tamoxifen. *Carcinogenesis* 16:1299-1305

Clarke R, van den Berg HW, Murphy RF (1990): Reduction of the Membrane Fluidity of Human Breast Cancer Cells by Tamoxifen and 17 beta-Estradiol. *J Natl Cancer Inst* 82:1702-1705

DeFriend DJ, Howell A (1994): Tamoxifen withdrawal responses - chance observations or clinical clues to antioestrogen resistance? *The Breast* 3:199-201

Fernö M, Baldetorp B, Borg A, Brouilett JP, Olsson H, Rochefort H, Sellberg G, Sigurdsson H, Killander D (1994): Cathepsin D, Both a Prognostic Factor for the Effect of Adjuvant Tamoxifen in Breast Cancer. *Europ J Cancer* 30A:2042-2048

Freitas I, Baronzio GF (1994): Neglected Factors in Cancer Treatment: Cellular Interactions and Dynamic Microenvironment in Solid Tumors. *Anticancer Res* 14:1097-1102

Graham ML, Smith JA, Jewett PB, Horwitz KB (1992): Heterogeneity of Progesterone Receptor Content and Remodelling by Tamoxifen Characterize Subpopulations of Cultured Human Breast Cancer Cells: Analysis by Quantitative Duel Parameter Flow Cytometry. *Cancer Res* 52:593-602

Horwitz KB (1995): Editorial: When Tamoxifen Turns Bad. *Endocrinol* 136:821-823

Howell A, Dodwell DJ, Anderson H (1992): Response after withdrawal of tamoxifen and progestogens in advanced breast cancer. *Ann Oncol* 3:611-617

Kellen JA (1994): Reversal of Multidrug Resistance in Cancer. CRC Press, Boca Raton, pp 93-125

King CM (1995): Tamoxifen and the induction of cancer. *Carcinogen* 16:1449-1454

Levy GB (1994): Merchandising science. *Amer Lab* 6:6-8

Mahfoudi A, Roulet E, Dauvois S, Parker MG, Wahli W (1995): Specific mutations in the estrogen receptor change the properties of antiestrogens to full agonists. *Proc Natl Acad Sci USA* 92:4206-4210

Markman M (1993): Why does a higher response rate to chemotherapy correlate poorly with improved survival? *J Cancer Res Clin Oncol* 119:700-701

Margolese R (1994): The challenge of breast cancer. *Lancet* 343:1086

Marsigliante S, Leo G, D'Elia M, Vinson GP, Greco S, Puddefoot J, Storelli C (1994): Relationships Between Tamoxifen Binding Proteins in Primary Breast Cancer Biopsies. *Europ J Ca* 30A:1694-1700

Mestdagh N, D'Hooghe MC, Lantoine D, Henichart JP (1995): Expression of a tumour-suppressor gene and of various proto-oncogenes in human and murine adriamycin-resistant and sensitive cell lines. *Int J Oncol* 6:1255-1260

Millon R, Nicora F, Muller D, Eber M, Klein-Soyer C, Abecassis J (1989): Modulation of human breast cancer cell adhesion by estrogens and antiestrogens. *Clin Expl Metastasis* 7:405-415

Pollak M (1995): Potential Impact of Genetic Testing on Cancer Prevention Trials, Using Breast Cancer as an Example. *J Natl Cancer Inst* 87:1557

Rajah TT, Pento JT (1995): The Mutagenic Potential of Antiestrogens at the *hprt* Locus in V79 Cells. *Res Comm Molec Pathol Pharmacol* 89:85-92

Shannon JA, Harnett PR (1994): Multiple responses to tamoxifen in advanced breast cancer - clinical and biological implications. *The Breast* 3:235-237

Index

Note: Frequently occurring terms, such as: Antiestrogens, Antioxidants, Breast cancer, Estrogens, Tamoxifen, Toremifene, and Receptors (ER, PR) have not been indexed.

Related Birkhäuser Titles

Alternative Mechanisms of Multidrug Resistance in Cancer
J.A. Kellen, Editor
ISBN 0-8176-3775-3
1995 296 pp.

Chemical Induction of Cancer: Modulation and Combination Effects:
An Inventory of the Many Factors Which Influence Carcinogenesis
J.C. Arcos, Editor; M.F. Argus & Y.-T. Woo, Associate Editors
ISBN 0-8176-3766-4
1995 744 pp.

Hormones and Cancer
W.V. Vedeckis, Editor
ISBN 0-8176-3797-4
1996 640 pp.

Epithelial-Mesenchymal Interactions in Cancer
I.D. Goldberg, E.M. Rosen, Editors
ISBN 3-7643-5117-9
1995 298 pp.

Molecular Oncology and Clinical Applications
A. Cittadini, R. Baserga, H.M. Pinedo, T. Galeotti, D. Corda, Editors
ISBN 0-8176-2915-7
1993 448 pp.